Psychiatric–Mental Health Nurse Practitioner Review and Resource Manual

2nd Edition

D0988910

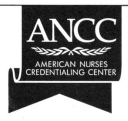

ANCC
AMERICAN NURSES
CREDENTIALING CENTER

Karen Guess, MSN, PMHNP, ANP-BC

Library of Congress Cataloging-in-Publication Data

Psychiatric-mental health nurse practitioner review and resource manual
/ [edited by] Karen Guess. -- 2nd ed.
    p. ; cm.
  Includes bibliographical references and index.
  ISBN-13: 978-0-9793811-2-6
  ISBN-10: 0-9793811-2-6
1. Psychiatric nursing--Examinations, questions, etc. 2. Psychology,
Pathological--Examinations, questions, etc. 3. Psychiatric
nurses--Examinations, questions, etc. 4. Nurse
practitioners--Examinations, questions, etc. I. Guess, Karen. II.
American Nurses Credentialing Center. Institute for Credentialing
Innovation.
  [DNLM: I. Psychiatric Nursing--methods. 2. Education, Nursing,
Continuing. WY 18.5 P974 2008]

  RC440.P7337 2008
  616.89'0231076--dc22   2008001691

1. Nursing--Examinations, questions, etc. 2. Surgical nursing--Examinations, questions, etc. I. American
Nurses Credentialing Center. Institute for Credentialing Innovation.

[DNLM: I. Education, Continuing, Nursing. 2. Perioperative Nursing--methods. WY 18.5 M489 2007]

Published by: American Nurses Credentialing Center
                  The Institute for Credentialing Innovation

                  8515 Georgia Avenue, Suite 400
                  Silver Spring, MD 20910-3492

                  www.nursecredentialing.org

ISBN 13: 978-0-9793811-2-6   ISBN 10: 0-9793811-2-6

© 2008 American Nurses Credentialing Center. All rights reserved.

Psychiatric–Mental Health Nurse Practitioner Review and Resource Manual, 2nd Edition

March 2008

Please direct your comments and/or queries to revmanuals@ana.org

The health care services delivery system is a volatile marketplace demanding superior knowledge, clinical skills, and competencies from all registered nurses. Nursing autonomy of practice and nurse career marketability and mobility in the new century hinge on affirming the profession's formative philosophy, which places a priority on a lifelong commitment to the principles of education and professional development. The knowledge base of nursing theory and practice is expanding, and while care has been taken to ensure the accuracy and timeliness of the information presented in the **Psychiatric–Mental Health Nurse Practitioner Review and Resource Manual, 2nd Edition,** clinicians are advised to always verify the most current national guidelines and recommendations and to practice in accordance with professional standards of care used with regard to the unique circumstances that apply in each practice situation. In addition, every effort has been made in this text to ensure accuracy and, in particular, to confirm that drug selections and dosages are in accordance with current recommendations and practice, including the ongoing research, changes to government regulations, and developments in product information provided by pharmaceutical manufacturers. However, it is the responsibility of each nurse practitioner to verify drug product information and to practice in accordance with professional standards of care. In addition, the editors wish to note that provision of information in this text does not imply an endorsement of any particular products, procedures, or services.

Therefore, the authors, editors, American Nurses Association (ANA), American Nurses Association's Publishing (ANP), American Nurses Credentialing Center (ANCC), and the Institute for Credentialing Innovation cannot accept responsibility for errors or omissions, or for any consequences or liability, injury, and/or damages to persons or property from application of the information in this manual and make no warranty, express or implied, with respect to the contents of the **Psychiatric–Mental Health Nurse Practitioner Review and Resource Manual, 2nd Edition.**

Published by: The Institute for Credentialing Innovation
                 8515 Georgia Avenue, Suite 400
                 Silver Spring, MD 20910-3492
                 www.nursecredentialing.org

Introduction to the Continuing Education Contact Hour Application Process for *Psychiatric–Mental Health Nurse Practitioner Review and Resource Manual*, 2nd Edition

The Institute for Credentialing Innovation now offers the continuing education (CE) contact hours for this manual online at www.NursingWorld.org, the American Nurses Association's Web site. This process involves answering approximately 25–30 questions that test knowledge of the information contained within this manual. The CE contact hours can be completed at any time and a certificate can be printed from the Web site immediately upon successful completion of the test.

The *Psychiatric-Mental Health Nurse Practitioner Review and Resource Manual, 2nd Edition* is designed to meet the following objectives:

1. Readers will be able to conduct a psychiatric history and mental status examination.

2. Readers will be able to diagnose common psychiatric disorders and develop a plan of care with both pharmacological and nonpharmacological treatment modalities.

3. Readers will be able to discuss rules, regulations, and advanced practice issues that may influence practice and the role of the nurse practitioner.

Upon completion of this manual *and* the online CE test, a nurse can receive a total of 23 CE contact hours at a price of $46, only $2 per CE. **The entire process—online test and evaluation form—must be completed by December 31, 2011 in order to receive credit.** To begin the process, please e-mail **revmanuals@ana.org.** Your patience with this process is greatly appreciated.

Inquiries or Comments

If you have any questions about the CE contact hours, please e-mail the Institute at revmanuals@ana.org. You may also mail any comments to Editor/Project Manager at the address listed below.

Duplicate CE Certificates

Once you have successfully passed the CE test on NursingWorld, you may go back and re-print your certificate as often as you wish.

The Institute for Credentialing Innovation
American Nurses Credentialing Center
Attn: Editor/Project Manager
8515 Georgia Avenue, Suite 400
Silver Spring, MD 20910-3492
Fax: (301) 628-5342

The American Nurses Association is accredited as a provider of continuing nursing education by the American Nurses Credentialing Center's Commission on Accreditation.
ANA is approved by the California Board of Registered Nursing, Provider Number 6178.

Contents

Psychiatric–Mental Health Nurse Practitioner Role, Scope of Practice, and Regulatory Process

Starting in the 1950s with the seminal work of two psychiatric nurses, June Mellow and Hildegard Peplau (1952), psychiatric nursing has been a well-established, well-recognized subspecialty of nursing. The emergence of the psychiatric–mental health nurse practitioner (PMHNP) role reflects the growth of the advanced practice role, the acceptance of a brain-based etiology of psychiatric disorders, and an awareness of the need to provide holistic nursing care that does not artificially separate mind and body (Stuart & Laraia, 2005).

The PMHNP role is built on fundamental, core advanced practice knowledge common to all nurse practitioners. This base of knowledge is expanded to include the very specific knowledge of the subspecialty of psychiatry. This chapter reviews the role of the PMHNP, the scope of practice, and the regulatory process.

Advanced practice nurses specializing in psychiatry are educationally prepared at the master's or doctoral level, possess in-depth knowledge and skills in the specialty area, and provide primary psychiatric care to individuals or families at risk for or currently experiencing a psychiatric disorder.

Advanced Practice Core Content

All nurse practitioners (NP) upon graduation are expected to meet a set of core competencies. Specialty competencies are then built upon these core competencies (National Organization of Nurse Practitioner Faculties, 2006).

Management of Health Status
- Health assessment
- Health history
- Physical exam
- Screening and diagnostic testing
- Diagnosing
- Prescribing meds and other treatment modalities
- Evaluating care outcomes.

Maintenance of Nurse–Client Relationship

- Displaying environment of trust and respect
- Maintaining healthy boundaries
- Engaging in therapeutic communication.

Teaching/Coaching

- Health promotion/disease prevention
- Risk reduction
- Coaching toward behavioral change.

Professional Role

- Serving as client advocate
- Utilizing information and technology in health care
- Using interdisciplinary collaboration and consultation
- Practicing ethically
- Showing leadership
- Undertaking professional development
- Participating in policy making.

Managing/Negotiating Health Care Delivery Systems

- Decision making with regard to cost, access, and efficacy
- Applying business strategies to practice
- Negotiating legislative change when needed.

Monitoring Quality of Care

- Evaluating quality of care
- Incorporating continuous quality improvement into practice.

Providing Culturally Sensitive Care

- Remaining culturally sensitive when assessing client's symptoms and his or her perceptions of symptoms.

Advanced Practice Specialized Content

The specialty competencies are specifically designed for entry-level psychiatric–mental health nurse practitioners. These competencies emphasize the uniqueness of psychiatric nursing and reflect the scope of practice of PMHNPs. As changes occur within the health care system, these competencies will also change (National Organization of Nurse Practitioner Faculties, 2003).

Health Promotion, Health Protection, Disease Prevention, and Treatment

- *Assessment*—Physical and mental health assessment, psychiatric evaluation including mental status evaluation, differentiating normal and abnormal symptomology, family system assessment

- **Reasons for Conducting a Physical Assessment in Psychiatry**
  - To identify general health status of client
  - To screen for general, nonpsychiatric disorders or problems
  - To ascertain differential diagnoses
  - To identify primary psychiatric disorder.

- *Diagnosis of Health Status*—Ordering/interpreting diagnostic tests, differential diagnoses, diagnosing psychiatric disorders, applying taxonomy systems to the diagnosis

  - **Neurobiological and Associated Taxonomies**
    - *International Classification of Diseases (ICD-9;* World Health Organization, 2007)
    - *Diagnostic and Statistical Manual of Mental Disorders (DSM-IV-TR;* American Psychiatric Association, 2000)
    - Health Insurance Portability and Accountability Act (HIPAA, P.L. 104-191) code sets
    - *Nursing Interventions Classification (NIC;* McCloskey & Bulechek, 2000)
    - *Nursing Outcomes Classification (NOC;* Johnson, Maas, & Moorhead, 2003)
    - North American Nursing Diagnosis Association (NANDA, 2000).

- *Plan of Care and Implementation of Treatment*—Applying etiological models to care of clients (e.g., neurobiological, psychosocial), using evidence-based standards of care and practice guidelines, using psychotherapy, prescribing psychotropic meds; managing psychiatric emergencies.

NP–Client Relationship
- Using therapeutic communication
- Promoting trust
- Maintaining professional boundaries.

Teaching/Coaching Function
- Psychopharmacological education
- Psychoeducation.

Professional Role
- Interdisciplinary collaboration
- Consultation
- Coordination of referrals
- Participation in professional organizations
- Research involvement and utilization
- Use of ethical/legal standards.

Managing and Negotiating Health Care Delivery Systems
- Using ethical principles to advocate for clients
- Participating in health policy.

Monitoring and Ensuring the Quality of Health Care Practice
- Consulting with others to improve quality of care
- Engaging in continuing education
- Staying current with research.

Cultural Competence
- Remaining culturally sensitive when assessing client's symptoms and his or her perceptions of symptoms.

History of the NP Role

The NP role was introduced in 1965 by Dr. Loretta C. Ford and Henry K. Silver, MD, at the University of Colorado (Mirr Jansen & Zwygart-Stauffacher, 2006). These individuals identified new roles in which experienced registered nurses with advanced education and skills were performing clinical duties traditionally reserved for physicians. Universities were slow to implement NP programs at the master's level. However, registered nurses embraced the new role and rushed into continuing education programs of varying length, quality, and focus to accomplish the necessary educational preparation for this new role.

- Proven competence brought an acceptance of the NP role in the health care system— Acceptance and recognition of the title and role by consumers and other health professionals.
- NP programs were accredited to achieve standardization and control over quality.
- NPs are recognized providers under many third-party insurance coverage plans (e.g., Medicare, Medicaid, CHAMPUS, federal programs funding school-based clinics, U.S. military, Veterans Administration).

Growth of the NP Role
Facilitating Factors for Growth
- Consumer demand for services
- Acceptance of the advanced practice nursing role
- Emergence of the PMHNP role
- Decreasing stigmatization
- Emphasis on integrated health care services.

Constraining Factors for Growth
- Growing competition in job market in general for NPs
- Reduction in salaries because of NP oversupply
- Reimbursement struggles with Medicare and private insurance companies
- Issue of overlapping scope of practice with other NPs
- Increased concerns over reimbursement fraud and abuse (e.g., issues of coding and billing for services).

Regulatory and Statutory Dimensions of the NP Role

State Legislative Statutes
- Grant *legal authority* for NP practice
- Are the *Nurse Practice Act* of every state
  - Provides title protection (who may be called a nurse practitioner)
  - Defines advanced practice
  - Is prevailing state law that defines scope of practice (what NPs may do)
  - Places restrictions on practice
  - Sets NP credentialing requirements (e.g., educational requirements, certification)
  - States grounds for disciplinary action:
    - Practicing without valid license
    - Falsification of records
    - Medicare fraud
    - Failure to use appropriate nursing judgment
    - Failure to follow accepted nursing standards
    - Failure to complete accurate nursing documentation.
- May specifically require that an NP develop a collaborative agreement with a physician
  - *Collaborative agreement*—Also known as a protocol that describes what types of drugs might be prescribed and defines some form of oversight board for NP practice.

Statutory Law
- Rules and regulations differ for each state
- May further define scope of practice and practice requirements
- May provide restrictions in practice unique to specific state.

Licensure
- A process by which an agency of state government grants permission to individuals accountable for the practice of a profession to engage in the practice of that profession
- Also prohibits all others from legally doing protected practice.

Credentialing
- Process used to protect the public by ensuring a minimum level of professional competence.

Certification
- Is a credential that provides title protection
- Determines scope of practice (i.e., who NPs can see and what NPs can treat)
- Is the process by which a professional organization or association certifies that an individual licensed to practice as a professional has met certain predetermined standards specified by that profession for specialty practice
- Assures the public that an individual has mastery of a body of knowledge
- Assures that the individual has acquired the skills necessary to function in a particular specialty
- Primary certifying body for psychiatric nursing is the American Nurses Association.

Scope of Practice

- Defines NP roles and actions
- Identifies competencies assumed to be held by all NPs who function in a particular role
- Has broad variations from state to state
- Advanced practice PMHNP standards are identified in *Scope and Standards of Psychiatric–Mental Health Clinical Nursing Practice* (ANA, 2000b).

Standards of Practice

- Gives authoritative statements regarding the quality and type of practice that should be provided
- Provides a way to judge the nature of care provided
- Reflects the expectation for the care that should be provided to clients with various illnesses
- Reflects professional agreement focused on the minimum levels of acceptable performance
- Can be used to legally describe the standard of care that must be met by a provider
- May be precise protocols that must be followed or more general guidelines that recommend actions.

Professional Role Responsibilities

Confidentiality

- Is the client's right to assume that information given to the health care provider will not be disclosed
- Is protected under federal statute through the Medical Record Confidentiality Act of 1996 (S. 1360)
- Pertains to oral and written client information
- Requires that the provider discuss confidentiality issues with clients, establish consent, and clarify any questions about disclosure of information
- Requires that provider obtain a signed medical authorization and consent form to release medical records and information when requested by the client or when requested by another health care provider.

Health Insurance Portability and Accountability Act (HIPAA)

- Is the first national comprehensive privacy protection act
- Guarantees clients four *fundamental rights:* (1) To be educated about HIPAA privacy protection, (2) to have access to their own medical records, (3) to request amendment to those aspects of their health information to which they object, and (4) to require their permission for disclosure of their personal information.

Exceptions to Guaranteed Confidentiality

- When appropriate individuals or organizations determine that the need for information outweighs the principle of confidentiality
  - If a client reveals an intent to harm self or others
  - To attorneys involved in litigation

- When records are released to insurance companies
- When answering court orders, subpoenas, or summons
- When meeting state requirements for mandatory reporting of diseases or conditions
- *Tarasoff* principle (1976)—Duty to warn potential victim of imminent danger of homicidal clients
- In cases of child abuse or elder abuse.

Informed Consent
- The communication process between the provider and the client that results in the client's acceptance or rejection of the proposed treatment
- An explanation of relevant information that enables the client to make an appropriate and informed decision
- The right of all competent adults or emancipated minors
  - *Emancipated minors*—Individuals ages 18 or younger who are married, parents, or self-sufficiently living away from the family domicile.

Elements of Informed Consent
- Nature and purpose of proposed treatment or procedure
- Risks or discomforts and benefits of treatment
- Risks and benefits of not undergoing treatment
- Alternative procedures or treatments
- Diagnosis and prognosis.

- Provider must document in the medical record that informed consent has been provided to client
- PMHNP is responsible for ensuring that the client is cognitively capable of giving informed consent.

Ethics
- An important aspect of the NP role that deals with moral duties, obligations, and responsibilities
- What is right vs. what is wrong
- Ethical principles that provide foundation and direction for complex decisions:
  - *Justice*—Doing what is fair; fairness in all aspects of care
  - *Beneficence*—Promoting well-being and doing good
  - *Nonmalfeasance*—Doing no harm
  - *Fidelity*—Being true and loyal
  - *Autonomy*—Doing for self
  - *Veracity*—Telling the truth
  - *Respect*—Treating everyone with equal respect.
- NP ethical behavior is defined in an ANA policy statement (*Code of Ethics for Nurses*, 2005) on ethics that provides guidelines related to delivering care that preserves client's dignity, autonomy, rights, and confidentiality.

Important Ethical Principles in Psychiatry
- Clients must be involved in decision making to the full extent of their capacity (mutual decision making)
- Clients have a right to treatment in the least restrictive setting

- Clients have a right to refuse treatment unless a legal process resulting in a mandatory court order for treatment has been obtained.

Ethical Dilemma
- Occurs in a situation in which there are two or more justifiable alternatives
- Occurs when the choice is made to promote good
- Which option sacrifices the fewest high-priority values (a harm reduction approach)?

Theoretical Approaches to Ethical Decision Making
- *Deontological Theory*—An action is judged as good or bad based on the act itself regardless of the consequences
- *Teleological Theory*—An action is judged as good or bad based on the consequence or outcome
- *Virtue Ethics*—Actions are chosen based on the moral virtues (e.g., honesty, courage, compassion, wisdom, gratitude, self-respect) or the character of the person making the decision.

Legal Considerations

Malpractice Insurance
- Provides financial protection against claims of malpractice
  - Coverage for negligent professional acts
  - Coverage for highly technical or professional skills required by health professionals, including NPs.
- Recommended universally for all NPs
- Does not protect NPs from charges of practicing outside their legal scope of practice
- Provides NPs own legal representation to advocate for them even if their agency also carries malpractice liability insurance protection.

Four Elements of Negligence That Must Be Established to Prove Malpractice
1. *Duty*—The NP had a duty to exercise reasonable care when undertaking and providing treatment to the client.
2. *Breach of Duty*—The NP violated the applicable standard of care in treating the client's condition.
3. *Proximate Cause*—There is a causal relationship between the breach in the standard of care and the client's injuries.
4. *Damages*—There are permanent and substantial damages to the client as a result of the breach in the standard of care.

Competency
- A legal—not a medical—concept
- A determination that a client can make reasonable judgments and decisions regarding treatment and other health concerns
- An individual is considered competent until a court rules the person to be incompetent
- If deemed incompetent, a court-appointed guardian will make health-related decisions for the individual.

Commitment
- Process of involuntarily forcing an individual to receive evaluation or treatment
- Process may differ from state to state
- Basic criteria include
  - Individual has a diagnosed psychiatric disorder
  - Individual is harmful to self or others as a consequence of the disorder
  - Individual is unaware or unwilling to accept the nature and severity of the disorder
  - Treatment is likely to improve functioning.

Involuntary Admission
- Admission to a hospital or other treatment facility that is involuntary
- Clients maintain all civil liberties except the ability to come and go as they please
- Amount of time clients can be kept against their wishes varies by state.

Voluntary Admission
- Admission to a hospital or other treatment facility that is voluntary
- Client maintains all civil liberties
- Client consents to potential confinement within the structure of a hospital setting.

Scholarly Activities

- As an NP, it is important to engage in scholarly activities:
  - Publishing
  - Lecturing/presenting
  - Preceptorship
  - Continuing education.

Mentoring
- A process in which a more experienced NP agrees to guide and support a junior colleague in the role, competencies, and skills
- Comprises mutual respect and an interactive process of learning
- Needs involvement by both the mentor and the mentee in the relationship.

Client Advocacy
- Standing up for clients' rights and empowering them to become their own advocate
- Helping clients receive available services
- Promoting mental health by participating in a professional organization:
  - American Psychiatric Nurses Association (APNA)
  - International Society of Psychiatric Nurses (ISPN)
- Coordinating quality and cost-effective care.

Case Management
- Is a system of controlled oversight and authorization of services and benefits provided to clients
- Consists of coordinating care, ensuring quality outcomes, monitoring plan of care, and doing advocacy
- Has overall goal to promote quality cost-effective outcomes.

Health Promotion/Disease Prevention Education
- Preventive care and screening practices essential aspects of the PMHNP role
- Screening for physical health problems in the psychiatric client
- Usually guided by Healthy People 2010 (U.S. Department of Health and Human Services, 2005), which identifies national health objectives, including behavioral health
- Mental health promotion and education includes
  - Teaching about interventions and ways to cope with specific stressors
  - Validating "normalcy" of feelings; ensuring clients that they are not "crazy"
  - Helping clients recognize and identify their feelings or behaviors
  - Helping clients identify resources in the community.

Public Health Principles
- *Primary prevention*—Aimed at decreasing the incidence (number of new cases) of mental disorders
  - Helping people avoid stressors or cope with them more adaptively
    - *Example:* Stress management classes for graduate students, smoking prevention classes, Drug Abuse Resistance Education (DARE).
- *Secondary prevention*—Aimed at decreasing the prevalence (number of existing cases) of mental disorders
  - Early case finding
  - Screening
  - Prompt and effective treatment
    - *Example:* Telephone hotlines, crisis intervention, disaster responses.
- *Tertiary prevention*—Aimed at decreasing the disability and severity of a mental disorder
  - Rehabilitative services
  - Avoidance or postponement of complications
  - *Example:* Day treatment programs; case management for physical, housing, or vocational needs; social skills training.

Risk Factors
- Predisposing characteristics that make it more likely that a person will develop a disorder
- *Biological risk factors*—History of mental illness in family, poor nutritional status, poor general health
- *Psychological risk factors*—Poor self-concept, external locus of control, poor ego defenses
- *Social risk factors*—Stressful occupation, low socioeconomic status, poor level of social integration.

Preventive Factors
- Factors that prevent or protect the individual from the disorder
- Coping mechanisms or resources that facilitate a healthy response to stress
- *Biological preventive factors*—Without a history of mental illness in the family, healthy nutritional status, good general health
- *Psychological preventive factors*—Good self-esteem or self-concept, internal locus of control, healthy ego-defenses
- *Social preventative factors*—Low-stress occupation, higher socioeconomic status, higher level of education.

Risk Assessment
- The continuous monitoring for high-risk situations
- Assessing individuals for nonhealthy behaviors.

Risk Management
- Activities or systems designed to recognize and intervene to reduce the risk of injury to clients
- Appropriate interventions that are implemented to reduce nonhealthy behaviors in clients and high risk situations
- Functions to recognize and intervene to reduce subsequent claims against health care providers.

Advance Directives
- Legally binding in all 50 states
- *Living will*—Document giving specific instructions while client is mentally competent that providers must follow if client becomes incompetent
  - Designates preferences for care if client becomes incompetent or terminally ill.
- *Durable power of attorney for health care*—Also known as *health care proxy*
  - Designates in writing an agent to act on behalf of an individual should he or she become unable to make health care decisions
  - Not limited to terminal illness, and also covers other aspects of illness, such as making financial decisions during an individual's illness
  - Should be considered as an aspect of relapse planning for clients with chronic psychiatric disorders.

Culturally Competent Care
- Treating clients from diverse cultures, viewing each client as a unique individual, and noting a potential relationship between the client's cultural experiences and his or her symptom presentation and perceptions
- Assumes that if the NP becomes more sensitive to cultural issues surrounding the client's symptoms and treatment, more comprehensive health care can be provided
- *Culture*— The learned beliefs and behaviors or the socially inherited characteristics that are common among all members of a group; may be a racial, social, ethnic, or religious grouping
- *Culture-bound syndromes*—Specific behaviors related to a person's culture and not linked to a psychiatric disorder
- Be cognizant of inaccurately judging a client's behavior as psychopathology when it is really related to his or her culture.

Cultural Influences
- *Family*—A group of adults and children who are usually related and whose adults participate in carrying out the essential functions of providing food, clothing, shelter, safety, and education of children
  - Concept broadened beyond the traditional husband–wife–children pattern
  - Family initially teaches the belief patterns, religion, culture, and mores of a society.
- *Ethnicity*—Self-identified race, tribe, or nation with which a person or group identifies and which greatly influences beliefs and behavior

- *Community*—A group of families often sharing the same race, tribe, or culture and who have beliefs or behavior not shared by others
- *Environment*—Includes both physical and psychosocial factors; the general circumstances of an individual's life:
  - Social contacts
  - Housing surroundings
  - Climate
  - Altitude
  - Temperature
  - Air pollution
  - Fluoride in water
  - Water contamination
  - Crime
  - Poverty
  - Transportation.

Research

- *Research utilization*—Process of synthesizing, disseminating, and using research-generated knowledge to make a change in practices; a subset of the broader evidence-based practice
- *Evidence-based practice*—The integration of best research evidence with clinical expertise and patient values and needs
- Research utilization and evidence-based practice are two models for reducing the gap between research findings and application to practice.

Research Utilization Process

- Critique research
- Synthesize the findings
- Apply the findings
- Measure the outcomes.

Evidence-Based Practice Model

- Develop a clinical question using the PICO method (Richardson, Wilson, Nishikawa, & Hayward, 1995)
  - P = patient, population of patients, problem
  - I = intervention
  - C = comparison (another treatment or therapy, placebo)
  - O = outcome.
- Systematically search for relevant research evidence
- Critique the research evidence
- Make an evidence-based decision regarding implementation
- Implement the change, depending on the above decision
- Evaluate the change.

Concepts in Interpreting Research Findings

- *Internal validity*—When the independent variable (the treatment) caused a change in the dependent variable (the outcome)
- *External validity*—When the sample is representative of the population and the results can be generalized
- *Descriptive statistics*—Used to describe the basic features of the data in the study; numerical values that summarize, organize, and describe observations; can be generated by either quantitative or qualitative studies

- Examples include
  - *Mean*—Average of scores
  - *Standard deviation*—Indication of the possible deviations from the mean
  - *Variance*—How the values are dispersed around the mean; the larger the variance, the larger the dispersion of scores.
- *Inferential statistics*—Numerical values that enable one to reach conclusions that extend beyond the immediate data alone; generated by quantitative research designs
  - Examples include
    - *t test*—Assesses whether the means of two groups are statistically different from each other
    - *Analysis of variance (ANOVA)*—Tests the difference among 3 or more groups
    - *Pearson's* r *correlation*—Tests the relationship between 2 variables
    - *Probability*—Likelihood of an event occurring; lies between 0 and 1; an impossible event has a probability of 0, and a certain event has a probability of 1
    - *p value*—Also known as *level of significance;* describes the probability of a particular result occurring by chance alone (if p = .01, there is a 1% probability of obtaining a result by chance alone).

Ethical Considerations in Research
- *Institutional review boards (IRBs)* ensure that
  - Risks to participants are minimized
  - Participant selection is equitable
  - Adverse events are reported and risks/benefits are reevaluated
  - Informed consent is obtained and documented
  - Data and safety monitoring plans are implemented when indicated
  - Overall, the IRB protects the rights and welfare of human research participants and has the authority to approve, require modifications, or disapprove of any research activities.
- All investigators or individuals involved in research studies must take and pass a test on protection of human participants—*The Belmont Report* (U.S. Department of Health, Education, and Welfare, 1979).

Critical Thinking
- Defined as the acquisition of knowledge with an attitude of deliberate inquiry
- Making clinical decisions based on evidence-based practice
- Decreases the difficulty of choosing from conflicting or multiple recommendations when diagnosing and treating clients.

Case Study

Karen is a newly graduated PMHNP. She worked as a psychiatric nurse for 5 years before going to graduate school. She is considering a job at the local community mental health center. The director of the center has told her that her role would consist of seeing mainly adult patients with serious, chronic, and persistent mental illness.

On occasions when the psychiatrist is "busy," Karen is told she may be expected to see a few children in addition to adults. The director expects Karen to provide medication management to well-known clients and occasionally to assist in diagnostic evaluations of new clients or clients in crisis. He also expects that she will "from time to time" meet the emergent medical needs of clients who have limited access to primary care providers, including the routine, ongoing care of nonpsychiatric disorders such as diabetes, hypertension, and chronic pain. Karen has many issues to consider before deciding to take or not take the position:

- Would she be legally authorized to treat both children and adults?

- What regulation, rule, or standard should she consult to determine if she is legally allowed to treat both children and adults?

- What regulation, rule, or standard should she consult to determine if she is legally allowed to treat both physical and psychiatric disorders?

- What is the role of professional psychiatric nursing organizations in assisting her to determine the scope of practice that is appropriate for her as a new graduate?

Karen decides not to take that job and instead has been working for about a year as a PMHNP in a nurse-managed primary mental health clinic. One day she is asked to assess a client who is clearly psychotic, experiencing hallucinations and delusions, and expressing verbal threats against many individuals at another clinical practice in town who had "malpracticed me." The client is adamant that he does not wish any treatment and that he is not ill. To care for this client, Karen has significant issues to consider:

- Is she able to treat the client if he is not consenting to care?

- What legal standards must be met if she is to involuntarily treat this client?

About 5 weeks later the above-mentioned client returns to the clinic for follow-up care. He is clinically stable, on medication, and showing no active symptoms. He is interested in developing a relapse prevention plan and asks Karen to assist him in this process. Karen has important issues to consider:

- Is the inclusion of a durable power of attorney an appropriate strategy in relapse planning for this client?

- What quality indicators should be considered in planning his care with the client?

- What risk management and liability issues should she consider?

Review Questions

1. The purpose of the American Nurses Association's *Scope and Standards of Psychiatric–Mental Health Clinical Nursing Practice* is to

   a. Define the role and actions for the NP

   b. Establish the legal authority for the prescription of psychotropic medications

   c. Define the legal statutes of the role of the PMHNP

   d. Define the differences between the physician role and the NP role

2. The trend in legal rulings on cases involving mental illness over the past 25 years has been to

   a. Encourage juries to find defendants not guilty by reason of insanity

   b. Protect the individual's freedoms or rights when he or she is committed to a mental hospital

   c. Place increasing trust in mental health professionals to make good and ethical decisions

   d. Decrease all the "red tape" associated with commitments so that commitments are faster and easier

3. A community has an unusually high incidence of depression and drug use among the teenage population. The public health nurses decide to address this problem, in part, by modifying the environment and strengthening the capacities of families to prevent the development of new cases of depression and drug use. This is an example of

   a. Primary prevention

   b. Secondary prevention

   c. Tertiary prevention

   d. Protective factorial prevention

4. Mrs. Kemp is voluntarily admitted to the hospital. After 24 hours she states she wishes to leave because "this place can't help me." The best nursing action that reflects the legal right of this client is

   a. To discharge the client

   b. Explain that the client cannot leave until the nurse can complete further assessment

   c. Allow the client to leave but have her sign forms stating she is leaving against medical advice

   d. Immediately start the paperwork to commit the client and to allow her to be treated against her wishes

References and Resources

American Nurses Association. (2000a). *Medicare and "incidental to" payment: Coverage of nursing services in hospital outpatient clinics and emergency departments.* Washington, DC: Author.

American Nurses Association. (2000b). *Scope and standards of psychiatric–mental health clinical nursing practice.* Washington, DC: Author.

American Nurses Association. (2005). *Code of ethics for nurses.* Washington, DC: ANA Code of Ethics Project Task Force.

American Psychiatric Association. (2000). *Diagnostic and statistical manual of mental disorders* (4th ed., text rev.). Washington, DC: Author.

Brownson, R. C., & Petitti, D. (2006). *Applied epidemiology: Theory to practice* (2nd ed.). London: Oxford University Press.

Buppert, C. (2003). *Nurse practitioners business practice and legal guide* (2nd ed.). Gaithersburg, MD: Aspen.

Burgess, A. W. (1998). *Advanced practice psychiatric nursing.* Stamford, CT: Appleton & Lange.

Cotroneo, M., Kurlowicz, L. H., Outlaw, F. H., Burgess, A. W., & Evans, L. K. (2001). Psychiatric mental health nursing at the interface: Revisioning education for the specialty. *Issues in Mental Health Nursing, 22,* 549–569.

Delaney, K., Chisholm, M., Clement, J., & Merwin, E. (1999). Trends in psychiatric mental health education. *Archives of Psychiatric Nursing, 13*(2), 67–73.

Edmunds, M. W., Horan, N. M., & Mayhew, M. S. (2000). *Adult nurse practitioner review manual.* Washington, DC: American Nurses Association.

Farnam, C., Zipple, A. M., Tyrell, W., & Chittiinanda, P. (1999). Health status risk factors of people with severe and persistent mental illness. *Journal of Psychosocial Nursing, 37,* 16–19.

Ford, L. C. (1992). Advancing nursing practice: Future of the nurse practitioner. In L. H. Aiken & C. M. Fagin (Eds.), *Charting nursing's future: Agenda for the 1990s.* Philadelphia: J. B. Lippincott.

Friedman, M. (2002). *Family nursing: Research, theory, and practice* (5th ed.). Stamford, CT: Appleton & Lange.

Harris, E., & Barraclough, B. (1999). Excess mortality of mental disorder. *British Journal of Psychiatry, 173,* 476–481.

Health Insurance Portability and Accountability Act (HIPAA). (1996). Public Law 104-191.

Institute for the Future. (2000). *Health and health care 2010: The forecast, the challenge.* San Francisco: Jossey-Bass.

Johnson, M., Maas, M., & Moorhead, S. (Eds.). (2003). *Nursing outcomes classification* (3rd ed.). St. Louis, MO: Mosby/Year Book

Macnee, C., & McCabe, S. (2000). Micro stressors: The impact of hassles and uplifts. In V. H. Rice (Ed.), *Handbook of stress and coping: Implications for nursing research, theory, and practice* (pp. 125–142). Thousand Oaks, CA: Sage.

McBride, A., & Austin, J. (1996). *Psychiatric mental health nursing: Integrating the behavioral and biological sciences.* Philadelphia: W. B. Saunders.

McCabe, S. (2000). Bringing psychiatric nursing into the twenty-first century. *Archives of Psychiatric Nursing, 14*(3), 109–116.

McCabe, S. (2002). The nature of psychiatric nursing: The intersection of paradigm, evolution, and history. *Archives of Psychiatric Nursing, 16*(2), 51–60.

McCabe, S., & Macnee, C. L. (2002). Weaving a new safety net of mental health care in rural America: A model of integrated practice. *Issues in Mental Health Nursing, 23,* 263–278.

McCloskey, J. C., & Bulechek, G. M. (Eds.). (2000). *Nursing interventions classification* (3rd ed.). St. Louis, MO: Mosby/Year Book.

Mellow, J. (1968). Nursing therapy. *American Journal of Nursing, 68,* 2365.

Mirr Jansen, M., & Zwygart-Stauffacher, M. (2006). *Advanced practice nursing: Core concepts for professional role development* (3rd ed.). New York: Springer Publishing.

Nagle, M., & Krainovich-Miller, B. (2001). Shaping the advanced practice psychiatric nursing role: A futuristic model. *Issues in Mental Health Nursing, 22,* 461–482.

National Organization of Nurse Practitioner Faculties. (2003). *Psychiatric mental health nurse practitioner competencies.* Washington, DC: National Panel for Nurse Practitioner Faculties.

National Organization of Nurse Practitioner Faculties. (2006). *Domains and core competencies of nurse practitioner practice.* Washington, DC: National Panel for Nurse Practitioner Faculties.

Nettina, S. M., & Knudtson, M. (2001). *The family nurse practitioner review manual.* Washington, DC: American Nurses Credentialing Center.

North American Nursing Diagnosis Association. (2000). *Nursing diagnosis: Definitions and classifications 1999–2000.* Philadelphia: Author.

Peplau, H. (1952). *Interpersonal relations in nursing.* New York: G. P. Putnam's Sons.

Richardon, W. S., Wilson, M. C., Nishikawa, J., & Hayward, R. S. (1995). The well-built clinical question: A key to evidence based decisions. *ACP Journal Club, 123*(3), A12–3.

Sadock, B., & Sadock, V. (2007). *Kaplan and Sadock's synopsis of psychiatry* (10th ed.). New York: Lippincott Williams & Wilkins.

Shea, C. A., Pelletier, L., Poster, E. C., Stuart, G. W., & Verhey, M. P. (1999). *Advanced practice nursing in psychiatric mental health care.* St. Louis, MO: Mosby.

Stuart, G. W., & Laraia, M. T. (2005). *Principles and practice of psychiatric nursing* (8th ed.). St. Louis, MO: Mosby.

Tarasoff v. The Regents at the University of California, Supreme Court of California. (1976).

U.S. Department of Health and Human Services. (2000). *Mental health: A report of the Surgeon General.* Washington, DC: Substance Abuse and Mental Health Service Administration, National Institute of Mental Health.

U.S. Department of Health and Human Services. (2005). *Healthy People 2010.* Washington, DC: Office of Disease Prevention and Health Promotion.

U.S. Department of Health, Education, and Welfare. (1979). *The Belmont Report.* Washington, DC: Author.

World Health Organization. (2007). *International classification of diseases* (9th rev.). Geneva: World Health Organization Assembly.

Notes:

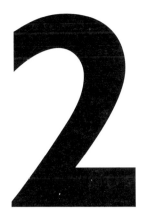

Theoretical Basis of Care

Whereas the psychiatric–mental health nurse practitioner (PMHNP) role is relatively new, psychiatric–mental health nursing has a long, well-established, and cherished tradition of advanced practice. As with all other specialty areas of nursing, advanced practice psychiatric nursing is theoretically grounded, and a wide array of theories form the basis of the PMHNP role. These theories help identify the foundational, core concepts of advanced-practice psychiatric nursing. The scope of practice for the PMHNP is based on an understanding of the foundational core concepts and the theories from which these concepts are drawn (Marriner-Tomey & Alligood, 2005).

This chapter reviews the foundational/core concepts and theories that underpin the PMHNP role. Four foundational concepts (see Table 2–1) are discussed, followed by a review of both the nursing and non-nursing theories on which the PMHNP role is based. The core concepts and theories form the basis of the care practices of the PMHNP. Therapeutic interventions derived from the theories also are addressed.

Foundational/Core Concepts for PMHNP Practice

Foundational/Core Concept 1: Mental Health
- Mental health can be seen as a dynamic, fluid state that is made up of many components.
- Mental health is best viewed as the totality of an individual's ability to function in and to interact with the world.

Factors That Compose Mental Health
- Ability to form age-appropriate interpersonal relationships
- Ability for productivity
  - School productivity for children or adolescents
  - Work productivity for adults
- Ability to display humor
- Capacity for flexibility
- Ability to form healthy self-concept

- Degree of self-esteem
- Ability to correctly evaluate reality, including one's own strengths and weaknesses
- Capacity to deal with conflict
- Utilization of a variety of coping strategies
- Capacity to accept responsibility for one's own actions
- Ability to think clearly
- Capacity for problem solving
- Judgment
- Reasoning
- Insight
- Capacity for self-defined spirituality
- Capacity for self-control and age-appropriate modulation of emotions and behavior.

Foundational/Core Concept 2: Mental Illness

- Mental illness is seen as a clinically significant behavioral or psychological syndrome or pattern causing distress, pain, or disability for the individual.
- Research from the American Psychological Association's Decade of the Brain (National Institute of Mental Health, 1990) has increasingly shown that common, well-identified mental disorders such as schizophrenia, major depression, bipolar disorders, attention deficit/hyperactivity disorder, and obsessive–compulsive disorder have an underlying biological basis.
- Brain-based focus has strengthened the belief that continuing to call these disorders "mental illness" continues a stigmatizing approach to patient care.
- The focus on mental illnesses as brain-based disorders has led to name changes.
  - Mental illnesses are now commonly referred to as *psychiatric disorders* and *behavioral health disorders*.
- Some of the factors identified as aspects of the complex etiology of common psychiatric disorders include

  - Genetic
  - Hormonal
  - Immune
  - Stress
  - Coping

  - Interpersonal
  - Demographic and geographic
  - Developmental history
  - Health practices and beliefs
  - Cultural.

Classifying Psychiatric Disorders

- Psychiatric disorders are classified using standard criteria of the *Diagnostic and Statistical Manual of Mental Disorders* (*DSM-IV-TR;* American Psychiatric Association, 2000).
- The *DSM-IV-TR* classifies mental illnesses on the basis of specific criteria that have been tested for reliability when used by mental health professionals.
- The *DSM-IV-TR* classification system uses a multiaxial approach (see Table 2–2) to diagnostic classifications that allows for holistic assessment.
- A client is assessed in five general areas, and each area is individually coded as an axis.
- Each axis represents a specific assessment, and when taken together the five axes represent the totality of an individual's psychosocial–biological functioning, not merely the assessment of a single psychiatric disorder.

Table 2–1. Core Concepts of the PMHNP Role

Core Concept	Definition
Mental health	The totality of an individual's ability to function in and interact with the world as indicated by a person's sense of self, level of growth, development, self-actualization, integration, autonomy, flexibility, perceptual capacities, and environmental mastery (Sadock & Sadock, 2007).
Mental illness Psychiatric disorders Behavioral health disorders	Any disruption in the usual constitutions of mental health; assumes an underlying psychopathology and can be defined as a clinically significant behavioral/psychological syndrome or pattern that occurs in an individual and that is associated with persistent distress or disability or with a significant increased risk of death, pain, disability, or an important loss of freedom (American Psychiatric Association, 2000).
Therapeutic relationship	The mutual interactive, interpersonal, relational experience between nurse and client that forms the context for care in which the nurse uses herself or himself to assist a client toward optimal health (Sadock & Sadock, 2007).
Growth and development	An overarching principle of normal adaptive changes—associated with human growth—that allows an individual to exhibit dynamic changes on both the cellular and social levels (Sadock & Sadock, 2007).

Table 2–2. DSM-IV-TR Multiaxial Classification Schema

Axis	Definition	Disorder Example
Axis I	Clinical disorders; other conditions that may be the focus of clinical attention	Mood disorders Anxiety disorders Psychotic disorders Disorders usually diagnosed in infancy, childhood, and adolescence (excluding mental retardation)
Axis II	Personality disorders Mental retardation Prominent maladaptive personality features Defense mechanisms	Borderline personality disorder Antisocial personality disorder Image-distorting defense mechanisms Diseases of the nervous system
Axis III	General medical condition potentially relevant to the management of Axis I or II disorders	Endocrine disorders Conditions originating in the perinatal period

Continued on the next page

Table 2–2. Continued

Axis	Definition	Disorder Example
Axis IV	Psychosocial and environmental problems	Problems with primary supports Problems related to social environment Housing problems Problems with access to health care
Axis V	Global assessment of functioning (GAF)	Clinician's judgment of the client's overall functioning coded on a scale of 0–100, with the higher number indicating higher functioning; also the highest GAF in the last year is stated

Adapted from American Psychiatric Association. (2000). *Diagnostic and statistical manual of mental disorders* (4th ed., text rev.). Washington, DC: Author.

Foundational/Core Concept 3: Therapeutic Relationship

- Assumes the client and nurse enter into a mutual, interactive, interpersonal relationship specifically to focus on the identified needs of the client.
- Therapeutic relationships are focused on the client's needs, goal directed, theory based, and open to supervision.

Characteristics of a Therapeutic Relationship

- Genuineness
- Acceptance
- Nonjudgmental attitude
- Authenticity
- Empathy
- Respect
- Professional boundaries.
- The therapeutic relationship is seen as having specific and sequential phases (see Table 2–3).
- Transference and countertransference are key concepts in the nurse–client relationship.
    - *Transference*—Displacement of feelings for significant people in the client's past onto the PMHNP in the present relationship
    - *Countertransference*—Represents the nurse's emotional reaction to the client based on her or his past experiences.

Table 2–3. Phases of a Therapeutic Nurse–Client Relationship

Phase	Nursing Action	Common Client Behavior
Introduction (Orientation)	Creating a trusting environment Establishing professional boundaries Establishing the length of anticipated interaction Providing diagnostic evaluation Setting mutually agreed-on treatment objectives	Initial hesitancy by the client to participate fully in assessment and treatment planning (approach avoidance)
Working (Identification and Exploitation)	Clarifying client expectations and mutually set goals Implementing treatment plan Monitoring health Undertaking preventive health care Measuring outcomes of care Evaluating outcomes of care Reprioritizing plan and objectives as indicated	Transference—client Countertransference—nurse Client resistance to care practices Client resistance to change
Termination (Resolution)	Reviewing client's progress toward objectives Establishing long-term plan of care Focusing on self-management strategies Disengaging from relationship Referring client to other services as needed	Client resistance to termination Regression Reemergence of symptoms or problems

Adapted from Keltner, N., Schwecke, L. H., & Bostrom, C. E. (2006). *Psychiatric nursing* (5th ed.). St. Louis, MO: Mosby.

Signs indicating the presence of countertransference in the PMHNP include
- Intense emotional reactions, positive or negative, on first contact with client
- Recurrent anxiety or uneasiness while dealing with client
- Uncharacteristic carelessness in interaction and follow-up with client
- Difficulty empathizing
- Resistance to others treating or interacting with client
- Preoccupation with or dreaming about client
- Running overtime with client or always cutting time short with client
- Depression or other strong emotions during or after interaction with client
- Feedback from others over involvement with client.

- The PMHNP is expected to monitor her or his reaction to clients to constantly assess for the presence of countertransference.
- If identified, countertransference is usually dealt with through the supervisory process and in talking to coworkers about the issues.
  - Provided in peer–peer or peer–supervisor relationship
  - Examines interpersonal dynamics inherent in the PMHNP's relationship with client.

Foundational/Core Concept 4: Growth and Development

- Assumes that growth, change, and development are part of the dynamic, constant life process of being human.
- Humans develop uniquely from simple to complex.
- The health states of individuals and families can be viewed over a continuum of development.
- Developmental stages and the milestones or tasks that accompany them give insight into age-appropriate behaviors, measure levels of comprehension for client teaching, and provide a context within which to evaluate assessment data (see Table 2–4).
  - *Example:* The mental status finding of concrete thinking in a 9-year-old client would be normal and expected; however, the same finding in a 29-year-old client is non-normative and suggestive of psychopathology (see Table 2–5 for typical age of onset for psychiatric disorders).

Table 2–4. Erik Erikson's (1902–1994) Stages of Human Development

Developmental Stage	Age	Developmental Task	Indications of Developmental Mastery	Indications of Developmental Failure
Infancy	0–1 year	Trust vs. mistrust	Ability to form meaningful relationships, hope about the future, trust in others	Poor relationships, lack of future hope, suspicious of others
Early childhood	1–3	Autonomy vs. shame and doubt	Self-control, self-esteem, willpower	Poor self-control, low self-esteem, self-doubt, lack of independence
Late childhood	3–6	Initiative vs. guilt	Self-directed behavior, goal formation, sense of purpose	Lack of self-initiated behavior, lack of goal orientation
School age	6–12	Industry vs. inferiority	Ability to work; sense of competency and achievement	Sense of inferiority; difficulty with working, learning

Table 2–4. Continued

Developmental Stage	Age	Developmental Task	Indications of Developmental Mastery	Indications of Developmental Failure
Adolescence	12–20	Identity vs. role confusion	Personal sense of identity	Identify confusion, poor self-identification in group settings
Early adulthood	20–35	Intimacy vs. isolation	Committed relationships, capacity to love	Emotional isolation, egocentrism
Middle adulthood	35–65	Generativity vs. self-absorption or stagnation	Ability to give time and talents to others, ability to care for others	Self-absorption, inability to grow and change as a person, inability to care for others
Late adulthood	>65	Integrity vs. despair	Fulfillment and comfort with life, willingness to face death, insight and balanced perspective on life's events	Bitterness, sense of dissatisfaction with life, despair over impending death

Adapted from B. Sadock & V. Sadock, 2007, *Kaplan and Sadock's synopsis of psychiatry* (10th ed.). New York: Lippincott Williams & Wilkins.

Table 2–5. Examples of Typical Age of Onset for Common Psychiatric Disorders

Disorder	Age of Onset
Mental retardation	Infancy—usually evident at birth
Attention-deficit/hyperactivity disorder	4–6 years
Schizophrenia	18–25 years for men; 25–35 years for women
Major depression	Late adolescence to young adulthood
Dementia	Most common after age 85

Adapted from B. Sadock & V. Sadock, 2007, *Kaplan and Sadock's synopsis of psychiatry* (10th ed.). New York: Lippincott Williams & Wilkins.

Foundational Theories Supporting PMHNP Role

Psychodynamic (Psychoanalytic) Theory (Sigmund Freud, 1856–1939)

- Focus on concepts of intrapsychic conflict among the structures of the mind
- Initially designed to explain neurosis, conditions of high anxiety such as phobias and hysteria

- Theory later expanded to include normal and abnormal development and personality development.

Basic Tenets of Psychodynamic Theory

- Psychoanalytic theory assumes that all behavior is purposeful and meaningful. All behavior has meaning.
- Referred to as the *Principle of Psychic Determinism;* even apparently meaningless, random, or accidental behavior is actually motivated by underlying unconscious mental content.
  - *Example:* A person forgets where he parked the car because he really does not wish to go wherever it was that he was headed.
- Most mental activity is unconscious—urges, feelings, and fantasies that would be unacceptable to the person's values if consciously experienced.
- Conscious behaviors and choices are affected by unconscious mental content.
- Past childhood experiences shape adult personality.
- Instincts, urges, or fantasies function as drives that motivate thoughts, feelings, and behaviors.
- Two types of normal drives: sexual drives (libido) and aggressive drives.
- Drives affect behavior as an individual attempts to deal with the associated feelings and seeks gratification through release of the tension the drive produces.
- Normally, different actions/behaviors are used at different ages to discharge tension from drives and to therefore seek gratification.
- Psychosexual stages of development have been identified to show the age-related behaviors commonly used for discharging drives and obtaining gratification (see Table 2–6).

Table 2–6. Freud's Psychosexual Stages of Development

Stage	Age	Primary Means of Discharging Drives and Achieving Gratification	Psychiatric Disorder Linked to Failure of Stage
Oral stage	0–18 months	Sucking, chewing, feeding, crying	Schizophrenia Substance abuse Paranoia
Anal stage	18 months– 3 years	Sphincter control, activities of expulsion and retention	Depressive disorders
Phallic stage	3–6 years	Exhibitionism, masturbation with focus on Oedipal conflict, castration anxiety, and female fear of lost maternal love	Sexual identity disorders
Latency stage	6 years– puberty	Peer relationships, learning, motor-skills development, socialization	Inability to form social relationships
Genital stage	Puberty forward	Integration and synthesis of behaviors from early stages, primary genital-based sexuality	Sexual perversion disorders

Adapted from B. Sadock & V. Sadock, 2007, *Kaplan and Sadock's synopsis of psychiatry* (10th ed.). New York: Lippincott Williams & Wilkins.

- *Three primary psychic structures* make up the mind and personality and are responsible for mental functioning:

The Id

- Contains primary drives or instincts, urges, or fantasies (hunger, sex, or aggression)
- Drives are largely unconscious, sexual or aggressive in content, and infantile in nature
- Operates on the pleasure principle; seeks immediate satisfaction
- Is present at birth and motivates early infantile actions
- The id says "I want."

The Ego

- Contains concept of *external reality*
- Rational mind; logical and abstract thinking
- Functions in adaptation
- Mediates between demands of drives and environmental realities
- Operates on the reality principle
- Begins to develop at birth as infant struggles to deal with environment
- Use of defense mechanisms
- The ego says "I think, I evaluate."

The Superego

- Is the ego-ideal
- Contains sense of conscience or right vs. wrong
- Also contains aspirations, ideals, and moral values
- Regulated by guilt and shame
- Begins to fully develop around age 6 as a child comes into contact with external authority figures such as schoolteachers, coaches, or religious figures
- The superego says "I should or ought."

- Psychic structures commonly come in conflict over what to do to achieve gratification.
- While exact nature of conflict is often unconscious, conflict is experienced consciously as anxiety.
- The function of anxiety is to alert conscious mind to presence of conflict.
- Conflict normally dealt with through use of defense mechanisms (see Table 2–7).
  - Are a function of the ego
  - Are unconsciously called into action
  - Are used to reduce anxiety
  - Become part of the personality
  - Maintain sense of safety
  - Promote self-esteem and a sense of well-being
  - May be used episodically or habitually
  - May be constantly used and become fixed as seen in neurosis.

Table 2–7. Defense Mechanisms

Defense Mechanism	Explanation
Denial	Avoidance of unpleasant realities by unconsciously ignoring their existence
Projection	Unconscious rejection of emotionally unacceptable personal attributes, beliefs, or actions by attributing them to other people, situations, or events
Regression	Return to more comfortable thoughts, behaviors, or feelings used in earlier stages of development in response to current conflict, stress, or threat
Repression	Unconscious exclusion of unwanted, disturbing emotions, thoughts, or impulses from conscious awareness
Reaction formation	Often called *overcompensation;* unacceptable feelings, thoughts, or behaviors are pushed from conscious awareness by displaying and acting on the opposite feeling, thought, or behavior
Rationalization	Justification of illogical, unreasonable ideas, feelings, or actions by developing an acceptable explanation that satisfies the person
Undoing	Behaviors that attempt to make up for or undo an unacceptable action, feeling, or impulse
Intellectualization	Attempts to master current stressor or conflict by expansion of knowledge, explanation, or understanding
Suppression	Conscious analog of repression; conscious denial of a disturbing situation, feeling, or event
Sublimation	Unconscious process of substitution of socially acceptable, constructive activity for strong unacceptable impulse
Altruism	Meeting the needs of others in order to discharge drives, conflicts, or stressors

Adapted from C.A. Shea, L. Pelletier, E. C. Poster, G. W. Stuart & M. P. Verhey, 1999, *Advanced practice nursing in psychiatric mental health care.* St. Louis, MO: Mosby.

Cognitive Theory (Jean Piaget, 1896–1980)

- Belief that human development evolves through cognition, learning, and comprehending.
- Belief that factors such as native endowment and biological and environmental factors set the course for a child's development.
- Piaget developed *four stages of cognitive development:*
  - *Sensorimotor* (Birth–2 years)—Critical achievement of this stage is *object permanence,* the ability to understand that objects have an existence independent of the child's involvement with them
  - *Preoperational* (2–7 years)—More extensive use of language and symbolism; magical thinking

- *Concrete operations* (7–12 years)—Begins to use logic; develops concepts of reversibility and conservation
  - *Reversibility*—Realization that one thing can turn into another and back again (e.g., water and ice)
  - *Conservation*—Ability to recognize that although the shape of an object may change, it will still maintain characteristics that enable it to be recognized as that object (e.g., clay)
- *Formal operations* (12 years–adult)—Ability to think abstractly; thinking operates in a formal, logical manner.

Interpersonal Theory (Harry Stack Sullivan, 1892–1949)

- Behavior occurs because of interpersonal dynamics.
- Interpersonal relationships and experiences influence one's personality development, which is called the *self-system* (the total components of personality traits).
- Understanding behavior requires understanding the relationships in the individual's life.
- *Two drives for individual's behavior:* drive for satisfaction (basic human drives such as sleep, sex, hunger) and drive for security (conforming to social norms of individual's reference group).
- Belief that when the individual's need for satisfaction and security is interfered with by the self-system, mental illness occurs.
- Belief that humans experience anxiety and behavior is directed towards relieving the anxiety, which then results in *interpersonal security.*
- Sullivan eveloped *stages of interpersonal development* (see Table 2–8).

Table 2–8. Stages of Interpersonal Development

Stage	Time Period	Developmental Task
Infancy	Birth–18 months	Oral gratification; anxiety occurs for the first time
Childhood	18 months–6 years	Delayed gratification
Juvenile	6–9 years	Forming of peer relationships
Preadolescence	9–12 years	Same-sex relationships
Early adolescence	12–14 years	Opposite-sex relationships
Late adolescence	14–21 years	Self-identity developed

Adapted from B. Sadock & V. Sadock, 2007, *Kaplan and Sadock's synopsis of psychiatry* (10th ed.). New York: Lippincott Williams & Wilkins.

Hierarchy of Needs Theory (Abraham Maslow, 1908–1970)

- Health model rather than illness model
- A hierarchical organization of needs
- Hypotheses that certain needs are more important than others
- An individual will attempt to meet more important needs before satisfying other needs.

Hierarchy of Needs

Survival Needs
- Water
- Air
- Food
- Sleep.

Safety and Security Needs
- Protection from harm—emotional and physical.

Love and Belonging
- Affection, intimacy, and companionship.

Self-Esteem
- Sense of worth.

Self-Actualization Needs
- Achieving one's potential
- Being all that one can be.

Health Belief Model (Marshall Becker, 1940–1993)
- Explains that healthy people do not always take advantage of screening or preventive programs because of certain variables:
  - Perception of susceptibility
  - Seriousness of illness
  - Perceived benefits of treatment
  - Perceived barriers to change
  - Expectations of efficacy.

Trans-Theoretical Model of Change
- States that change such as in health behaviors occurs in six predictable stages (Prochaska, Norcross, & DiClemente, 1992):
  - *Pre-contemplation*—The individual has no intention to change.
  - *Contemplation*—The individual is thinking about changing—is aware that there is a problem but not committed to changing.
  - *Preparation*—The individual has made the decision to change—is ready for action.
  - *Action*—The individual is engaging in specific overt actions to change.
  - *Maintenance*—The individual is engaging in behaviors to prevent relapse.

Self-Efficacy/Social Learning Theory (Albert Bandura, 1925–)
- Behavior is the result of cognitive and environmental factors.
- Individuals learn by observing others, relying on role modeling.

- *Self-efficacy* is the perception of one's ability to perform a certain task at a certain level of accomplishment.
- Behavioral change and maintenance are a function of outcome expectations and efficacy expectations.

Nursing Theories

Theory of Cultural Care (Madeline Leininger, 1925–)
- Regardless of the culture, care is the unifying focus and the essence of nursing.
- Health and well-being can be predicted through cultural care.

Theory of Self-Care (Dorothy Orem, 1914–2007)
- *Self-care*—Activities that maintain life, health, and well-being.

Human Becoming Theory (Rosemarie Parse)
- Individuals freely choose personal meaning in situations.

Health Promotion Theory (Nola Pender, 1941–)
- Explains behavior that enhances health and prevents disease.

Therapeutic Nurse–Client Relationship Theory/Interpersonal Theory (Hildegard Peplau, 1909–1999)
- First significant psychiatric nursing theory
- Based in part on interpersonal theory (Sullivan)
- Sees nursing as an interpersonal process in which all interventions occur within the context of the nurse–client relationship
- The therapeutic nurse–client relationship is central or core to nursing
- Developed *phases of the nurse–client relationship* (see Table 2–3):
  - Orientation phase
  - Working phase (identification, exploitation)
  - Termination phase (resolution).

Theory of Adaptation (Sister Callista Roy, 1939–)
- Promotion of adaptive responses is the goal of nursing.
- Behavior represents the individual trying to adapt to internal or environmental forces.

Caring Theory (Jean Watson)
- Caring is an essential component of nursing.
- "Carative factors" guide the core of nursing and should be implemented in health care.
- Carative factors are those aspects of care that potentiate therapeutic healing and relationships.

Case Study

Thomas Jones is a 19-year-old college freshman. During the second week of classes, he presented to the student health services clinic of the college he attends seeking help for "shyness." As the PMHNP working the day Mr. Jones presented for care, you are responsible for assessment and care planning with this client.

As you are working with him, he gives a chief complaint of feeling uncomfortable around all of the strangers he is meeting and of a desire to return home and drop out of school. There are several issues for you to consider as you begin to work with Mr. Jones:

- Chronologically, what stage of development should Mr. Jones be experiencing?

- What are the tasks of this stage?

- How would you assess the actual developmental issues that he is experiencing?

- What factors do you need to consider to determine if he is experiencing normative or non-normative behaviors?

- What characteristics do you as the PMHNP need to display to establish a therapeutic relationship with him?

Mr. Jones reported that he has not been sleeping well, has experienced a decrease in appetite, and just wants to talk to someone about his problems in adjusting to school. In planning the follow-up care for Mr. Jones, you have important issues to consider:

- What would be the goal of continued work with Mr. Jones?

- If you were to start therapy with him, what kind of therapy would you consider?

- Would you consider him to have a mental illness?

Review Questions

1. The *DSM-IV-TR* is the most common classification system used to identify and diagnose mental illness. The one aspect of an illness not discussed in the *DSM-IV-TR* is:

    a. Complications of the common disorders

    b. Symptoms of common disorders

    c. Lab tests useful in diagnosing common disorders

    d. Etiology of common disorders

2. Mrs. French has been in individual therapy for 3 months. She has shown much growth and improvement in her functioning and insight and is to discontinue services within the next few weeks. In the next session, after you discuss service termination, she suddenly begins to demonstrate the original symptoms that had brought her to treatment initially. She is now hesitant to discharge, wants to continue services, and is

displaying an increase in regressive defense mechanisms. The best explanation for Mrs. French's behavior is

a. An exacerbation of her symptoms related to stress
b. The normal cyclic nature of chronic mental health symptoms
c. A sign of normal resistance to termination seen in the termination phase of the nurse–client relationship
d. A sign of pathological attachment to the therapist that must be addressed

3. An example of a mature, healthy defense mechanism is

a. Denial
b. Rationalization
c. Repression
d. Suppression

4. A man thinks to himself that his wife is ugly as he sees her at the breakfast table one morning. He doesn't tell her his thinking because he doesn't want to hurt her feelings. Later in the day he gets a sudden unexplainable urge to send his wife flowers. The best explanation for his unconscious action is

a. Undoing
b. Suppression
c. Denial
d. Repression

References and Resources

American Nurses Association. (2000). *Scope and standards of psychiatric–mental health clinical nursing practice.* Washington, DC: Author.

American Psychiatric Association. (2000). *Diagnostic and statistical manual of mental disorders* (4th ed., text rev.). Washington, DC: Author.

Burgess, A. W. (1998). *Advanced practice psychiatric nursing.* Stamford, CT: Appleton & Lange.

Erikson, E. H. (1963). *Childhood and society.* New York: Basic Books.\Freud, S. (1934). *The ego and the id.* New York: W. W. Norton.

Freud, S. (1936). *The problem of anxiety.* New York: Basic Books.

Haley, J. (1996). *Learning and teaching therapy.* New York: Guilford Press.

Keltner, N., Schwecke, L. H., & Bostrom, C. E. (2006). *Psychiatric nursing* (5th ed.). St. Louis, MO: Mosby.

Kerr, M., & Bowen, M. (1989). *Family evaluation: An approach based on Bowen theory.* New York: W. W. Norton.

Marriner-Tomey, A., &Alligood, M. (2005). *Nursing theorists and their work* (6th ed.). St. Louis, MO: Mosby.

Marsh, D. (1998). *Serious mental illness and the family: The practitioner's guide.* New York: John Wiley and Sons.

Minuchin, S., & Fishman, H. (1981). *Family therapy techniques.* Cambridge, MA: Harvard University Press.

Mohr, W. (2000). Partnering with families. *Journal of Psychosocial Nursing, 38,* 15–19.

National Institute of Mental Health (NIMH). (1990). *Decade of the brain.* Washington, DC: Author.

Peplau, H. (1952). *Interpersonal relations in nursing.* New York: Putnam.

Prochaska, J., & DiClemente, C. (1984). *The transtheoretical approach: Crossing traditional boundaries therapy.* Homewood, IL: Dow Jones Irwin.

Prochaska, J., Norcross, J., & DiClemente, C. (1992). In search of how people change: Applications to addictive behaviors. *American Psychologist, 47*(9), 1102–1112.

Sadock, B., & Sadock, V. (2007). *Kaplan and Sadock's synopsis of psychiatry* (10th ed.). New York: Lippincott Williams & Wilkins.

Shea, C. A., Pelletier, L., Poster, E. C., Stuart, G. W., & Verhey, M. P. (1999). *Advanced practice nursing in psychiatric mental health care.* St. Louis, MO: Mosby.

Sherman, C. (2000). Assessment is good opportunity to change family dynamics. *Clinical Psychiatric News, 3,* 25–29.

Stuart, G. W., & Laraia, M. (2004). *Principles and practice of psychiatric nursing.* St. Louis, MO: Mosby.

Sullivan, H. S. (1953). *Interpersonal theory of psychiatry.* New York: Basic Books.

Yalom, I. (2005). *The theory and practice of group psychotherapy* (5th ed.). New York: Basic Books.

Notes:

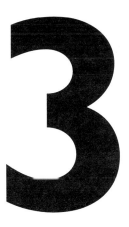

Neuroanatomy, Neurophysiology, and Behavior

A tremendous expansion of knowledge about the brain has occurred in the past two decades. As more has been learned about the brain and its complex functioning, the assessment and treatment of psychiatric disorders have been altered dramatically. Increasingly, the links among genetics, altered brain anatomy and physiology, and the symptoms of psychiatric disorders have been identified (Sadock & Sadock, 2007).

This growing knowledge base will continue to alter the treatment of psychiatric disorders. As new knowledge is disseminated, it is helping diminish the stigma long associated with psychiatric illness.

This chapter reviews the basics of neuroanatomy and physiology that provide the scientific rationale for many of the psychiatric–mental health nurse practitioner (PMHNP) care practices, including psychopharmacological interventions described elsewhere in this review book. PMHNPs need a solid grounding in neurobiology. Increasingly, the roles of the PMHNP require the application of this knowledge to clinical practice.

The Nervous System

- All human thoughts, feelings, and actions are seated in and start with actions of the nervous system.
- Necessary for the PMHNP's role functioning is an understanding of the following basic neuroanatomy and physiology:
  - Neurodeficits that underlie psychiatric disorders
  - Actions of and client responses to psychopharmacological treatment agents.
- The nervous system's primary function is to transfer and exchange information.

The Neuron ("Nerve Cells")
- The basic cellular unit of the nervous system
- The microprocessor of the brain responsible for conducting impulses from one part of the body to another
- Components of the neuron:
  - *Cell body*—Also known as soma; made up of the nucleus and cytoplasm within the cell membrane

- *Stem or axon*—Transmits signals *away* from the neuron's cell body to connect with other neurons and cells
- *Dendrites*—Collect incoming signals from other neurons and send the signal *toward* the neuron's cell body.

Nervous System

- Composed of two separate, interconnected divisions:
  - *Central nervous system (CNS)*
    - Composed of the spinal cord and the brain.
  - *Peripheral nervous system (PNS)*
    - Composed of the peripheral nerves that connect the CNS to receptors, muscles, and glands
    - Includes the cranial nerves just outside the brain stem
    - Composed of the somatic nervous system and the autonomic nervous system
      - *Somatic nervous system*—Conveys information from the CNS to skeletal muscles; responsible for voluntary movement
      - *Autonomic nervous system*—Regulates internal body functions to maintain homeostasis; conveys information from the CNS to smooth muscle, cardiac muscle, and glands; responsible for involuntary movement; divided into the sympathetic nervous system and the parasympathetic nervous system
        - *Sympathetic nervous system*—The excitatory division; prepares the body for stress (fight or flight); stimulates or increases activity of organs
        - *Parasympathetic nervous system*—Maintains or restores energy; inhibits or decreases activity of organs.

Neuroanatomy and the Brain

- Brain tissue is categorized as either white matter or gray matter.
  - *White matter* is the myelinated axons of neurons.
  - *Gray matter* is composed of nerve cell bodies and dendrites; it is the working area of the brain and contains the synapses or area of neuronal connection.
- *Outermost surface of the brain*—Structured to contain grooves and dips of corrugated wrinkles within the brain tissue to provide anatomical landmarks or reference points
  - Functions to increase the brain's surface area
    - Increases working area and cell communication area.
  - Grooves and dips named by size and depth
    - *Sulci*—Small shallow grooves
    - *Fissures*—Deeper groves extending into the brain.
  - *Gyri* are the raised tissue areas.

Distinct Anatomical Areas of the Brain

- The brain is subdivided into the cerebrum and the brain stem.

Cerebrum

- Largest part of the brain, which is divided into two halves, the right and left cerebral hemispheres

- *Left hemisphere*—Dominant in most people; controls most right-sided body functions
- *Right hemisphere*—Controls most left-sided body functions
- Normal functioning requires effective coordination of two hemispheres
- Both hemispheres connected by a large bundle of white matter, the *corpus callosum,* an area of sensorimotor information exchange between the two hemispheres
- Each hemisphere is divided into four major lobes, which work in an interactive and integrated manner, with each having a distinct function:
    1. *Frontal Lobe*—Largest and most developed lobe. Functions include
        - *Motor function*—Responsible for controlling voluntary motor activity of specific muscles
        - *Premotor area*—Coordinates movement of multiple muscles
        - *Association cortex*—Allows for multimodal sensory input to trigger memory and lead to decision making
        - *Seat of executive functions*—Working memory, reasoning, planning, prioritizing, sequencing behavior, insight, flexibility, judgment, impulse control, behavioral cueing, intelligence, abstraction
        - *Language (Broca's area)*—Expressive speech
        - *Personality variables*—The most focal area for personality development
        - Problems in the frontal lobe can lead to personality, emotional, and intellectual changes.

    2. *Temporal Lobe*—Functions include
        - *Language (Wernicke's area)*—Receptive speech or language comprehension
        - *Primary auditory area*
        - *Memory*
        - *Emotion*
        - *Integration area*—Integrates vision with other sensory information
        - Problems in the temporal lobe can lead to visual or auditory hallucinations, aphasia, and amnesia.

    3. *Occipital Lobe*—Functions include
        - *Primary visual cortex*
        - *Integration area*—Integrates vision with other sensory information
        - Problems in the occipital lobe can lead to visual field defects, blindness, and visual hallucinations.

    4. *Parietal Lobe*—Functions include
        - *Primary sensory area*
        - *Taste*
        - *Reading and writing*
        - Problems in the parietal lobe can lead to sensory–perceptual disturbances and agnosia.

- Cerebrum includes important areas of brain, including cerebral cortex, limbic system, thalamus, hypothalamus, and basal ganglia.

- *Cerebral Cortex*
    - Controls wide array of behaviors.
    - Controls the *contralateral* (opposite) side of the body: The right hemisphere controls the left side of the body, and the left hemisphere controls the right side of the body.
    - Sensory information is relayed from thalamus and then processed and integrated in the cortex.
    - Responsible for much of the behavior that makes us human: speech, cognition, judgment, perception, and motor function.

- *Limbic System*
    - Essential system for the regulation and modulation of emotions and memory.
    - Composed of the hypothalamus, thalamus, hippocampus, and amygdala.
        - *Hypothalamus*—Plays key roles in various regulatory functions such as appetite, sensations of hunger and thirst, water balance, circadian rhythms, body temperature, libido, and hormonal regulation
        - *Thalamus*—Sensory relay station except for smell; modulates flow of sensory information to prevent overwhelming the cortex; regulates emotions, memory, and related affective behaviors
        - *Hippocampus*—Regulates memory and converts short-term memory into long-term memory
        - *Amygdala*—Responsible for mediating mood, fear, emotion, and aggression; also responsible for connecting sensory smell information with emotions.

- *Basal Ganglia*—Also known as the *corpus striatum*
    - Serves as a complex feedback system to modulate and stabilize somatic motor activity (information conveyed from the CNS to skeletal muscles).
    - Plays a role in movement initiation; complex motor functions with association connections.
    - Functions in learning and automatic actions such as walking or driving a car.
    - Contains extrapyramidal motor system or nerve track.
    - Functions in involuntary motor activities (e.g., muscle tone, posture, coordination of muscle movement and common reflexes).
    - Many psychotropic medications can affect the extrapyramidal motor nerve track, causing involuntary movement side effects.
    - Contains both the caudate and the putamen.
    - Problems in the basal ganglia can lead to bradykinesia, hyperkinesias, and dystonia.

Brain Stem

- Includes the midbrain, pons, medulla, cerebellum, and reticular formation system.
- Is made up of cells that produce neurotransmitters.
- *Midbrain*—Houses the ventral tegmental area and the substantia nigra (areas of dopamine synthesis)
- *Pons*—Houses the locus ceruleus (area of norepinephrine synthesis)

- *Medulla*—Together with the pons, contains autonomic control centers that regulate internal body functions
- *Cerebellum*—Responsible for maintaining equilibrium; acts as a gross movement control center (e.g., control movement, balance, posture)
    - Each hemisphere of cerebellum has *ipsalateral* control (same side of body).
    - Problems with the cerebellum can lead to ataxia (uncoordinated and inaccurate movements).
    - Rhomberg test is important for detecting deficiencies in cerebellar functioning.

- *Reticular formation system*—The primitive brain
    - Receives input from cortex; an integration area for input from post sensory pathways
    - Innervates thalamus, hypothalamus, and cortex
    - Regulation functions include
        - Involuntary movement
        - Reflex
        - Muscle tone
        - Vital sign control
        - Blood pressure
        - Respiratory rate.
    - Is critical to consciousness and ability to focus mentally, to be alert and pay attention to environmental stimuli.

Neurophysiology and the Brain

- Two classes of cells are in the nervous system: glia and neurons.
    - *Glia*—Structures that form the myelin sheath around axons and provide protection and support
    - *Neurons*—Nerve cells responsible for conducting impulses from one part of the body to another.

- Components of a neuron include
    - *Cell body*—Also known as *soma;* made up of the nucleus and cytoplasm within the cell membrane
    - *Dendrites*—Receive information to conduct impulse *toward* the cell body
    - *Axon*—Sends or conducts information *away* from cell body.

- *Synapse or synaptic cleft*—The connection site and area of communication between neurons where neurotransmitters are released
    - The synapse converts an electrical signal (action potential) from the presynaptic neuron into a chemical signal (neuron transmitter) that is transferred to the postsynaptic neuron.
    - Neurotransmitters are released at the synaptic cleft as the result of an electrical activity (action potential).
        - Two phases of an action potential include
            - *Depolarization*—The initial phase of the action potential; an excitatory response; influx of sodium and calcium ions into the cell
            - *Repolarization*—The restoration phase; an inhibitory response; potassium leaves cell or chloride enters cell.

- Problems in either the structure or chemistry of the synapse interrupt normal flow of impulses and stimuli, contributing to symptoms commonly seen in psychiatric disorders.
- *Neurotransmitters*—Chemicals synthesized from dietary substrates; communicate information from one cell to another
    - The neurotransmitter will be released from the presynaptic neuron, cross the synapse, and then bind to a specific finite receptor on the postsynaptic neuron.
    - Specific criteria must be met for a molecule to be classified as a neurotransmitter (see Table 3–1).

Table 3–1. Classification Nomenclature for Neurotransmitters

Criteria

1. Neurotransmitter must be present in the nerve terminal.

2. Stimulation of neuron must cause release of neurotransmitter in sufficient quantities to cause an action to occur at postsynaptic membrane.

3. Effects of exogenous transmitter on post synaptic membrane must be similar to those caused by stimulation of presynaptic neuron.

4. A mechanism for inactivation or metabolism of the neurotransmitter must exist in the area of the synapse.

5. Exogenous drugs should alter the dose–response curve of the neurotrans-mitter in a manner similar to the naturally occurring synaptic potential.

Adapted from B. Sadock & V. Sadock, 2007, *Kaplan and Sadock's synopsis of psychiatry* (10th ed.). New York: Lippincott Williams & Wilkins.

Categories of Neurotransmitters

Monoamines, amino acids, cholinergics, peptides

Monoamines
- "Biogenic amines": dopamine, norepinephrine, epinephrine, serotonin
    - *Dopamine*—Known as a *catecholamine;* produced in the substantia nigra and the ventral tegmental area; precursor is tyrosine; removed from the synaptic cleft by monoamine oxidase (MAO) enzymatic action
    - *Four dopaminergic pathways*—Mesocortical, mesolimbic, nigrostriatal, tuberoinfundibular (see Chapter 9)
    - *Norepinephrine*—Also known as a *catecholamine;* produced in the locus ceruleus of the pons; precursor is tyrosine; removed from the synaptic cleft and returned to storage via an active reuptake process
    - *Epinephrine*—Also known as a *catecholamine;* produced by the adrenal glands; epinephrine system referred to as the adrenergic system

- *Serotonin*—Known as an *indole;* produced in the raphe nuclei of the brain stem; precursor is tryptophan; removed from the synaptic cleft and returned to storage via an active reuptake process.

Amino Acids

- Glutamate, γ-aminobutyric acid (GABA), glycine, aspartate
  - *Glutamate*—Universal excitatory neurotransmitter; major neurotransmitter involved in process of kindling; significant in bipolar and seizure disorders
  - *GABA*—Universal inhibitory neurotransmitter; site of action of benzodiazepines, alcohol, barbiturates, and other CNS depressants
  - *Glycine*—Another inhibitory neurotransmitter, which works with GABA
  - *Aspartate*—Another excitatory neurotransmitter, which works with glutamate.

Cholinergics

- Acetylcholine
  - *Acetylcholine*—Synthesized by the basal nucleus of Meynert; precursors are acetylcoenzyme A and choline.

Neuropeptides

- Nonopioid type (substance P, somatostatin); opioid type (endorphins, enkephalins, dynorphins)
  - Modulate pain; decreased amount of neuropeptides is thought to cause substance abuse.
- See Table 3–2 for identification of neurotransmitters' role in symptom expression in common psychiatric disorders.

Table 3–2. Common Psychiatric Disorders and Neurotransmitters Implicated in the Complex Pathophysiology of Disorders

Neurotransmitter	Psychiatric Disorder	Suspected Deficit
Acetylcholine	Alzheimer's disease	Decrease
	Impaired memory	Decrease
Dopamine	Schizophrenia	Increase
	Substance abuse	Decrease
	Parkinson's	Decrease
Norepinephrine	Depression	Decrease
Serotonin	Depression	Decrease
	Obsessive–compulsive disorder	Decrease
	Schizophrenia	Decrease
$\acute{A}$-aminobutyric acid (GABA)	Anxiety disorders	Decrease
Glutamate	Bipolar affective disorder	Increase
	Psychosis from ischemic neurotoxicity	Increase
Opioid neuropeptides	Substance abuse	Decrease

Adapted from Thibodeau, G., & Patton, K. (2006). *Anatomy and physiology* (6th ed.). St. Louis, MO: Mosby.

Recovery and Degradation of Neurotransmitters

- After the neurotransmitter reaches the postsynaptic neuron, it may then diffuse off its receptor to be destroyed by enzymes or to be transported back to the presynaptic neuron for reuse.
- *Enzymatic destruction* occurs either in the cytosol or in the synapse. The neurotransmitter can be destroyed by the enzymes MAO in the cytosol or catechol-O-methyl transferase (COMT) in the synapse.
- *Reuptake pumps* can remove the neurotransmitter from acting in the synapse. The neurotransmitter will be reloaded into the presynaptic neuron and will be recycled.

The function of neurotransmitters can be found in Table 3–3.

Table 3–3. Comparison of Common CNS Neurotransmitters

Neuro-transmitter	Receptors	General Function	Symptoms of Deficit	Symptoms of Excess
Dopamine	D_1-like D_2-like	Thinking Decision making Reward-seeking behavior Fine muscle action Integrated cognition	*Mild* Poor impulse control Poor spatiality Lack of abstractive thought *Severe* Parkinson's Endocrine alterations Movement disorders	*Mild* Improved creativity Ability to generalize Improved spatiality *Severe* Disorganized thinking Loose association Tics Stereotypic behavior
Norepine-phrine	α1 α2	Alertness Focused attention Orientation Primes "fight–flight" Learning Memory	Dullness Low energy Depressive affect	Anxiety Hyperalertness Increased startle Paranoia Decreased appetite
Serotonin	5HT1a 5HT1d 5HT2 5HT2a 5HT3 5HT4	Regulation of sleep Pain perceptions Mood states Temperature Regulation of aggression Libido Precursor for melatonin	Irritability Hostility Depression Sleep dysregulation Loss of appetite Loss of libido	Sedation Increased aggression Hallucinations (rare)
Acetylcholine	Nicotinic Muscarinic	Attention Memory Thirst	Lack of inhibition Decreased memory Euphoria	Over-inhibition Anxiety Depression

Table 3–3. Continued

Neuro-transmitter	Receptors	General Function	Symptoms of Deficit	Symptoms of Excess
		Mood regulation REM sleep Sexual behavior Muscle tone	Antisocial action Speech decrease Anticholinergic symptoms	Somatic complaints Self-consciousness Drooling
GABA	GABAa GABAb	Reduces arousal Reduces aggression Reduces anxiety Reduces excitation	Irritability Hostility Tension and worry Anxiety Seizure activity	Reduced cellular excitability Sedation Impaired memory
Glutamate	AMPA MNDA	Memory Sustained automatic functions	Poor memory Low energy Distractible	Kindling Seizures
Peptides: Opioid type	μ mu κ kappa ε epsilon δ delta σ sigma	Modulate emotions Reward-center function Consolidation of memory Modulate reactions to stress	Hypersensitivity to pain and stress Decreased pleasure sensation Dysphoria	Insensitivity to pain Catatonic-like movement disturbance Auditory hallucinations Decreased memory

Adapted from B. Sadock & V. Sadock, 2007, *Kaplan and Sadock's synopsis of psychiatry* (10th ed.). New York: Lippincott Williams & Wilkins.

Neuroimaging Assessment and Diagnostic Procedures

Techniques that permit observation of the brain can be divided into three categories: structural imaging, functional imaging, and structural/functional imaging.

Structural Imaging

Provides evidence of size and shape of anatomical structures.
- Common structural imaging tests include
  - *Computed tomography (CT)*—Provides a three-dimensional view of the brain structures; differentiates structures based on density; provides suggestive evidence of brain-based problems but no specific testing for psychiatric disorders
    - *Advantages:* Widely available, relatively inexpensive
    - *Disadvantages:* Lack of sensitivity, cannot differentiate white matter from gray matter and cannot view structures close to the bone tissue; underestimation of brain atrophy; inability to image sagittal and coronal views.

- *Magnetic resonance imaging (MRI)*—Provides a series of two-dimensional images that represent the brain.
  - *Advantages:* Can view brain structures close to the skull and can separate white matter from gray matter; readily available; resolution of brain tissue superior to CT scanning
  - *Disadvantages:* Expensive; many contraindications to its use (e.g., patients with pacemakers, patients on ventilators, patients with any metallic implants such as orthopedic screws or plates); patients with claustrophobia often are unable to complete study because of design of machinery (an enclosed tubelike structure with a confining environment).

Functional Imaging

Technique that measures function of areas of the brain and bases the resulting assessment on blood flow to the brain; may use radioactive pharmaceuticals to cross the blood–brain barrier; mainly used for research purposes

- Common functional imaging tests include
  - *Electroencephalograpphy (EEG) and evoked potentials testing*—Least expensive tests that convey information on electrical functioning of the CNS
  - *Magnetoencephalography (MEG)*—Similar to the EEG but detects different electrical activities; often used in a complementary fashion with EEG testing; more useful in diagnosing psychiatric disorders than EEG because it better measures auditory, visual, and sensory stimuli
  - *Single photon emission computed tomography (SPECT)*—Provides information on the cerebral blood flow; limited availability; expensive but less than positron emission tomography
  - *Positron emission tomography (PET)*—Provides images of the brain when positron-emitting radionuclei interact with an electron; expensive procedure that requires extensive resources and support team.

Structural/Functional Imaging

The newest imaging; attempts to examine structure in conjunction with function
- Mainly research tools at present
- Available tests include
  - *Functional MRI (fMRI)*
  - *Three-dimensional event-related functional MRI (3fEMRI)*
  - *Fluorine magnetic spectroscopy*
  - *Dopamine D$_2$ receptor binding.*

Case Study

Ms. Franklin is a 24-year-old sales clerk. She has a strong family history of mental illness and is worried that she may experience some problems in her life because of her family history. She presents to her local primary care provider complaining of the following symptoms:

- Hyperalertness
- Increased startle response

- Concern that people are staring at her and watching what she eats
- Decreased appetite
- Sedation
- Impaired memory.

Ms. Franklin is trying to determine if these experiences are normal or are the beginning of a mental illness. She wants to have a brain scan done to determine the answer. She also is getting married soon and wants to know what the risk is that her future children will experience mental illness, as she believes it runs in her family. In working with Ms. Franklin, the PMHNP must consider many issues.

- Are the symptoms described by Ms. Franklin consistent with a psychiatric disorder?
- Do psychiatric disorders run in families, as Ms. Franklin believes?
- Do the symptoms as described by Ms. Franklin link with any known neuroanatomical or neurophysiological deficit?
- Is a brain scan warranted for Ms. Franklin?
- Can the risk of Ms. Franklin's children developing psychiatric disorders be determined?

Review Questions

1. The role of neurotransmitters in the CNS is to function as

   a. A communication medium
   b. A gatekeeper for transmissions
   c. A building block for amino acids
   d. An agent to break down enzymes

2. Serotonin is produced in which of the following locations?

   a. Locus ceruleus
   b. Nucleus basalis
   c. Raphi nuclei
   d. Substantia nigra

3. A client presents with complaints of changes in appetite, feeling fatigued, problems with sleep–rest cycle, and changes in libido. The neuroanatomical area of the brain responsible for the normal regulation of these functions is the

   a. Thalamus
   b. Hypothalamus
   c. Limbic system
   d. Hippocampus

4. In considering whether or not to order an MRI for a client with suspected psychiatric disorders, which of the following would be a contraindication to this diagnostic test?

   a. Prosthetic limb
   b. History of head trauma
   c. Pacemaker
   d. Pregnancy

References and Resources

Alexander, E., Chen, K., Pietrini, P., Rapoport, S. I., & Reiman, E. M. (2002). Longitudinal PET evaluation of cerebral metabolic decline in dementia: A potential outcome measure in Alzheimer's disease treatment studies. *American Journal of Psychiatry, 159,* 238–245.

Amen, D. G. (1998). Brain SPECT imaging in psychiatry. *Primary Psychiatry, 5,* 83–87.

American Nurses Association. (2000). *Scope and standards of psychiatric–mental health clinical nursing practice.* Washington, DC: Author.

Carlson, N. R. (2006). *Physiology of behavior* (9th ed.). Boston: Allyn & Bacon.

Doyle, A. E., Roe, C. M., & Faraone, S. V. (2001). The genetics of attention deficit hyperactivity disorder. *Primary Psychiatry, 8*(9), 65–71.

Dubin, M. W. (2002). *How the brain works.* Williston, VT: Blackwell Science.

Goff, D., & Coyle, J. (2001). The emerging role of glutamate in the pathophysiology and treatment of schizophrenia. *American Journal of Psychiatry, 158,* 1367–1377.

Gribbin, J. (2002). *How the brain works: A beginner's guide to the mind and consciousness.* New York: Dorling Kindersley.

Gross-Isseroff, R., Bigeon, A., Voet, H., & Weizman, A. (1998). The suicide brain: A review of postmortem receptor transporter binding studies. *Neuroscience Biobehavioral Review, 22,* 653.

Gur, R. (2002). Functional imaging is fulfilling some promises. *American Journal of Psychiatry, 159,* 693–694.

Keltner, N. L., Folks, D. G., Palmer, C. A., & Powers, R. E. (1998). *Psychobiological foundations of psychiatric care.* St. Louis, MO: Mosby.

McCabe, S. (2001a). The biological foundations of psychiatric nursing. In M. A. Boyd (Ed.), *Psychiatric nursing* (2nd ed., pp. 94–126). Philadelphia: Lippincott Williams & Wilkins.

McCabe, S. (2001b). Psychopharmacology and other biological treatments. In M. A. Boyd (Ed.), *Psychiatric nursing* (2nd ed., pp. 128–175). Philadelphia: Lippincott Williams & Wilkins.

McLeod, T. M., Lopez-Figueroa, A., & Lopez-Figueroa, M. O. (2001). Nitric oxide, stress, and depression. *Psychopharmacology Bulletin, 35,* 24–41.

Mohr, W. K., & Mohr, B. (2001). Brain, behavior, connections, and implications: Psychodynamics no more. *Archives of Psychiatric Nursing, 15,* 171–181.

Mujica-Parodi, L. R., Corcoran, C., Greenberg, T., Saceim, H. A., & Malaspina, D. (2002). Are cognitive symptoms of schizophrenia mediated by abnormalities in emotional arousal? *CNS Spectrums, 7*(1), 58–69.

Raemaekers, M., Johannus, M. J., Cahn, W., Van der Geest, J. N., van der Linden, J. A., Kahn, R. S., et al. (1999). Neuronal substrate of the saccadic inhibition deficit in schizophrenia investigated with 3-dimensional event-related functional MRI. *Archives of General Psychiatry, 59,* 313–320.

Raine, T., Lencz, T., Bihrle, S., LaCasse, L., & Colletti, P. (2000). Reduced gray matter volume and reduced autonomic activity in antisocial personality disorder. *Archives of General Psychiatry, 57,* 119–129.

Sadock, B., & Sadock, V. (2007). *Kaplan and Sadock's synopsis of psychiatry* (10th ed.). New York: Lippincott Williams & Wilkins.

Schindler, K. M., Pato, M. T., Torre, C. D., Valente, J., Azevedo, M. H., Coelho, I., et al. (2001). Candidate genes for schizophrenia: Further evaluation of KCNN3. *Primary Psychiatry, 8*(9), 51–53.

Shihabuddin, L. S., Ray, J., & Gage, F. H. (1999). Stem cell technology for basic science and clinical applications. *Archives of Neurology, 6,* 29–32.

Stahl, S. M. (2000). *Essential psychopharmacology: Neuroscientific basis and practical applications* (2nd ed.). New York: Cambridge University Press.

Stuart, G. W., & Laraia, M. T. (2004). *Principles and practice of psychiatric nursing* (8th ed.). St. Louis, MO: Mosby.

Thibodeau, G., & Patton, K. (2006). *Anatomy and physiology* (6th ed.). St. Louis, MO: Mosby.

Young, G. B., & Pigott, S. E. (1999). Neurobiologic basis of consciousness. *Archives of Neurology, 56,* 153–157.

Notes:

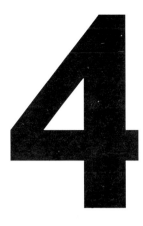

Assessment of Acute and Chronic Disease States

This chapter reviews the role of psychiatric–mental health nurse practitioners (PMHNPs) in assessment. It reviews the process of history taking, physical exam, mental status exam, differential diagnosis, and the appropriate use of diagnostic and laboratory testing in providing competent nursing care for patients and families experiencing psychiatric disorders. The chapter specifically highlights the PMHNP role in assessing and diagnosing common psychiatric disorders.

Statistics for Psychiatric Disorders

General Incidence and Demographics

- *Epidemiology*—The study of the distribution, incidence, prevalence, and duration of disease
- *Incidence rate*—The number of new cases occurring over a specified time (usually 1 year)
- *Prevalence rate*—The number of existing cases of a disorder at a specified time
  - One in four adults will be diagnosed with a psychiatric disorder within their lifetime.
  - An estimated 26.2% of Americans ages 18 and older have a diagnosable psychiatric disorder in a given year. On the basis of census data (National Institute of Mental Health, 2006), this translates to 57.7 million Americans with a psychiatric disorder in any given year.
  - The leading cause of disability in the United States and Canada is mental illness.
  - Psychiatric disorders have common, frequently occurring comorbidities; that is, individuals often have more than one psychiatric disorder at a given time. Also, individuals often have a psychiatric disorder and another common health disorder at a given time.
  - Four of the 10 leading causes of disability in Americans are psychiatric disorders: major depression, bipolar disorder, schizophrenia, and obsessive–compulsive disorder.

Assessment of Psychiatric Disorders

General Considerations

- Interviewing is the primary form of assessment and data collection.
- The psychiatric assessment process is a structured, organized, and systematic process that includes multiple components: patient history, physical examination, mental status examination, and diagnostic and laboratory examinations.

Fundamentals of Interviewing

- Psychiatric interviewing requires many skills on the part of the PMHNP:
  - Openness
  - Respect for the client and family
  - Appropriate use of therapeutic communication
  - Ability to establish rapport with the client
  - Subjective and objective data collection skills using all senses
  - Critical thinking to identify the needs of the client.
- The psychiatric assessment process is a focused, goal-directed, interactional process between the PMHNP and the client and family.

Primary Goals of the Assessment Process

- To gather intentional specific data
- To identify the health needs of the client
- To plan for care
- To evaluate outcomes of care
- To evaluate ongoing health needs of the client.

- Assessment requires the PMHNP to form an *effective relationship with the client by*
  - Learning about the client's interest and motivation for care
  - Having open and respectful engagement with the client using a nonjudgmental approach
  - Exploring the client's current emotional status
  - Validating assumptions about the emotional status of the client
  - Displaying empathy
  - Instilling hope that the client's concern can be addressed
  - Developing a sense of partnership with the client and family.

- The *initial assessment* of the client focuses on the process of differential diagnostic assessment.
- *Subsequent assessments* with the client focus on monitoring client outcomes, general health status, and modifying care practices based on clinical outcomes.

Therapeutic Communication Considerations

- Therapeutic communication techniques (see Table 4–1) need to be used in all interactions with the client and family.

Active Listening

- Paying attention to nonverbal communication (e.g., loss of eye contact, shift in body posture, increase in fidgeting or restlessness, clenched fists, bouncing legs)

- Maintaining an open and engaging posture (i.e., positioning oneself at patient's eye level, being relaxed and unhurried, leaning slightly forward)
- Maintaining eye contact that is matched to client's comfort level and cultural background.

Facilitative Communication Techniques

- Are intended to foster greater disclosure by the client
- Allow the client to pace the conversation
- Avoid interrupting the client unnecessarily
- Avoid nonstop questions directed at the client
- Use open-ended questioning initially
- Avoid much self-disclosure by the PMHNP
- Use encouraging vocalizations such as "go on" or "tell me more"
- Request clarification when needed
- Summarize key points to ensure congruency of understanding
- Follow up with directive and closed questions for confirmatory data assessment.

- *Paraphrasing*—Repeating the client's thoughts or feelings with similar words
- *Confrontation*—Pointing out to a client something that he or she is not paying attention to, is missing, or is denying
- *Silence*—May be constructive; may allow clients to contemplate, cry, or just sit in an accepting and supportive environment.

Table 4–1. Therapeutic Communication Techniques

Technique	Example
Broad opening	"How are things for you?" "What brings you here today?" "What's happened since we last saw each other?"
Accepting	"I can imagine that it has been very difficult for you." (nodding)
Summarizing	"So what you are most concerned about is ..." "So let me see if I understand ..."
Reflection	CLIENT: "I keep worrying about what will happen next." PMHNP: "You're worried about the future."
Focusing	"Could we talk about the suicidal thoughts a little more?" "Tell me more about when this all started."
Validating	"It sounds like you are saying ..." "So I am hearing you say ..."
Exploring	"How does the depression affect your husband?" "Tell me what was happening in your life when the voices started."
Clarifying	"Could you explain to me how that mattered?" "I'm not sure I understand. Could you tell me how that happened?"

Continued on the next page

Table 4–1. Continued

Sequencing	"Which came first …" "Was that before or after you were in the hospital?"
Recognizing	"I notice that you are looking very sad today." "I see that you still have some trouble with tremors in you hands."
Theming	"We have talked for a while now, and I've noticed that we are mainly talking about how you feel unsupported by your family."

- Always compare the client's current symptoms with his or her premorbid symptoms.
- Ask how the client was functioning 6 months ago.

Other Assessment and Planning Considerations

Milieu Considerations
- The interview location should be conducive to data collection (a comfortable, private, and quiet low sensory stimulus area), which will decrease anxiety and promote a sense of safety and security for the client.
- The milieu also needs to be public enough to access equipment, supplies, or assistance as needed.

Cultural Considerations
- *Culture*—The pattern of behavior of a group (racial, social, ethnic, religious grouping) that includes the thoughts, customs, beliefs, values, or communication patterns of that particular group
- *Cultural competence*—Viewing the client as a unique individual and providing care that is sensitive to issues related to culture, race, gender, and sexual orientation.
- Demonstrating respectfulness of diversity
    - *Types of diversity*—Age, gender, sexual orientation, race, ethnicity, language, disability, religion, social class, education, occupation
    - Being aware of the need to modify the interview to match cultural differences (e.g., behavioral etiquette, inappropriate or taboo topics, gender differences, differences in affective expressions)
    - Accommodating the interview style to cultural needs (e.g., language, family structure, health beliefs, health practices).

Focal Areas for Assessment of Cultural Issues
- *Family roles*—Who is the primary caretaker? Who makes most of the decisions?
- *Family customs*
- *Religious beliefs*
- *Beliefs about death and dying*
- *Dietary preferences*
- *Meaning of nonverbal gestures*
- *Physical space.*

- It's important to be aware of the various cultural perspectives of mental health.

✓ Keep in mind that cultural factors may affect the expression of mental disorders. Be aware of incorrectly judging a person's behavior as psychopathology, when it is in fact culturally related.

- *Culture-Bound Syndromes*—Those specific behaviors related to a person's culture and not linked to a psychiatric disorder
- *Acculturation*—The process by which the person acquires the culture of the society that he or she inhabits
- When intervening in psychiatric situations that are affected by cultural influences,
  - *L*isten with empathy
  - *E*xplain your perceptions of the client's problem
  - *A*cknowledge similarities and differences in perceptions between the two cultures
  - *R*ecommend treatment
  - *N*egotiate treatment.

Age Considerations

- *Assessment in children*
  - Modify language use based on the age of the child.
  - Exhibit nurturing behavior.
  - Use play and fantasy in the interview process.
  - Allow more time for the assessment.
  - Use a direct and clear questioning style for adolescents.

- *Assessment in elderly people*
  - Allow more time for the assessment.
  - Allow the client to pace the conversation.
  - Allow time for rapport building before asking sensitive questions.
  - Allow time for the client to reminisce and share past history.

Collateral Sources of Data

- Sometimes comparing what the client says with what other family members, friends, peers, or significant others say about situations or previous treatment can be helpful.
- Using collateral sources of data can be useful with individuals with
  - Impaired insight
  - Cognitive deficits
  - Substance abuse problems
  - Unstable behavior
  - Children and adolescents.

Nature of Symptom Presentation of Psychiatric Disorders

- Generally, psychiatric symptoms are nonspecific. Ensure that the assessment has been broad and holistic. Identify *clusters* and *patterns* emerging in assessment data rather than looking for discrete signs or symptoms.

- Symptoms of psychiatric disorders often are best observed in the behavioral manifestation of the client and may not initially be recognized by the client or family as symptoms. It often is helpful to specifically ask the client if a particular sign or symptom has been present. Use nonmedical words, avoid jargon, and be aware of the regional or cultural vocabulary used to describe common psychiatric symptoms.
- Many symptoms of common psychiatric disorders have a *somatic component*.
    - The client initially may be reluctant to view a symptom as an indication of a psychiatric disorder.
    - Sensitivity is needed in forming questions.
    - The stigmatizing nature of psychiatric disorders often will initially limit client disclosure.

- The presence of certain active symptoms in the client may increase the difficulty of obtaining assessment data. The following assessment techniques may be used when certain symptoms are present:
    - *Anger*
        - Take time to establish rapport.
        - Extend courtesy and respect.
        - Use humor to defuse the situation.
        - Get quickly to the client's agenda and expectations for assessment.
        - Be clear and honest about the goal of assessment and how the data will be used.
        - Use limit setting when needed.

    - *Psychosis*
        - Frequently reestablish reality for the client.
        - Use clear and concise language.
        - Avoid word choices that the patient can interpret in concrete ways.
        - Avoid unnecessary physical touch.

    - *Suspiciousness*
        - Explain carefully to the client any physical touch that is necessary before initiating it with him or her.
        - Be clear and honest about the goals of assessment and how the data will be used.
        - Acknowledge the client's suspiciousness.

    - *Controlling features*
        - Provide the client with information about what is happening and will happen.
        - Focus initially on intellectual aspects to match the client's control needs.
        - Allow the client to control aspects of interview as appropriate.

    - *Dependent features*
        - Set limits as needed.
        - Allow time for and show patience during interview process.
        - Express an interest in dealing with the client.
        - Maintain professional boundaries.

    - *Anxiety*
        - Attend to milieu considerations.
        - Notice that the client may have a decreased ability to process information.
        - Repeat questions as needed.
        - Refocus the client as needed.

Components of the PMHNP Assessment Process

History

- *Elements of a psychiatric history*
    - *Identifying demographic information*—Age, gender, marital status, race, referral source.

- *Chief complaint*
    - The client's presenting problem
    - The client's explanation, regardless of how bizarre or irrelevant it is, should be recorded verbatim and placed in quotation marks.

- *History of present illness (HPI)*
    - Provides a comprehensive and chronological picture of events leading up to the current moment in the client's life
    - Is the most helpful part in making a diagnosis and the most important aspect of the history
    - Requires ascertaining information about the presenting problem:
        - *Palliative*—What makes it better?
        - *Provocative*—What makes it worse?
        - *Quality*—How and where does the presence of the complaint affect the client's quality of life?
        - *Radiation*—Is the problem radiating to other areas of the client's life, such as work?
        - *Severity*—How much does the client's complaint affect day-to-day life? On a scale of 0 to 10 with 0 least severe and 10 most severe, rate the severity of the problem.
        - *Timing*—Is this a new complaint? How long has it been a problem? Is there any particular time of day the complaint occurs?

- *Goals for the HPI*
    - To develop rapport
    - To record at least one-half of the mental status exam (MSE)
    - To keep track of cues for further exploration of facts or feelings
    - To develop and devise a preliminary diagnosis.

- *Past psychiatric history*
    - Important to determine the course and severity of the disorder
    - Entails past mental disorders, any remissions or exacerbations, family psychiatric history, past treatments and responses, past suicidal or homicidal ideations or attempts.

- *Past medical history*
    - Important to distinguish between organic and psychiatric disorders
    - Gives a chronological history of medical problems.

- *Social history*
    - Home situation
    - Family constellation/marital history, children, dependents
    - Work/school situation
    - Social network/relationship with others

- Typical pattern of activity
- Spirituality
- Recent stressors
- Legal history.
- *Family history* (family of origin and nuclear family)
  - Structure
  - Health history, cause of death if deceased, psychiatric disorders and treatments
  - Family risk factors
  - Conflicting and supportive relationships, cutoffs
  - Family strengths.
- *Developmental history*
  - Maternal history of pregnancy
  - Adverse perinatal events
  - History of delivery.
- Important aspects to include in *developmental/social history for child/adolescent:*
  - Relevant birth and infancy history (e.g., temperament, motor development)
  - Cognitive development (e.g., school performance, milestones)
  - Emotional development (e.g., self-esteem, self-efficacy, sense of right/wrong)
  - Losses, including divorce
  - Abuse, including neglect
  - Sexual activity, birth control, and pregnancies
  - Childhood illnesses
  - Childhood psychiatric disorders, learning disabilities
  - Secondary sexual characteristics (e.g., onset of puberty, onset of menses)
  - Parental pressures
  - Sense of personal identity.
- *Key principles of child development*
  - Development proceeds along a predictable pathway marked by milestones.
  - Children mature and develop at different rates.
  - Development may be affected by many factors, such as abuse or poverty.
- *Clues to developmental/behavioral problems in children*
  - Enuresis/encopresis
  - Night terrors
  - Thumb sucking
  - Frequent tantrums
  - Excessive isolation
  - Fire setting
  - Cruelty to animals
  - Frequent school truancy.
- *Functional assessment*
  - Looks at the degree to which the individual's abilities/performance match the demands of his or her life
  - Determines the impact of the illness on the overall functioning
  - Is used to differentiate depression from dementia in elderly people
  - Is used to track client improvement or decline from his or her baseline

- Includes activities of daily living (ADLs) and instrumental activities of daily living (IADLs)
  - *ADLs*—Basic self-care skills, such as eating, bathing, dressing, and toileting
  - *IADLs*—Activities needed for independent functioning, such as shopping, cooking, taking medications, driving, housekeeping.
- *History taking during crisis*
  - Determine as the first priority the status of the emergency and assess danger to the client and others
  - Always be alert to risk of impending violence
  - Attend to the safety of the physical surroundings
  - Focus on the presenting complaint or problem and obtain a supplemental history from others if necessary
  - Assess drug or alcohol use, mental status, current meds, and past effective coping skills
  - Be straightforward, calm, honest, and nonthreatening.

Physical Exam

- *Reasons to study or be familiar with the physical exam in psychiatry*
  - To be able to detect underlying medical problems
  - To be familiar with a screening neurological exam and to be able to rule out neurological problems that may manifest as symptoms of a psychiatric problem
  - To be able to differentiate normal vs. abnormal signs and symptoms
  - To know when to refer.
- Done by the PMHNP in the context of his or her primary psychiatric care role
- Goals of identifying the presence of psychiatric disorders, determining general health status, and screening for nonpsychiatric disorders
- Focuses on the physical assessment required to accomplish differential diagnoses to determine client health needs
- Specifically focuses on assessing for disorders or conditions that explain client presentation
  - Psychiatric disorders
  - Nonpsychiatric disorders.
- Not intended to replace the role of the primary health care provider for the client
  - The PMHNP should assist the client to establish a primary care provider.
- Avoids highly personal or intrusive procedures that may make the formation of a therapeutic alliance more difficult (e.g., Pap smear, male genital exam, rectal exam, breast exam), but it is important to be familiar with these exams and to be able to differentiate normal vs. abnormal
- Requires the PMHNP to have depth of knowledge regarding the common *health* disorders that can mimic symptoms of a psychiatric disorder
  - Differential diagnostic considerations.
- Requires the PMHNP to have depth of knowledge regarding the common *psychiatric* disorders that can mimic or produce symptoms of other disorders
  - Differential diagnostic considerations
  - Comorbid condition and clinical management issues.

- Generally, if client health disorders are determined to be nonpsychiatric, the client is referred to primary care providers other than the PMHNP.
- Because of the brain-based nature of psychiatric disorders, the PMHNP role requires the ability to perform an in-depth neurological exam.

Neurological Exam

- *Reflexes* (i.e., biceps, triceps, brachioradialis, patellar, Achilles, plantar)
  - Grade reflexes and note symmetry between right and left sides.
  - Check primitive reflexes in infants (i.e., head lag, flexion, rooting, grasping, moro, glabellar, Babinski).
  - A positive Babinski (i.e., fanning of toes and dorsiflexion of the great toe) is normal in infants up to age 2.

- *Cranial nerves*
  - *Olfactory*—1st
    - Test sense of smell and ensure patency of the nasal passages.
    - Have the client close eyes, and test each nostril separately while the other is occluded by asking the client to identify familiar odors.

  - *Optic*—2nd
    - Test vision using Snellen chart or other suitable chart depending on the client's acuity and ability to cooperate.
    - Examine the inner aspect of the eyes with the ophthalmoscope.
    - Test peripheral vision using the confrontation test.

  - *Oculomotor*—3rd
    - This is the motor nerve to the five extrinsic eye muscles. Test together with cranial nerve 4 (trochlear) and cranial nerve 6 (abducens) (see below).
    - Test the extraocular movements (EOMs).
    - Check the equality of pupils, their reaction to light, and their ability to accommodate.
    - Test the corneal light reflex (i.e., when shining a light at the bridge of the nose, the light should appear symmetrically in both eyes).

  - *Trochlear*—4th
    - Use the same process as cranial nerve 3 (oculomotor) and cranial nerve 6 (abducens).

  - *Trigeminal*—5th (Motor Division)
    - Palpate the masseter muscles with the fingertips while the client clenches his or her teeth.
    - Look for disparity in tension between the two muscles, which can indicate paralysis on the weak side.
    - Look for tremor of the lips, involuntary chewing movements, and spasm of the masticatory muscles.

  - *Trigeminal*—5th (Sensory Division)
    - Test tactile perception of the facial skin by touching with a wisp of cotton.
    - Test corneal reflex with wisp of cotton.
    - Test superficial pain of the skin and mucosa with pinpricks.
    - Test the sense of touch in the oral mucosa.

- *Abducens*—6th
  - Use the same process as cranial nerve 3 (oculomotor) and cranial nerve 4 (trochlear).
- *Facial*—7th (Motor Division)
  - Inspect the face in repose for evidence of flaccid paralysis.
  - Test by asking the patient to elevate eyebrows, wrinkle forehead, close eyes, frown, smile, and puff cheeks.
- *Facial*—7th (Sensory Division)
  - Test taste for sugar, vinegar, and salt.
- *Acoustic*—8th
  - Check hearing with the audiometer or by the whisper test.
  - Check for hearing loss using the Weber and the Rinne tests.
- *Glossopharyngeal*—9th
  - Test together with cranial nerve 10 (vagus; see below).
- *Vagus*—10th
  - Test for elevation of the uvula by having the patient open his or her mouth and say "ah."
  - Test the gag reflex by touching the back of the throat with a tongue blade.
- *Accessory*—11th
  - Test the strength of the sternocleidomastoid and trapezius muscles against resistance of your hands.
- *Hypoglossal*—12th
  - Look for tremors and other involuntary movement when the client protrudes his or her tongue.

Coordination and Fine-Motor Skills

- *Equilibrium*—Check by administering the Romberg test: Have the client stand up straight with feet together, arms by sides, and eyes closed. Only slight swaying is normal, and the client will be able to sustain this pose for approximately 5 seconds. More than slight swaying suggests cerebellar ataxia or vestibular dysfunction.
- *Diadochokinesia*—Ability to perform rapid alternating movements (e.g., patting knees alternating palm and back of hands, touching thumb to each finger); the client should be able to smoothly execute these movements and maintain the rhythm.
- *Dyssynergia*—Finger-to-nose test, heel-to-knee test.
- *Handwriting*.
- *Gait*—Observe client walking.

Sensory Functions

- *Pain*—Check sensation to pain with safety pinprick and compare on each side of body.
- *Temperature*—Check temperature if sensation to pain is abnormal.
- *Superficial touch*—Test with wisp of cotton.
- *Two-point discrimination*—Apply pins to skin simultaneously; ask the client if he or she feels one or two pinpricks.
- *Stereognosis*—Tests the ability to distinguish forms by placing objects in the client's hands while his or her eyes are closed.

- *Graphesthesia*—Tests the ability to identify figures, letters, or words by tracing the figure on the skin of the palm of the hand.

Motor Functions
- *Muscle mass*—Measure muscle mass to check for atrophy or hypertrophy.
- *Muscle tone*—Tension is present when the muscle is resting.
- *Muscle strength*—Check muscular strength against resistance.
- Be aware of abnormal muscle movements.

Neurological Soft Signs
- *Dysdiadochokinesia*—Inability to perform rapid alternating movements; result of a lesion to the posterior lobe of the cerebellum.
- *Astereognosis*—Inability to discriminate between objects based on touch alone; result of a lesion in the parietal lobe.
- *Choreiform movements*
- *Tics*
- *Agraphesthesia*—Inability to recognize letters or numbers "drawn" on the client's hand with a pointed object.
- *Facial grimacing*
- *Impaired fine-motor skills*
- *Abnormal blinking*
- *Abnormal motor tone.*
- ✓ Be alert for extrapyramidal symptoms (e.g., Parkinsonism, dystonia, akathisia) in the client taking antipsychotics.

Vital Signs
- Measure height, weight, blood pressure (on children ages 2 or older), pulse, respirations, temperature, and head circumference (during the first 2 years).
- Use growth charts for infants and children.
  - Greater than 85th percentile for body mass index (BMI) places a child at increased risk for being overweight.

- Use BMI charts.
  - Normal—20–25
  - Overweight—26–29
  - Obese—30–35.

- High BMI is a risk factor for diabetes, heart disease, stroke, hypertension, osteoarthritis, and some forms of cancer.
- ✓ Be alert for high BMI if the client also is being prescribed psychotropic meds with a propensity for weight gain, especially second-generation antipsychotics, Depakote, and Remeron.

- If a client is presenting with elevated temperature and also is taking psychotropic meds, such as Tegretol or Clozaril, be alert for agranulocytosis.

Skin, Nails, Head, and Hair
- Note the color and integrity of the skin and if lesions are present.
- Note whether the skin is well hydrated, dry, or scaly.

- Assess skin turgor.
- Palpate the skin's temperature.
- Note any unusual moles or other lesions.
- Look at hair texture and distribution.
- Determine the quality of the nails, noting splitting, clubbing, or onychomycosis.
- Check capillary refill.
- Examine head, scalp, sutures, and fontanelles (if infant).
- Check cranial nerve 7 (facial nerve) for symmetry (have client smile, frown, wrinkle forehead, puff cheeks).
✓ Be alert for Steven Johnson's syndrome (life-threatening rash), especially if the client is taking Tegretol or Lamictal.
- Cancerous moles can be detected by using the acronym ABCDE—*A*symmetry, *B*order irregularity, *C*olor variation, *D*iameter greater than 6 millimeters, and *E*levation.

Eyes
- Check visual acuity using the Snellen chart (tests cranial nerve 2–optic nerve).
- Test peripheral vision using the confrontation test (tests cranial nerve 2–optic nerve).
- Note the symmetry of eyes and the appearance of orbits, eyelids, and brows.
- Inspect the sclera.
- Assess corneal sensation with wisp of cotton (tests cranial nerves 5 and 7).
- Assess papillary reaction to light and accommodation (tests cranial nerves 3, 4, and 6).
- Assess the six cardinal fields of gaze (extraocular movements; tests cranial nerves 3, 4, and 6).
- Assess corneal light reflex. Light reflections should appear symmetrically in both pupils (tests cranial nerves 3, 4, and 6).
- Examine the inner aspect of the eyes with the ophthalmoscope (tests cranial nerve 2).
✓ Be aware that many psychotropics can cause blurry vision (an anticholinergic side effect).
- Seroquel may cause cataracts.

Ears
- Check for configuration, position, and alignment of auricles.
- Test auditory acuity (cranial nerve 8) with the whisper test or audiometer.
- Inspect external auditory canals with otoscope for redness, swelling, or excess cerumen.
- Tympanic membrane should be translucent pearly gray without retractions or bulges.

Nose and Sinuses
- Note the appearance of the external nose and whether it is smooth, intact, symmetric, midline, has discharge, or is flaring
- Assess nasal patency.
- Assess sense of smell.
- Inspect internal nasal cavity for patency and septal deviation.
- Palpate maxillary and frontal sinuses.

Neck
- Palpate the lymph nodes (preauricular, postauricular, tonsillar, submandibular, submental, anticervical) for swelling or masses.
- Palpate thyroid (usually not palpable except in very thin people).
- Palpate/auscultate carotid pulse and note any bruits.

Back

- Inspect skin and respiratory pattern on posterior chest.
- Palpate cervical, thoracic, lumbar, and sacral spine.
- Palpate thoracic expansion.
- Percuss posterior chest for tympany.
- Auscultate posterior chest for vesicular or bronchovesicular sounds and note any adventitious breath sounds.

Thorax and Lungs

- Assess respiratory rate, depth, regularity, and ease of respirations.
- Note anterior/posterior (AP) diameter, which should be less than the transverse diameter.
- Percuss anterior chest for resonance and note the quality and symmetry of percussion notes.
- Auscultate anterior chest for lung sounds; normal breath sounds include vesicular over peripheral lung, bronchovesicular over first and second intercostal spaces at the sternal border, and bronchial over the trachea.

Breasts

- Inspect breasts in different positions: with client arms relaxed and by side, with arms elevated above head, and with hands on hips. Look for dimpling, retractions, and orange-peel appearance.
- Palpate breasts for lumps, including Tail of Spence.
- Palpate axillary and epitrochlear lymph nodes.
- Palpate supraclavicular lymph nodes (also known as Sentinel or Virchow nodes).
- ✓ Be aware that typical antipsychotics as well as second-generation antipsychotics may cause galactorrhea.

Heart

- Inspect, palpate, and auscultate the carotid pulse.
- Palpate peripheral pulses and check for symmetry (carotid, brachial, radial, femoral, popliteal, pedal, and posterior tibial).
- Assess heart rate, rhythm, amplitude, and contour.
- Assess anatomic location of the apical pulse.
- Palpate precordium for pulsations, thrills, heaves, and lifts.
- Auscultate heart sounds with bell and diaphragm and note characteristics of the first and second heart sounds.
- Assess for jugular venous distention (JVD).
- ✓ Be alert for possible electrocardiogram (EKG) changes if the client is taking tricyclic antidepressants or antipsychotics.
- ✓ Be aware that lithium and anorexia nervosa can cause peripheral edema.

Abdomen

- Inspect the contour of the abdomen, scars, abdominal aortic pulsations, and the umbilical cord in the newborn.
- Auscultate for bowel sounds and the abdominal aorta for bruits.
- Percuss the abdomen and note areas of tympany and dullness. It is normal to hear tympany over the small and large intestines and dullness over organs and a distended bladder.

- Percuss the size of liver and spleen.
- Palpate the abdomen for masses and tenderness. Also palpate the liver and spleen, which are not normally palpable (sometimes the liver can be palpable in thin clients).

Musculoskeletal
- Assess client's posture for alignment of extremities and spine and for symmetry of body parts.
- Test muscle strength of upper and lower extremities.
- Note symmetry of muscle mass, tone, and strength.
- Assess active range of motion in neck and upper and lower extremities, and note any presence of pain with movement.
- Palpate muscles and joints to elicit pain, deformities, crepitus, and passive range of motion.
- Check for hip dysplasia in infants.
- Check for scoliosis in children and adolescents.

Common Indicators of Physical Child Abuse
- History of unexplained multiple fractures
- Burns, hand, or bite marks
- Injuries at various stages of healing
- Evidence of neglect
- Bruising on padded parts of body.

Mental Status Examination (MSE)

- The MSE is the examiner's observations of the client at the time of the interview.
- The MSE is part of the overall process of the psychiatric assessment. It does not stand alone but is used in conjunction with the history, physical exam, and diagnostic and laboratory findings.
- Performing the MSE is a key role function of the PMHNP; the MSE should be performed on every client.
- The MSE is a systematic method of evaluating a patient's behavioral, emotional, and cognitive functioning.

  - *Goals*
    - Establish a baseline of a client's emotional and cognitive functioning.
    - Identify a client's behavioral–psychiatric needs.
    - Monitor a client's functioning and symptom levels over time.
    - Function as a screening tool for at-risk clients.
    - Readily identify clients experiencing psychotic symptoms (secondary goal).

  - *Structure*
    - *Appearance*
      - Assess the client's overall appearance related to age or culture.
      - Assess the client's hygiene and grooming.
      - Assess the client's appropriateness of clothing to age, weather, or occasion.
      - Assess the client's posture and mannerisms.

- *Behavior*
  - Describe the client's general behavior.
  - Assess the client's motor behavior.
  - Describe the client's attitude—cooperative, confrontative, or evasive.
- *Mood*
  - Sustained emotional state of the individual; internal feelings that influence behavior.
  - Mood is recorded as the subjective state of emotions as described by the individual.
- *Affect*
  - Variation of emotional expression in facial expression, body language, nonverbal communication, and voice intonation
  - Recorded as the objectively observed state of emotions as determined by the PMHNP.
- *Thought process* (see Table 4–2)
  - How the client is thinking: stream of thought; continuity and logic in thought.
  - Ability to correctly identify abnormalities is essential to effective differential diagnosing of client needs.
  - Note problems with word finding and thought blocking.
  - ✓ Keep in mind that thought processes can be assessed during the interview before completing the MSE.
- *Thought content* (see Table 4–3)
  - What the client is thinking about: ideas, obsessions, and preoccupations.
  - Ability to correctly identify abnormalities is essential to effective differential diagnosing of client needs.

Table 4–2. Common Findings of Thought Disorder

Finding	Description
Flight of ideas	Speech pattern characterized by accelerated speech and rapid shifts in topic
	Often disorganized and difficult to follow, but syntax and vocabulary remain intact
Loose association (derailment)	Shift in thinking in which ideas move from one apparently unrelated topic to another
	Person remains unaware of the juxtaposed topics
Poverty of content	Vague, repetitive, and abstractive form of speech that contains many words but little information
Neologisms	Word inventions or unusual application of current words that, while having personal significance to the person, have no apparent meaning for the listener
Circumstantiality	Inclusion of unnecessary detail and parenthetical information into the conversation

Table 4–2. Continued

Finding	Description
Tangentiality	Shifts in topics that often start as related shifts but progressively move farther away from the original topic
Clanging	Form of loose association in which topics change on the basis of sounds of words rather than meaning of words
Word salad	Form of very disorganized speech in which syntax is lost and word use is random and idiosyncratic
Perseveration	Persistent repetition of words or phrases
Confabulation	Fabrication of facts and details to fill gaps in memory
Blocking	Sudden stoppage of speech attributed to losing thought or forgetting what was being talked about
Echolalia	Echoing of words or phrases just spoken by another

Table 4–3. Abnormalities of Thought Content

Abnormality	Description
Hallucination	False sensory perception without stimuli present; can be tactile, olfactory, gustatory, auditory, or visual; can be pervasive or episodic
Delusion	False belief firmly maintained despite evidence to the contrary
Illusion	False perception of a real external stimulus
Homicidal ideation	Thoughts of wishes or intentions to kill someone else
Suicidal ideation	Thoughts of wishes or desires to kill one's self
Hopelessness	Belief that things will not improve and that nothing can be done
Helplessness	Belief that one will not be able to change the course of events, affect a situation, or alter the outcome of things
Anhedonia	Inability to derive pleasure from ordinarily pleasurable activities
Somatic preoccupation	Preoccupation with bodily functions, processes, and sensations that may not be based in any realistic alteration in body functioning
Depersonalization	Feeling self far away, disconnected
Derealization	Sense that one's environment has changed and is different from the way it had been before

Types of Delusions

- *Religious*—Having an unrealistic or special relationship with God
- *Grandiose*—Believing in one's special powers or mission
- *Persecution*—Believing that others are conspiring against the person or have malevolent intentions toward him or her
- *Of reference*—Other people's thoughts, words, or actions refer to the individual (e.g., thought insertion, thought withdrawal, thought broadcasting, thought control)
  - Thought insertion—Delusion that thoughts are being placed into a person's mind by another person or force
  - Thought withdrawal—Delusion that thoughts are being removed by another person or force
  - Thought broadcasting—Delusion that others can hear a person's thoughts or a person's thoughts are being broadcast over the air
  - Thought control—Delusion that a person's thoughts are being controlled by another person or force.
- *Somatic*—False beliefs involving functioning of the body.

Structured (Tested) Data Set of the MSE

- Data collected through use of standardized questions; in general, a well-established way to assess for impairment in tested area of functioning
- Narrower range of possible findings
- Requires a degree of client cooperation to complete
- Includes the following:
  - *Orientation*—Person, time, and place
  - *Attention*—Attentive or distractible
  - *Concentration*
    - Digit span testing
    - Serial-number testing
    - Backward-spelling testing.

  - *Memory*
    - Long-term testing
    - President testing
    - Event testing
    - Short-term testing
    - Three-object testing
    - Immediate recall testing
    - Number-string testing.

  - *Abstraction* (used only if client is ages 12 or older)
    - Proverb testing
    - Similarity testing.

  - *Insight*—Client's recognition of need for treatment; can be impaired in delirium, dementia, psychosis, frontal-lobe syndrome, substance abuse/dependence
  - *Judgment*—Is client making realistic decisions on the basis of his or her age, knowledge, assets, and liabilities?

- • Personal welfare testing
- • Social welfare testing.

- Delirium and dementia will show a clouded or wandering sensorium.
- When testing cognition, depressed clients will usually say "I don't know," and clients with dementia will usually confabulate.

Mini-Mental Status Exam (MMSE)

- The MMSE is a brief instrument designed to assess a client's cognitive functioning, which can assist in diagnosing an organic component of his or her symptoms.
- Education and intelligence can skew the results.

  - *Orientation*
  - *Time*—Year, season, month, date, day
  - *Place*—Name of this place, floor, city, county, state.

  - *Registration (Memory)*
  - Repeat three objects, such as apple, table, and penny, immediately after PMHNP and have client recall the same three objects in 5 minutes.

  - *Attention and Calculation*
  - Subtract serial 7s from 100
  - Spell "world" backward.

  - *Recall*
  - Recall three objects previously named.

  - *Naming*
  - Show client items such as a watch and pencil and have him or her name them.

  - *Repeat*
  - Repeat the words "no ifs, ands, or buts."

  - *Three-Stage Verbal Command*
  - "Take this paper in your right hand."
  - "Fold it in half."
  - "Put it on the floor."

  - *Written Command*
  - Print on blank paper the sentence "Close your eyes" and have the client follow the directions.

  - *Write a Sentence*
  - Have client write a sentence with a subject, verb, and logical progression of thought.

  - *Intersecting Pentagons*
  - Copy intersecting pentagons on a piece of paper.

MMSE Scoring
- 25–30—Normal
- 21–24—Mild cognitive impairment
- 16–20—Moderate cognitive impairment
- Less than 15—Severe cognitive impairment
- Below 24—Possible indicator of dementia.

Diagnostic and Laboratory Testing

- Assessment of diagnostic and laboratory testing is an essential element of the PMHNP role. It is important for the PMHNP to know when to order such tests, how to interpret the findings, and how to appropriately alter care based on the findings.

- Reasons to assess diagnostic and laboratory testing in psychiatry
  - To assist in the establishment of a diagnosis; as knowledge of underlying pathophysiology grows, diagnostic and laboratory testing use will grow as well
  - Used to rule out other disorders such as medical causes of psychiatric symptoms; helpful in differential diagnostic assessment
  - Used to determine if a client's symptoms are better explained by a nonpsychiatric disorder or by factors such as drug use/abuse
  - Routine ongoing monitoring such as general health screening, monitoring drug levels of certain psychiatric meds, and assessment and monitoring for complications of psychiatric disorders or adverse effects of drugs.

Thyroid Function Tests
- Function of thyroid gland is to take iodine from the circulating blood, combine it with the amino acid tyrosine, and convert it to the thyroid hormones T3 and T4.
- It also stores T3 and T4 until they are released into the bloodstream under the influence of TSH released from the pituitary gland.
- Only a small amount of T3 and T4 are bound to protein.
- The free portion of the thyroid hormones is the true determinant of thyroid status.

Free Thyroxine T4 (FT4) (Normal Values 0.8–2.8 mg/dl)
- FT4 composes a small portion of the total thyroxine, is available to the tissues, and is the metabolically active form of this hormone.
- FT4 test is commonly done to determine thyroid status, to rule out hypo- and hyperthyroidism, and to evaluate thyroid therapy.
  - ***Increased levels***
    - Graves disease
    - Thyrotoxicosis due to T4
    - Hashimoto's thyroiditis
    - Acute thyroiditis.

  - ***Decreased levels***
    - Primary hypothyroidism
    - Secondary hypothyroidism (pituitary insufficiency)
    - Tertiary hypothyroidism (hypothalamic failure)
    - Thyrotoxicosis due to T3

- Renal failure
- Cushing's disease
- Cirrhosis.
- *Interfering factors*
  - Values can be increased during treatment with heparin, aspirin, and propranolol.
  - Values can be decreased during treatment with lasix or methadone.

Thyroid-Stimulating Hormone (TSH) (Normal Values 2–10 mu/L)

- Stimulation of the thyroid gland by TSH causes release and distribution of stored thyroid hormones.
  - When T4 and T3 are high, TSH secretion decreases.
  - When T4 and T3 are low, TSH secretion increases.
  - In primary hypothyroidism, TSH levels rise because of low levels of thyroid hormone.
  - If the pituitary gland fails, TSH is not secreted and blood levels of TSH fall.

- TSH level is commonly tested to establish the diagnosis of primary hypothyroidism.
  - *Increased levels*
    - Primary hypothyroidism
    - Thyroiditis.

  - *Decreased levels*
    - Hyperthyroidism
    - Secondary and tertiary hypothyroidism.

  - *Interfering factors*
    - Values can be decreased during treatment with T3, aspirin, corticosteroids, and heparin.
    - Values can be increased during drug therapy with lithium.

Systemic Effects of Hypothyroidism (Decreased T4, Increased TSH)

- May mimic symptoms of unipolar mood disorders
  - Confusion
  - Decreased libido
  - Impotence
  - Decreased appetite
  - Memory loss
  - Lethargy
  - Constipation
  - Somatic discomfort including aching and joint stiffness
  - Slowed speech and thinking
  - Headaches
  - Slow or clumsy movements
  - Syncope
  - Weight gain
  - Fluid retention
  - Muscle aching and stiffness
  - Slowed reflexes
  - Sensory disturbances, including hearing
  - Cerebellar ataxia
  - Loss of amplitude in EKG.

Systemic Effects of Hyperthyroidism (Increased T4, Decreased TSH)

- May mimic symptoms of bipolar affective disorders
  - Motor restlessness
  - Emotional lability
  - Short attention span
  - Increase in appetite
  - Abdominal pain
  - Excessive sweating

- Compulsive movement
- Fatigue
- Tremor
- Insomnia
- Impotence
- Weight loss

- Flushing
- Elevated upper eyelid leading to decreased blinking, staring, fine tremor of eyelid
- Tachycardia
- Dysrhythmias.

Electrolytes

- Measured as a part of routine screening in acute and critical illness or where there is a known or suspected disorder associated with fluid, electrolyte, or acid/base balance.

Calcium (Ca++) (Normal Values 8.8–10.5 mg/dl)

Abnormal values

- <7.0 mg/dl—associated with tetany
- >11.0 mg/dl—associated with hyperparathyroidism
- >13.5 mg/dl—associated with hypercalcemic coma and metastatic cancer.
- Most Ca (99%) is located in bone, and the remainder is in the plasma and body cells.
- Of the Ca in the plasma, 50% is bound to plasma proteins, and 40% is in the free or ionized form. The remaining fraction circulates in the blood.
- Ca is the major cation for the structure of bones and teeth.

Functions

- Enzymatic cofactor for blood clotting
- Required for hormone secretion
- Required for function of cell receptors
- Required for plasma membrane stability and permeability
- Required for transmission of nerve impulses and the contraction of muscles.
- Ca balance is mediated by interactions among three hormones: parathyroid hormone, vitamin D, and calcitonin.
- Acting together, these substances determine the amount of dietary Ca absorbed and the renal reabsorption and excretion of Ca by the kidney.

  - *Increased levels*
    - Acidosis
    - Hyperparathyroidism
    - Cancers (e.g., bone, leukemia, myeloma)
    - Drugs (e.g., thiazide diuretics, hormones, vitamin D, Ca)
    - Vitamin D intoxication
    - Addison's disease
    - Hyperthyroidism.

  - *Decreased levels*
    - Alkalosis
    - Hypoparathyroidism
    - Renal failure
    - Pancreatitis
    - Inadequate dietary intake of calcium, vitamin D
    - Drugs, including barbiturates, anticonvulsants, acetazolamide, adrenocorticosteroids.

- *Interfering factors*
    - Values are higher in children due to growth and active bone formation.
    - Values can be increased by excessive ingestion of milk or during treatment with lithium, thiazide diuretics, alkaline antacids, or vitamin D.
    - Values can be decreased during treatment with anticonvulsants, aspirin, calcitonin, corticosteroids, heparin, laxatives, diuretics, albuterol, and oral contraceptives.

Systemic Effects of Hypocalcemia (Ca <8.5 mg/dl)

- Increase in neuromuscular excitability
- Confusion
- Parathesias around the mouth and in the digits
- Muscle spasms in the hands and feet
- Hyperreflexia
- Convulsions
- Tetany
- Continuous severe muscle spasm
- EKG changes: prolonged QT interval
- Intestinal cramping
- Hyperactive bowel sounds.

Systemic Effects of Hypercalcemia (Ca >12.0 mg/dl)

- Fatigue
- Weakness
- Nausea
- Constipation
- Behavioral changes
- Impaired renal function
- Lethargy
- Anorexia
- EKG changes: shortened QT interval, depressed T-waves
- Bradycardia
- Heart block.

Sodium (Na⁺) (Normal Values 135–148 mEq/L)

- Na^+ accounts for 90% of the extracellular fluid cations and is the most powerful cation in the extracellular fluid.
- It regulates osmolality (interstitial and intravascular fluid volume).
- It works with potassium and calcium to maintain neuromuscular irritability for conduction of nerve impulses.
- It regulates acid/base balance.
- It participates in cellular chemical reactions and membrane transport.
- It regulates renal retention and excretion of water.
- It maintains systemic blood pressure.

    - *Increased levels*
        - Hypovolemia
        - Dehydration
        - Diabetes insipidus
        - Excessive salt ingestion
        - Gastroenteritis
        - Drugs such as adrenocorticosteroids, methydopa, hydralazine, or cough medication.

    - *Decreased levels*
        - Addison's disease
        - Renal disorder
        - GI fluid loss from vomiting, diarrhea, nasogastric suction, ileus
        - Diuresis
        - Drugs such as lithium, vasopressin, or diuretics.

Systemic Effects of Hyponatremia (Na <135 mEq/L)

- Lethargy
- Headache
- Confusion
- Apprehension
- Seizures
- Coma
- Hypotension
- Tachycardia
- Decreased urine output
- Weight gain
- Edema
- Ascites
- Jugular vein distention.

Systemic Effects of Hypernatremia (Na >147 mEq/L)

- Convulsions
- Pulmonary edema
- Thirst
- Fever
- Dry mucous membranes
- Hypotension
- Tachycardia
- Low jugular venous pressure
- Restlessness.

Magnesium (Mg) (Normal Values 1.3–2.1 mEq/L)

- Mg is a major intracellular cation; 40%–60% is stored in bone and muscle, with 30% in cells.
- A small amount is in the serum, where one-third is bound to plasma proteins and the rest is in ionized form.
- Regulation of Mg metabolism is primarily by the kidney.
- Low serum levels cause renal conservation of Mg.
- Mg is a cofactor in intracellular enzymatic reactions.
- Mg is a cause of neuromuscular excitability.

  - *Increased levels*
    - Addison's disease
    - Adrenalectomy
    - Renal failure
    - Diabetic ketoacidosis
    - Dehydration
    - Hypothyroidism
    - Hyperthyroidism.

  - *Decreased levels*
    - Hyperaldosteronism
    - Hypokalemia
    - Diabetic ketoacidosis
    - Malnutrition
    - Alcoholism
    - Acute pancreatitis
    - GI loss from vomiting, diarrhea, nasogastric suction, and fistula
    - Malabsorption syndrome
    - Pregnancy-induced hypertension.

  - *Interfering factors*
    - Hemolysis of a sample leads to falsely elevated levels.
    - Numerous drugs can alter levels.
    - Values can be increased by drugs such as antacids, laxatives containing Mg, salicylates, and lithium.
    - Values can be decreased by drugs such as thiazide diuretics, calcium gluconate, insulin, amphotericin B, neomycin, aldosterone, and ethanol.

Systemic Effects of Hypomagnesemia (Mg <1.5 mEq/L)

- Depression
- Irritability
- Confusion
- Nystagmus

- Increased reflexes
- Muscle weakness
- Ataxia

- Tetany
- Convulsions.

Systemic Effects of Hypermagnesemia (Mg >2.5 mEq/L)
- Nausea and vomiting
- Muscle weakness
- Depressed skeletal muscle contraction and nerve function

- Respiratory depression
- Hypotension
- Bradycardia.

Chloride (Cl) (Normal Values 98–106 mEq/L)
- Cl is the major anion in the extracellular fluid.
- It provides electroneutrality in relation to Na^+ (see above).
- Transport of Cl is passive and follows the active transport of sodium so that increases or decreases in Cl are proportional to changes in Na^+.

  - **Increased levels**
    - Acidosis
    - Hyperkalemia, hypernatremia
    - Dehydration
    - Renal failure

    - Cushing's disease
    - Hyperventilation
    - Anemia.

  - **Decreased levels**
    - Alkalosis
    - Hypokalemia
    - Hyponatremia
    - Overhydration
    - Burns

    - GI loss from vomiting, diarrhea, nasogastric suction, and fistula
    - Diuresis
    - Addison's disease.

  - **Interfering factors**
    - Elevated serum triglyceride levels and myeloma proteins may lead to falsely decreased levels.
    - Values can be increased by potassium chloride, acetazolamide, methyldopa, diazoxide, and guanethidine.
    - Values can be decreased by ethacrynic acid, lasix, thiazide diuretics, and bicarbonate.
- No specific symptoms are associated with Cl increase or decrease.

Potassium (K^+) (Normal Values 3.5–5.1 mEq/L)
- K^+ is the major intracellular electrolyte.
- Total body K^+ is about 4,000 mEq, with most of it located in the cells.
- Intracellular concentration of K^+ is 150–160 mEq/L; extracellular concentration is 3.5–4.5 mEq/L.
- As the predominant intracellular ion, K^+ regulates intracellular fluid osmolality and provides the balance for intracellular electrical neutrality.
- K^+ is required for glycogen deposition in liver and skeletal muscle cells.
- K^+ maintains resting membrane potential and assists in transmission and conduction of nerve impulses, maintenance of normal cardiac rhythms, and skeletal and smooth muscle contraction.

- K⁺ balance is regulated by the kidney, aldosterone levels, insulin secretion, and changes in pH.
  - *Increased levels*
    - Acidosis
    - Insulin deficiency
    - Hypoaldosteronism
    - Dehydration
    - Addison's disease
    - Acute renal failure
    - Infection.
  - *Decreased levels*
    - Alkalosis
    - Excessive insulin
    - GI loss
    - Laxative abuse
    - Burns
    - Trauma
    - Surgery
    - Cushing's disease
    - Hyperaldosteronism
    - Thyrotoxicosis
    - Anorexia nervosa
    - Diet deficient in meat and vegetables.
  - *Interfering factors*
    - False elevations can occur with vigorous pumping of the hand during venipuncture, hemolysis of the sample, or high platelet counts during clotting.
    - False decreases are seen in anticoagulated samples left at room temperature.
    - Values can be decreased by drugs such as lasix, ethacrynic acid, thiazide diuretics, insulin, aspirin, prednisone, cortisone, gentamycin, lithium, and laxatives.
    - Values can be increased by drugs such as amphotericin B, tetracycline, heparin, epinephrine, K⁺ sparing diuretics, and isoniazid.
    - Chronic marijuana use can elevate K⁺ level.

Systemic Effects of Hyperkalemia (K⁺ >5.5 mEq/L)

- Muscle weakness
- Paralysis
- Tingling of lips and fingers
- Restlessness
- Intestinal cramping
- Diarrhea
- EKG changes—narrow and taller T-waves
  - Mild hyperkalemia—shortened QT interval
  - Severe hyperkalemia—depressed ST segment, prolonged PR interval, widened QRS complex leading to cardiac arrest.

Systemic Effects of Hypokalemia (K⁺ <3.5 mEq/L)

- Impaired carbohydrate metabolism
- Impaired renal function
- Polyuria
- Polydipsia
- Skeletal muscle weakness
- Smooth muscle atony
- Cardiac dysrhythmias
- Paralysis and respiratory arrest.

Liver Function Tests

- Used to monitor liver disease or damage caused by hepatotoxic drugs, as confirmed by elevated levels.

Alanine Amnotransferase (ALT) (Normal Values 5–35 U/L)

- Formerly known as glutamic–pyruvic transaminase (SGPT), ALT is an enzyme produced by the liver that acts as a catalyst in the transamination reaction necessary for amino acid production.
- ALT is found in liver cells in high concentrations and in moderate amounts in body fluids, heart, kidneys, and skeletal muscles.
- When liver damage occurs, serum levels of ALT rise to as much as 50 times normal.

  - ***Pronounced elevated levels (>300 U/L)***
    - Liver disease or damage, such as hepatic cancer, hepatitis, or infectious mononucleosis.

  - ***Moderately elevated levels (100–300 U/L)***
    - Biliary tract obstruction
    - Recent cerebrovascular accident
    - Muscle injury from IM injections, trauma, infection, and seizures
    - Muscular dystrophy
    - Acute pancreatitis
    - Intestinal injury
    - Myocardial infarction
    - Congestive heart failure
    - Renal failure
    - Severe burns.

  - ***Interfering factors***
    - Uremia and hemodialysis can cause falsely decreased levels.
    - Values can be increased with acetaminophen, allopurinol, aspirin, ampicillin, carbamazepine, cephalosporins, codeine, digitalis, indomethacin, heparin, isoniazid, methotrexate, methyldopa, oral contraceptives, phenothiazines, propranolol, tetracycline, and verapamil.

Aspartate Amino Transferase (AST) (Normal Values 5–40 U/L)

- Previously known as serum glutamate oxaloacetate transaminase (SGOT), AST measures the level of the enzyme that catalyzes the reversible transfer of an amino between the amino acid, aspartate, and alphaketoglutamic acid.
- AST exists in large amounts in both liver and myocardial cells and in smaller but significant amounts in skeletal muscles, kidneys, the pancreas, and the brain.
- Serum AST rises when there is cellular damage to the tissues in which the enzyme is found.

  - ***Pronounced elevation (>5x normal)***
    - Acute hepatocellular damage   •   Shock
    - Myocardial infarction   •   Acute pancreatitis.

  - ***Moderate elevation (3–5x normal)***
    - Biliary tract obstruction   •   Chronic hepatitis
    - Cardiac arrhythmias   •   Muscular dystrophy

- Congestive heart failure
- Liver tumors
- Dermatomyositis.

- *Slight elevation (2–3x normal)*
  - Pericarditis
  - Cirrhosis, fatty liver
  - Pulmonary infarction
  - Delirium tremens
  - Cerebrovascular accident
  - Hemolytic anemia.

- *Interfering factors*
  - Numerous drugs may elevate levels, such as antihypertensives, cholinergic agents, anticoagulants, digitalis, erythromycin, isoniazid, methyldopa, oral contraceptives, opiates, salicylates, hepatotoxic meds, and verapamil.
  - Exercise can cause increased levels.

Gamma Glutamyl Transpeptidase (GGT) (Normal Values 10–38 IU/L)

- GGT is an isoenzyme of alkaline phosphatase and assists with the transfer of amino acids and peptides across cellular membranes.
- Hepatobiliary tissues and renal tubular and pancreatic epithelium contain large amounts of GGT.
- Other sources of GGT include the prostate gland, brain, and heart.
- GGT is used to evaluate and monitor clients with known or suspected alcohol abuse, as levels rise even after ingestion of small amounts of alcohol.
- Also used to evaluate elevated alkaline phosphatase of uncertain etiology.
- Pronounced early rises of GGT are found in hepatic disease.
- Modest elevation in GGT occurs in cirrhosis and pancreatic or renal disease.

  - *Elevated GGT*
    - Hepatobiliary tract disorders
    - Hepatocellular carcinoma
    - Hepatocellular degeneration such as cirrhosis
    - Hepatitis
    - Pancreatic or renal cell damage or neoplasm
    - Congestive heart failure
    - Acute myocardial infarction (after 4–10 days)
    - Hyperlipoproteinemia
    - Diabetes mellitus with hypertension
    - Seizure disorder
    - Significant alcohol ingestion.

  - *Interfering factors*
    - Alcohol, barbiturates, and phenytoin can elevate GGT levels.
    - Late pregnancy, oral contraceptives, and clofibrate can lower GGT levels.

Case Study

Veronica, a 22-year-old college student, presents to the clinic for assistance with complaints of frequent headaches, generalized body aches, difficulty concentrating, and insomnia. She has been losing weight over the past few weeks and is unable to study or concentrate in class. She states that she feels "sick" but denies any other recent illnesses. She has an unremarkable history, has no chronic illnesses, and takes no routine medications. She is a moderate social drinker and does not smoke. Recent stressors include a heavy course load and a recent disappointment at failing to be accepted for membership in a sorority on campus. She denies family history for mental illness and talks at great length about why she believes she is "sick, not crazy." There are many issues to consider in assessing this patient.

- What additional assessments would you make at this time?

- What specific diagnostic and laboratory tests would you order, and why?

- What, if any, specific physical findings would you look for?

- What communication strategies would you use to facilitate assessment of this client?

- What milieu considerations would precede your interactions with her?

Review Questions

1. The concept of target symptom identification is best explained as

   a. Identification of the major clinical presentation of the client
   b. Identification of specific, precise, and individualized symptoms reasonably expected to improve with medication
   c. Identification of the secondary messenger system syndrome
   d. Intentional modulation of synaptic pathways

2. Mr. Johnson is a newly admitted client to an inpatient psychiatric hospital. The PMHNP on call at the facility plans to perform the initial intake assessment and diagnostic process. Mr. Johnson asks to please talk in his room because, he says, "People make me nervous." His room is at the end of the hallway and is the farthest away from the nursing station. The PMHNP's action should be based on awareness that the best location to do the assessment is

   a. In Mr. Johnson's room, because it is the least noisy and most comfortable for him, thus facilitating data collection
   b. In the dayroom, which is full of people, to observe his interactions with other individuals
   c. In a quiet place but public enough to get assistance with client care should it be required during the assessment
   d. In the treatment room with the door closed, a neutral location

3. In assessing a client, you ask him the meaning of the proverb "People who live in glass houses shouldn't throw stones." He replies, "Because it will break the windows." The correct interpretation of this finding is

   a. Client has a probable mood disorder
   b. Client has a probable anxiety disorder
   c. Client has limited intellectual ability
   d. Unable to interpret the finding without knowing the client's age

4. The PMHNP is planning to work with a client using an individual therapy model of care. During the first session, the client makes the following statement: "This is the third time my son has run away. I've grounded him, taken away his bike, even tried cutting his allowance and locking him in his room. What should I do now?" The most therapeutic response for the PMHNP to make is

    a. "I wonder if locking him in his room was abusive."
    b. "Maybe that depends on what you are trying to accomplish."
    c. "Perhaps talking to his friends and teachers would help."
    d. Remain silent

5. Mrs. Shea has come to the mental health center seeking treatment for depression. She has a history of a suicide attempt by overdose 1 month ago. She was started on imipramine (TCA) after that event but stopped taking the medication 1 week later because it "did no good." The PMHNP meets with Mrs. Shea to plan care with her. Which of the following is the most appropriate initial action?

    a. Asking Mrs. Shea how to help her
    b. Providing client teaching about the long time frame for TCAs to work
    c. Contracting with Mrs. Shea for six sessions of individual therapy
    d. Providing Mrs. Shea with feedback about how suicide might affect her family

References and Resources

American Nurses Association. (2000). *Scope and standards of psychiatric–mental health clinical nursing practice.* Washington, DC: Author.

American Psychiatric Association. (1995). *Practice guidelines for psychiatric evaluation of adults.* Washington, DC: Author.

American Psychiatric Association. (2000a). *Diagnostic and statistical manual of mental disorders* (4th ed., text rev.). Washington, DC: Author.

American Psychiatric Association. (2000b). *Practice guidelines for the treatment of patients with major depressive disorder.* Washington, DC: Author.

American Psychiatric Association, Work Group on Eating Disorders. (2000). Practice guidelines for the treatment of patients with eating disorders. *American Journal of Psychiatry, 157*(Suppl. 1), 1–39.

Bakerman, S. (2002). *ABCs of interpretive laboratory data* (4th ed.). Greenville, NC: Interpretive Laboratory Data.

Bickley, L. S. (2007). *Bate's guide to physical examination and history taking* (9th ed.). Philadelphia: Lippincott.

Bryson, S. E., & Smith, I. M. (1998). Epidemiology of autism: Prevalence, associated characteristics, and service delivery. *Mental Retardation and Developmental Disabilities Research Reviews, 4,* 97–103.

Clinical Evidence Organization. (2000). *Clinical evidence international sourcebook.* London: BMJ Publishing Group.

Davidson, J. R. (2000). Trauma: The impact of post-traumatic stress disorder. *Journal of Psychopharmacology, 14*(Suppl. 1), S5–S12.

Faulkner, G. (2000). *Behavioral outcomes and guidelines sourcebook.* New York: Faulkner & Gray.

Fombonne, E. (1998). Epidemiology of autism and related conditions. In F. R. Volkmar (Ed.), *Autism and pervasive developmental disorders* (pp. 32–63). Cambridge, England: Cambridge University Press.

Haddow, J. E., Palomaki, G. E., Allan, W. C., Williams, J. R., Knight, G. J., & Gagnon, J. (1999). Maternal thyroid deficiency during pregnancy and subsequent neuropsychological development of the child. *New England Journal of Medicine, 341,* 549–555.

Hoyert, D. L., Kochanek, K. D., & Murphy, S. L. (1999). *Deaths: Final data for 1997–99* (National Vital Statistics Report 47[19], DHHS Publication No. 99-1120). Hyattsville, MD: National Center for Health Statistics.

Margolin, G., & Gordis, E. B. (2000). The effects of family and community violence on children. *Annual Review of Psychology, 51,* 445–479.

National Institute of Mental Health. (2006). *The numbers count: Mental disorders in America.* Last accessed August 15, 2007, from www.nimh.nih.gov.

O'Reilly, D. J. (2000). Thyroid function tests: Time for reassessment. *British Medical Journal, 320,* 1332–1334.

Pop, V. J., Kuijpens, J. L., van Baar, A. L., Verkerk, G., van Son, M. M., & de Vijlder, J. J. (1999). Low maternal free thyroxine concentrations during early pregnancy are associated with impaired psychomotor development in infancy. *Clinical Endocrinology, 50,* 149–155.

Sadock, B., & Sadock, V. (2007). *Kaplan and Sadock's synopsis of psychiatry* (10th ed.). New York: Lippincott Williams & Wilkins.

Schatsburg, A., Cole, J., & DeBattista, C. (2007). *Manual of clinical psychopharmacology* (6th ed.). Washington, DC: American Psychiatric Association.

Shea, C. A., Pelletier, L., Poster, E. C., Stuart, G. W., & Verhey, M. P. (1999). *Advanced practice nursing in psychiatric mental health care.* St. Louis, MO: Mosby.

Strub, R. (2000). *The mental status examination in neurology.* Philadelphia: Oxford University Press.

Stuart, G. W., & Laraia, M. T. (2004). *Principles and practice of psychiatric nursing* (8th ed.). St. Louis, MO: Mosby.

Weissman, M. M., Bland, R. C., & Canino, G. J. (1999). Prevalence of suicide ideation and suicide attempts in nine countries. *Psychological Medicine, 29*(1), 9–17.

Wolraich, M. L., Hannah, J. N., Baumgaertel, A., & Feurer, I. D. (1998). Examination of *DSM-IV* criteria for attention deficit/hyperactivity disorder in a countywide sample. *Journal of Developmental and Behavioral Pediatrics, 19,* 162–168.

Notes:

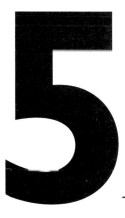

Pharmacological Principles

Psychopharmacology, one of the most active and developing areas of research, is the use of psychotropic medication to treat psychiatric disorders (Sadock & Sadock, 2007). Psychiatric–mental health nurse practitioners (PMHNPs) must have a thorough understanding of the art of prescribing—of the pharmacokinetic and pharmacodynamic actions. The basic pharmacological principles are discussed in this chapter.

Concepts in Pharmacological Management

- *Pharmacology*—Study of what drugs do and how they do it
- *Pharmacokinetics*—Study of what the body does to drugs; includes absorption, distribution, metabolism, and excretion
- *Pharmacodynamics*—Study of what drugs do to the body; target sites for drug actions include receptors, ion channels, enzymes, and carrier proteins.

Pharmacokinetics

- *Absorption*—Method and rate at which drugs leave the site of administration
    - With oral medications, absorption normally occurs in the small intestine and then is ultimately metabolized by the liver.

- *Distribution*—Occurs after the drug leaves the systemic circulation and enters the interstitium and cells
    - Drugs are redistributed in organs according to the fat and protein content of the organ.
    - Most psychotropic medications are lipophilic and highly protein bound. Only the unbound (free) portion of the drug is active. Therefore, individuals with low protein (albumin) levels, as found in patients with malnutrition, wasting, or aging, can potentially experience toxicity (see below) from an increased amount of free drug.

- *Metabolism*—Process by which the drug becomes chemically altered in the body.
- *First-pass metabolism*—Process by which the drug is metabolized by P450 enzymes in the intestines and liver before going to the systemic circulation.
- *Elimination*—Process by which the drug is removed from the body.

- *Half-life (T¹/2)*—Time needed to clear 50% of the drug from the plasma.
  - The half-life also determines the dosing interval and the length of time to reach a steady state.
- *Steady state*—Point at which the amount of drug eliminated between doses is approximately equal to the dose administered.
  - Drugs usually are administered once every half-life to achieve a steady state.
  - It takes approximately five half-lives to achieve a steady state and five half-lives to completely eliminate a drug.

Alterations in Pharmacokinetics

- Hepatic cytochrome P450 enzyme interactions can induce or inhibit the metabolism of certain drugs, thus changing their desired concentration levels.

  - *Common Enzyme Inducers*
    - Tegretol
    - Antifungals
    - Rifampin
    - Dilantin
    - Phenobarbital
    - Trileptal or Topamax (weak inducers).

  - *Common Enzyme Inhibitors*
    - Tagamet
    - Erythromycin
    - Biaxin
    - Fluoroquinolones
    - Prozac
    - Paxil.

- Enzyme inducers can decrease the serum level of other drugs that are substrates of that enzyme, thus possibly causing subtherapeutic drug levels.
- Enzyme inhibitors can increase the serum level of other drugs that are substrates of that enzyme, thus possibly causing toxic levels.
- Liver disease will affect liver enzyme activity and first-pass metabolism, resulting in possible toxic plasma drug levels.
- Kidney disease or drugs that reduce renal clearance, such as nonsteroidal anti-inflammatory drugs (NSAIDs), may increase serum concentration of drugs that are excreted by the kidneys (lithium).
- Elderly people are more sensitive to psychotropics because of their decreased intracellular water, protein binding, low muscle mass, decreased metabolism, and increased body fat concentration.
  - ✓ Remember that most psychotropics are lipophilic and highly protein bound. Thus, because elderly people have more body fat and less protein, they are more likely to develop toxicity.

Pharmacodynamics

- Target sites for drug actions include *receptors*. Several types of pharmacodynamics involving receptors are
  - *Agonist effect*—Bind to receptors and activate a biological response
  - *Inverse agonist effect*—Cause the opposite effect of agonists; do not bind to receptor
  - *Partial agonist effect*—Do not fully activate the receptors
  - *Antagonist effect*—Bind to the receptor but do not activate a biological response
- Another site for drug actions are *ion channels,* which exist for many ions such as sodium, potassium, chloride, and calcium and can be open at some times and closed at

other times. Neurotransmitters or drugs may be excitatory or inhibitory depending on the type of ion channel they gate.

- *Excitatory response*—Depolarization; involves the opening of sodium and calcium channels with these ions going into the cell
- *Inhibitory response*—Repolarization; involves the opening of chloride channels with chloride going into the cell, potassium leaving, or both.

- Another site for drug actions are *enzymes,* which are important for drug metabolism and play an important role in the chemical alteration of the drug. Some drugs will inhibit the action of a particular enzyme, thus increasing the availability of the neurotransmitter. An example is monoamine oxidase inhibitors (MAOIs).
- Another site for drug actions are *carrier proteins* or *reuptake pumps,* which transport neurotransmitters out of the synapse and back into the presynaptic neuron to be recycled or reused. Some drugs will inhibit reuptake pumps such as selective serotonin reuptake inhibitors (SSRIs), thus increasing the synaptic availability of the neurotransmitter.

Other Terminology

- *Potency*—Relative dose required to achieve certain effects
- *Therapeutic index*—Relative measure of the toxicity or safety of a drug; ratio of the median toxic dose to the median effective dose
    - Drugs with a high therapeutic index (Depakote, 50–125) have a high margin of safety; that is, the therapeutic dose and the toxic dose are far apart.
    - Drugs with a low therapeutic index (Lithium, 0.5–1.2) have a low margin of safety, that is, the therapeutic dose and the toxic dose are close together.
- *Tolerance*—Process of becoming less responsive to a particular drug as it is administered over time.

PMHNP Role of Pharmacological Management

Pharmacological Management Process
- Make a diagnosis and identify the target symptoms.
- Consider the phase of illness (e.g., acute, relapse, recurrence).
- Assess prior personal and family history of response to certain medications.
- Identify potential interactions between the current prescribed medications.
- Identify cultural implications of certain drugs.
- Discuss the risks and benefits of the treatment.
- Document informed consent and client's understanding of target symptoms, benefits, risks, and alternatives to treatment.
- Monitor response and side effects.

Follow-Up and Role of the PMHNP
- Use of standards of care.
- Assist in determining length of treatment.
- Do relapse planning.
- It is helpful and advisable to use standardized clinical rating scales to establish the client's baseline and to monitor progress or decompensation over time. Screening tests also will aid in making a diagnosis and ruling out other disorders.

- *Common screening tests for mood disorders include*
  - Beck Depression Inventory (BDI; Beck, Ward, Mendelson, Mock, & Erbaugh, 1961)
  - Mood Disorder Questionnaire (MDQ; Hirschfeld & Holzer, 2003)
  - Positive and Negative Symptom Scale (PANSS; Kay & Fiszbein, 1987)
  - Brief Psychosis Rating Scale (BPRS; Overall & Gorham, 1962).

- It is important to recognize the large body of evidence-based data supporting the combined use of pharmacological and nonpharmacological treatments as offering psychiatric clients the best possibility for significant clinical improvement.

- Nonadherence is a common problem with all chronic illness, including psychiatric disorders, and should be a continuous focus of concern for the PMHNP.

- Common medications used in the clinical management of psychiatric disorders and usually prescribed by the PMHNP are identified in Table 5–1.

- A Drug Enforcement Administration (DEA) number is required for prescription of controlled substances.

  - **Schedule of Controlled Drugs**
    - *Schedule I*
      - Nonmedicinal substances
      - High abuse potential
      - Used for research purposes only
      - Not legally available by prescription
      - Examples include heroin and marijuana.

    - *Schedule II*
      - Medicinal drugs in current use
      - High potential for abuse and dependency
      - Written prescription allowed
      - No telephone orders allowed
      - No refills allowed on prescription
      - Examples include morphine sulfate, codeine, fentanyl, methadone, Dilaudid, Oxycontin.

    - *Schedule III*
      - Medicinal drugs with less abuse potential than Schedule II drugs
      - Still greater potential for abuse than Schedule IV drugs
      - Telephone orders if followed by written prescription
      - Prescription must be renewed every 6 months
      - Refills limited to five
      - Examples include appetite suppressants, butalbital, testosterone.

    - *Schedule IV*
      - Medicinal drugs with less abuse potential than Schedule III drugs
      - Examples include Darvon, Talwin, benzodiazepines (e.g., Xanax, Librium, Klonopin, Valium, Tranxene, Ativan), Provigil, Phenobarbital, Ambien, Lunesta, Restoril, Darvocet.

    - *Schedule V*
      - Medicinal drugs with lowest abuse potential
      - Handled in manner similar to noncontrolled drugs
      - Examples include Imodium, Buprenex, Robitussin with codeine, Phenergan with codeine.

Other Pharmacological Considerations

- It is vital to be aware of the teratogenic nature of many psychotropic agents. It is important to discuss the risks vs. the benefits of medications during pregnancy.
  - Possible risks of psychotropic medications during pregnancy include
    - Feeding difficulties
    - Transient agitation or sedation
    - Premature labor
    - Drug discontinuation symptoms
    - Teratogenic effects of certain psychotropics.
  - Possible risks of not taking psychotropic medications during pregnancy include
    - Recurrence of symptoms
    - Adverse effects on mother–infant bonding
    - Poor maternal self-care.

Food and Drug Administration (FDA) Pregnancy Ratings for Medications
- **A**—Controlled studies show no risk
- **B**—No evidence of risk in humans
- **C**—Risk cannot be ruled out
- **D**—Positive evidence of risk
- **X**—Absolutely contraindicated in pregnancy.

Teratogenic Risks of Common Psychiatric Medications
- Benzodiazepines—Floppy baby syndrome, cleft palate
- Tegretol (carbamazepine)—Neural tube defects
- Eskalith (Lithium)—Epstein anomaly
- Depakote (divalproex sodium)—Neural tube defects, specifically spina bifida
- ✓ Remember that *some* common medications can induce depression or mania.

Medications That Can Induce Depression
- Beta blockers
- Steroids
- Interferon
- Accutane
- Some retroviral drugs
- Neoplastic drugs
- Benzodiazepines
- Progesterone.

Medications That Can Induce Mania
- Steroids
- Antidepressants in individuals with bipolar disorder
- Isoniazid (INH)
- Antabuse.
- ✓ Remember that *some medications may **possibly** cause a false urinary drug screen result.*
- **Positive Amphetamines**
  - Stimulants (e.g., Adderall, Ritalin)
  - Wellbutrin
  - Prozac
  - Trazadone
  - Ranitidine
  - Serzone

- Nasal decongestants
- Pseudoephedrine.

- **Positive Alcohol**
  - Valium.

- **Positive Benzodiazepines**
  - Zoloft (sertraline).

- **Positive Cocaine**
  - Amoxicillin
  - Most antibiotics
  - NSAIDs.

- **Positive Heroin or Morphine**
  - Quinolones
  - Rifampin
  - Codeine
  - Poppy seeds.

- **Positive Methadone or PCP**
  - Nyquil
  - Dextromethorphan.

Table 5–1. Medications Commonly Used in the Clinical Management of Psychiatric Disorders

---

Medications Used to Treat Schizophrenia and Other Psychotic Disorders

Typical antipsychotics	Haldol (haloperidol), Haldol Decanoate
	Loxitane (loxapine)
	Mellaril (thioridazine)
	Moban (molindone)
	Navane (thiothixene)
	Prolixin (fluphenazine), Prolixin Decanoate
	Serentil (mesoridazine)
	Stelazine (trifluoperazine)
	Thorazine (chlorpromazine)
	Trilafon (perphenazine)
Second-generation antipsychotics	Abilify (aripiprizole)
	Clozaril (clozapine)
	Geodon (ziprasidone)
	Invega (paliperidone)
	Risperdal (risperidone)
	Seroquel (quetiapine)
	Zyprexa (olanzapine)

Medications Used to Treat Mood Disorders and Bipolar Affective Disorders

Mood stabilizers	Depakene (valproic acid)
	Depakote (divalproex sodium)

Table 5–1. Continued

Equetro (carbamazepine ER)
Eskalith, Lithobid, Lithonate, Lithotabs (lithium carbonate)
Keppra (levetiracetam)
Lamictal (lamotrigine)
Neurontin (gabapentin)
Tegretol (carbamazepine)
Topamax (topiramate)
Tripleptal (oxcarbazepine)

Medications Used to Treat Mood Disorders, Unipolar Affective Disorders, and Depressive Disorders

Tricyclics (TCA)	Anafranil (clomipramine)
	Asendin (amoxapine)
	Elavil (amitriptyline)
	Norpramin (desipramine)
	Pamelor (nortriptyline)
	Sinequan (doxepin)
	Surmontil (trimipramine)
	Tofranil (imipramine)
	Vivactil (protriptyline)
Serotonin selective reuptake inhibitors (SSRIs)	Celexa (citalopram)
	Lexapro (escitalopram)
	Luvox (fluvoxamine)
	Paxil (paroxetine)
	Pexeva (paroxetine mesylate)
	Prozac (fluoxetine)
	Zoloft (sertraline)
Monamine oxidase inhibitors (MAOIs)	EMSAM (selegiline transdermal)
	Nardil (phenelzine)
	Parnate (tranylcypromine sulfate)
Other agents	Cymbalta (duloxetine)
	Desyrel (trazodone)
	Effexor (venlafaxine)
	Remeron (mirtazapine)
	Serzone (nefazodone)
	Wellbutrin (bupropion)

Medications Used to Treat Anxiety Disorders

Benzodiazepines (BNZs)	Ativan (lorazepam)
	Klonopin (clonazepam)
	Librium (chlordiazepoxide)
	Serax (oxazepam)
	Tranxene (clorazepate)
	Xanax (alprazolam)

Continued on the next page

Table 5–1. Continued

Anxiolytics	BuSpar (buspirone)
Other agents	Inderal (propranolol)
	Tenormin (atenolol)

Medications Used to Treat Attention-Deficit Disorder/Attention-Deficit Hyperactivity Disorder (ADHD)

Stimulants	Adderall (amphetamine, dextroamphetamine)
	Focalin (dexmethylphenidate)
	Dexedrine (dextroamphetamine)
	Ritalin (methylphenidate)
	Concerta (methylphenidate)
	Vyvanse (lisdexamfetamine dimesylate)
Other agents	Antidepressants such as Norpramine, Effexor, and Wellbutrin are also used in the clinical management of ADHD.

Case Study

Jane, a 74-year-old client who the PHMNP has been seeing for depression, presented at her appointment with complaints of tremors, diaphoresis, headache, and nausea over the past week. She is currently being prescribed Amitriptyline (50 mg q HS), which was increased at her last visit, and Zoloft (100 mg qd). She denies depression but admits to increased confusion and memory problems.

- What is your biggest pharmacological concern at this point with the combination of medication the client is being prescribed?

- What is your plan of action?

- What pharmacokinetics should you keep in mind when treating elderly people?

Review Questions

1. Sarah presents for her initial intake appointment with complaints of depression. She is being treated for hypertension and asthma by her primary care provider. Knowing that certain medications may cause or exacerbate depression, you obtain a complete medication history. Which of the following medications is known to exacerbate or cause depression?

    a. Prilosec
    b. Propranolol
    c. Synthroid
    d. Biaxin

2. When treating elderly people, you should keep in mind that they are more sensitive to issues of drug toxicity because of which of the following reasons?

    a. Decreased body fat

    b. Increased liver capacity

    c. Decreased protein binding

    d. Increased muscle concentration

3. Which known teratogenic effects can be caused by the common psychotropic medications Depakote and Lithium?

    a. Depakote—Epstein anomaly; Lithium—Cleft palate

    b. Lithium—Epstein anomaly; Depakote—Spina bifida

    c. Depakote—Limb malformations; Lithium—Seizure disorder

    d. Lithium—Spina bifida; Depakote—Mental retardation

4. The study of what the body does to drugs is called

    a. Pharmacodynamics

    a. Pharmacology

    a. Pharmacokinetics

    a. Distribution

References and Resources

American Psychiatric Association. (2000). *Practice guidelines for the treatment of patients with major depressive disorder.* Washington, DC: Author.

Antai-Otong D. (Ed). (2003). *Psychiatric nursing: Biological and behavioral concepts.* New York: Delmar.

Beck, A. T., Ward, C. H., Mendelson, M., Mock, J., & Erbaugh, J. (1961). An inventory for measuring depression. *Archives of General Psychiatry, 4,* 561–571.

Boyd, M. A. (2002). *Psychiatric nursing: Contemporary practice* (2nd ed.). Philadelphia: Lippincott.

Dipiro, J. T., Talbert, R. L., & Yee, G. C. (Eds.). (2002). *Pharmacotherapy: A pathophysiological approach* (5th ed.). New York: McGraw-Hill.

Fuller, M., & Sajatovic, M. (2005). *Lexi-Comp's psychotropic drug information handbook (mental health).* Cleveland, OH: Lexi-Comp.

Hirschfeld, R., & Holzer, C. (2003). Validity of the mood disorder questionnaire: A general population study. *American Journal of Psychiatry, 160,* 178–180.

Kay, S. R., & Fiszbein, A. (1987). The positive and negative syndrome scale for schizophrenia. *Schizophrenia Bulletin, 13,* 261–275.

Overall, J. E., & Gorham, C. R. (1962). The brief psychiatric rating scale. *Psychological Reports, 10,* 790–812.

Rapuri, S., Ramaswamy, S., Madaan, V., Rasimas, J., & Krahn, L. (2006). "WEED" out false positive urine drug screens. *Current Psychiatry, 5*(8), 107–110.

Sadock, B., & Sadock, V. (2007). *Kaplan and Sadock's synopsis of psychiatry* (10th ed.). New York: Lippincott Williams & Wilkins.

Schatsburg, A., Cole, J., & DeBattista, C. (2007). *Manual of clinical psychopharmacology* (6th ed.). Washington, DC: American Psychiatric Publishing, Inc.

Stahl, S. (2006). *Essential psychopharmacology: The prescriber's guide.* New York: Cambridge University Press.

Notes:

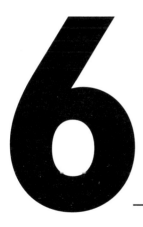

Nonpharmacological Treatment

This chapter discusses nonpharmacological interventions such as individual psychotherapies, group therapy, family therapies, and complementary/alternative therapies. Because medications alone do not treat an individual's environmental or interpersonal stressors and his or her responses to these stressors, an integrated approach is the most beneficial in treating mental illnesses. Although individuals seek counseling for self-discovery, the most common issues for individual therapy are

- Losses
- Interpersonal conflicts
- Symptomatic presentations such as panic, phobias, and negativity
- Unfulfilled expectations at life transitions
- Characterological issues such as narcissism or aggressiveness.

Confidentiality may be broken when there is increased potential for self-harm or harm to others, situations of child or elder abuse, in cases of abuse of people with disabilities, when the therapist determines that the individual needs hospitalization, when information is being made an issue in court, and when individuals request that their information be released to a third party.

Individual Therapy

Psychoanalytic Therapy
- Originated by Sigmund Freud (1856–1939), who believed that behavior is determined by unconscious motivations and instinctual drives (see also Chapter 2)
- Promotes change through the development of greater insight and awareness of maladaptive defenses
- Attends to past developmental and psychodynamic factors, which shape present behaviors.

Cognitive Therapy
- Originated by Aaron Beck (born 1921)
- Purports that external events do not cause anxiety and responses that are maladaptive, but rather the individual's expectations, perceptions, and interpretations of these events cause anxiety

- Allows clients to view reality more clearly through an examination of their central distorted cognitions
- Goal is to change clients' irrational beliefs, faulty conceptions, and negative cognitive distortions.

Behavioral Therapy
- Originated by Arnold Lazarus (born 1932)
- Focuses on changing maladaptive behaviors by participating in active behavioral techniques such as exposure, relaxation, problem solving, and role playing.

Dialectical Behavioral Therapy
- Originated by Marsha Linehan (born 1943)
- Commonly used with individuals with borderline personality disorder
- Focuses on emotional regulation, tolerance for distress, self-management skills, interpersonal effectiveness, and mindfulness, with an emphasis on treating therapy-interfering behaviors.

  - *Goals*
    - Decrease suicidal behaviors
    - Decrease therapy-interfering behaviors
    - Decrease emotional reactivity
    - Decrease self-invalidation
    - Decrease crisis-generating behaviors
    - Decrease active passivity
    - Increase realistic decision making
    - Increase accurate communication of emotions and competencies.

Existential Therapy
- Originated by Viktor Frankl (1905–1997)
- A philosophical approach in which reflection on life and self-confrontation are encouraged
- Emphasizes individual's accepting freedom and making responsible choices
- A basic dimension of humans includes finding meaning and purpose in life—"Why am I here? What is my purpose?"
- Goals are to live authentically and to focus on the present and on personal responsibility.

Humanistic Therapy
- Originated by Carl Rogers (1902–1987); also known as *person-centered therapy*
- Concepts include self-directed growth and self-actualization; people are born with the capacity to direct themselves toward self-actualization
- Each individual has the potential naturally through which he or she can actualize and find meaning.

Eye Movement Desensitization and Reprocessing (EMDR)
- A form of behavioral therapy
- Originated by Francine Shapiro
- Involves integrating the use of rhythmic eye movements to treat traumatic stress and memories
- Most commonly used in posttraumatic stress disorder

- *Desensitization phase:* The individual visualizes the trauma, verbalizes the negative thoughts or maladaptive beliefs, and remains attentive to physical sensations. This process occurs for a limited time while the individual maintains rhythmic eye movements. He or she is then instructed to block out negative thoughts; to breathe deeply; and then to verbalize what he or she is thinking, feeling, or imagining.
- *Installation phase:* The individual installs and increases the strength of the positive thought that he or she has declared as a replacement for the original negative thought.
- *Body scan:* The individual visualizes the trauma along with the positive thought and then scans his or her body mentally to identify any tension within.

Group Therapy

Benefits
- Increases insight about oneself
- Increases social skills
- Is cost-effective
- Develops sense of community.
- Irvin Yalom (born 1931) was the first person to put a theoretical perspective on group work and identified 10 curative factors that differentiate group therapy from individual therapy.
  1. *Instillation of hope*—Participants develop hope for creating a different life. Members are at different levels of growth; thus they gain hope from others that change is possible.
  2. *Universality*—Participants discover that others have similar problems, thoughts, or feelings and that they are not alone.
  3. *Altruism*—This results from sharing oneself with another and helping another.
  4. *Increased development of socialization skills*—New social skills are learned, and maladaptive social behaviors are corrected. The group can provide a "natural laboratory."
  5. *Imitative behaviors*—Participants are able to increase their skills by imitating the behaviors of others.
  6. *Interpersonal learning*—Interacting with others increases adaptive interpersonal relationships.
  7. *Group cohesiveness*—Participants develop an attraction to the group and other members as well as a sense of belonging.
  8. *Catharsis*—Participants experience catharsis as they openly express their feelings, which were previously suppressed.
  9. *Existential factors*—Groups enable participants to deal with the meaning of their own existence.
  10. *Corrective refocusing*—Participants reexperience family conflicts in the group, which allows them to recognize and change behaviors that may be problematic.

Group Phases
- *Pregroup phase*—The leader considers the direction and framework of the group.
  - Purpose
  - Goals

- Membership criteria
- Membership size
- Pregroup interview
- Informed consent.

- *Forming phase*—Members are concerned about self-disclosure and being rejected. Goals and expectations are identified, and boundaries are established. The development of trust and rapport is very important.
- *Storming phase*—Members are resistant and may begin to use testing behaviors. Issues related to inclusion, control, and affection begin to surface. Leaders' tasks are to allow expression of both positive and negative feelings, assist the group in understanding the underlying conflict, and examine nonproductive behaviors.
- *Norming phase*—Resistance to the group is overcome by members. A strong attraction to the group and others emerges. Open and spontaneous communication occurs, and the group norms are established.
- *Performing phase*—The group's work becomes more focused. There is creative problem solving, and solutions begin to emerge. Experiential learning takes place. Group energy is directed toward completion of goals.
- *Mourning phase*—Preparation is being made to end the group. (The work of termination begins during the first stage of the group.) Both members and leaders express their feelings about each other and termination. A discussion and overview of what has been learned, as well as what issues still need to be worked on, takes place.

Reminiscence Therapy
- Characterized by a progressive return of memories of past experiences
- Used with elderly individuals
- Enables participants to search for meaning in their lives and strive for some resolution of past interpersonal and intrapsychic conflicts.

Family Therapies

Family System Concepts
- A *system* is any unit structured on feedback—the family.
- The process by which all family members operate together is referred to as the *family system.*
- Family systems theory is based on the idea that one could not understand any family member (part) without understanding how all family members operate together (system).
- The family system operates based on a set of rules that may be overt or covert.
- *Boundaries*—Barriers that protect and enhance the functional integrity of families, individuals, and subsystems. System boundaries can be physical or psychological.
- *Types of Boundaries*
  - *Clearly defined boundaries*—Maintain individual's separateness and emphasize belongingness
  - *Rigid/inflexible boundaries*—May lead to distant relationships and disengagement
  - *Diffuse boundaries*—Blurred and indistinct boundaries; lead to enmeshment

- *Circular Causality*—An ongoing feedback loop; a series of actions and reactions that maintain a problem. Individuals and emotional problems are best understood within the context of relationships and through assessing interactions within an entire family.
- *Family Homeostasis*—Tendency of families to resist change to maintain homeostasis.
- *Morphogenesis*—Family's tendency to adapt to change when changes are necessary.
- *Morphostasis*—Family's tendency to remain stable in the midst of change.

Family Systems Therapy

- Originated by Murray Bowen (1913–1990), who believed that an individual's problematic behavior may serve a function or purpose for the family or be a symptom of dysfunctional patterns.
- Focus is on chronic anxiety within families.
- Treatment goals are to increase the family members' awareness of their function within the family and to increase levels of *self-differentiation* (the level at which one's sense of self-worth is not dependent on external relationships, circumstances, or occurrences).
  - *Triangles*—Dyads that form triads to decrease stress; the lower the level of family adaptation, the more likely a triangle will develop
  - *Nuclear family emotional system*—Level of differentiation of the parents usually equal to the level of differentiation of the entire family
  - *Multi-transmission process*—Dysfunction present over several generations
  - *Family projection process*—Parents transmitting their own level of differentiation onto the most susceptible child
  - *Emotional cutoffs*—Attempting to break contact with the family of origin
  - *Sibling position*—Influences interactions and personality characteristics.

Structural Family Therapy

- Originated by Salvador Minuchin, who placed emphasis on how, when, and to whom family members relate in order to understand and then change the family's structure.
- Individual's symptoms are rooted in the context of family transaction patterns. The symptom is a function of the health of the whole family and is maintained by structural problems in the system.
- Main treatment goal is to produce a structural change in the family organization to more effectively manage problems—changing transactional patterns and family structure.
  - *Family structure*—Invisible set of functional demands that organize the way members interact with each other, made up of subsystems (e.g., marital, parental, sibling), coalitions (e.g., two members joining forces against a third member), and boundaries
  - *Structural mapping* (genogram)—Mapping relationships using symbols to represent overinvolvement, conflict, coalitions, and so forth
  - *Hierarchies*—Distribution of power.

Experiential Therapy

- Originated by Virginia Satir (1916–1988)
- Behavior is determined by personal experience and not by external reality.

- Focus is on being authentic, freedom of choice, human validation, and experiencing the moment.
- Treatment goals are to develop authentic, nurturing communication and increased self-worth of each family member; overall goal is growth rather than reduction of symptoms alone.
- Does not focus on particular techniques.

Strategic Therapy

- Originated by Jay Haley (1923–2007)
- Focus is that symptoms are viewed as metaphors and reflect problems in the hierarchal structure. Symptoms are a way to communicate metaphorically within a family.
- Treatment goal is to help family members behave in ways that will not perpetuate the problem behavior.
- Interventions are problem focused. Strategic therapy is more symptom focused than structural therapy.
- Strategic family therapists are concerned mainly with those techniques that change the sequence of interactions that is maintaining the problem.
- Techniques are straightforward directives, paradoxical directives, and reframing belief systems.
  - *Straightforward directives*—Tasks that are designed in expectation of the family member's compliance
  - *Paradoxical directives*—A negative task that is assigned when family members are resistant to change and the member is expected to be noncompliant (use this technique with caution).
  - *Reframing belief systems*—Problematic behaviors are relabeled to have more positive meaning (e.g., *jealousy* reframed to *caring*).

Solution-Focused Therapy

- Originated by Steve deShazer, Bill O'Hanlon, and Insoo Berg
- Focus is to rework solutions that have previously worked in the present situation.
- Treatment goal is effective resolution of problems through cognitive problem solving and use of personal resources and strengths.
- Techniques include the use of miracle questions, exception-finding questions, and scaling questions.
  - *Miracle questions*—"If a miracle were to happen tonight while you were asleep, and tomorrow morning you awoke to find that the problem no longer existed, what would be different?" "How would you know the miracle took place?" "How would others know?"
  - *Exception-finding questions*—Directing individuals to a time in their life when the problem did not exist, which helps them move toward solutions by assisting them in searching for any exceptions to the pattern. "Was there a time when the problem did not occur?"
  - *Scaling questions*—"On a scale of 1–10, with 10 being very anxious and depressed, how would you rate how you are feeling now?" This is useful to highlight small increments of change.

Complementary/Alternative Therapies (CAMs)

- CAMs deal with the connection between the mind and the body and are viewed as holistic health care (dealing with the biopsychosocial and spiritual components of the individual).
    - *Complementary therapies*—Used in addition to traditional medical practices
    - *Alternative therapies*—Used in place of traditional medical practices.

Why Individuals Use CAMs
- Desire for more control over decision making
- Decreased insurance coverage, therefore making the use of CAMs cheaper
- Preference for natural rather than synthetic medications
- Increased cost of prescriptions and services
- Failure of conventional medications.

Types
- Progressive muscle relaxation
- Visual imagery
- Meditation
- Yoga
- Biofeedback
- Herbal products
- Acupressure/acupuncture
- Massage
- Art/dance therapy
- Aromatherapy
- Macrobiotics
- Reflexology
- Any of the CAMs can be integrated into standard psychotherapeutic practice.

Acupressure/Acupuncture
- Based on the basic tenet of Chinese medicine that vital energy (*chi*) flows along specific pathways that have many points which, when manipulated by either hands or needles, corrects imbalances. This occurs by stimulating energy flow or by removing blockages to energy flow.
- Thought to produce effects by regulating the nervous system and aiding the activity of endorphins and immune system cells at different sites in the body.
- Also thought to alter brain chemistry by changing the release of neurohormones and neurotransmitters.

Biofeedback
- A process providing an individual with visual or auditory information about the autonomic physiological functions of his or her body, such as blood pressure, muscle tension, and brain wave activity.
- The individual learns consciously to control these processes, which were previously regarded as involuntary.

Uses

- Stress-related symptoms (e.g., anxiety)
- Pain
- Insomnia
- Neuromuscular problems (e.g., migraines, muscular tension, tension headaches, Raynaud's disease, urinary incontinence)
- Neurobehavioral disorders
- Enhancement of healing
- Athletic and work performance.

Desired Outcome

- Positive change in baseline measures
- Demonstrated skill at self-regulation
- Improvement in symptoms
- Use of skills in daily life
- Reduction of muscle bracing
- Increased sense of self-efficacy.

Aromatherapy

- Therapeutic use of plants or oils to obtain many therapeutic effects, such as analgesic, psychological, and antimicrobial benefits
- In psychiatry, olfactory stimulation used to elicit feelings or memories during psychotherapy.

Herbal Products

- Originated in China; the oldest system of medicine
- Relies on plants to cure illnesses and maintain health
- Similar to most prescription medications, plants contain active compounds that produce physiological effect
- Food and Drug Administration (FDA) approval not required, thus no uniform standards for quality control or potency
- Common herbs and interactions include
  - *Omega-3 Fatty Acids*
    - Used for attention-deficit/hyperactivity disorder, dyslexia, cognitive impairment, dementia, cardiovascular disease, asthma, lupus, and rheumatoid arthritis
    - Interacts with Coumadin, increasing anticoagulant effect (individuals cautioned to stop using before surgery).
  - *Sam-e*
    - Used for depression, osteoarthritis, and liver disease
    - May cause hypomania, hyperactive muscle movements, and possible serotonin syndrome.
  - *Tryptophan*
    - Used for depression, obesity, insomnia, headaches, and fibromyalgia
    - High concentrations in turkey
    - Increased risk of serotonin syndrome with serotonin reuptake inhibitors (SSRIs), monoamine oxidase inhibitors (MAOIs), and St. John's wort.

- *Vitamin E*
  - Used for enhancing the immune system and protecting cells against effects of free radicals
  - Used for neurological disorders, diabetes, and premenstrual syndrome
  - Interacts with Coumadin, increasing anticoagulant effect; antiplatelet drugs; and statins, increasing additive effect and risk of rhabdomyolysis.

- *Melatonin*
  - Used for insomnia, jet lag, shift work, and cancer
  - Sets timing of circadian rhythms and regulates seasonal responses
  - Interacts with aspirin, nonsteroidal anti-inflammatory drugs (NSAIDs), beta blockers, corticosteroids, valerian, kava kava, and alcohol
  - Can inhibit ovulation in large doses.

- *Fish Oil*
  - Used for bipolar disorder, hypertension, lowering triglycerides, and decreasing blood clotting
  - Interacts with Coumadin, aspirin, NSAIDs, garlic, and ginkgo
  - May alter glucose regulation.
  - Most herbals are secreted in breast milk and are contraindicated during lactation and should be avoided during pregnancy
  - Common herbals with psychoactive effects include.

- *Black cohosh*—Menopausal symptoms, premenstrual syndrome, dysmenorrhea
- *Belladonna*—Anxiety
- *Catnip*—Sedation
- *Chamomile*—Sedation, anxiety
- *Ginkgo*—Delirium, dementia, sexual dysfunction caused by SSRIs
- *Ginseng*—Depression, fatigue
- *Valerian*—Sedation.

Massage
- Believed to increase blood circulation, improve lymph flow, improve musculoskeletal tone, and have tranquilizing effect on the mind.

Meditation
- Consciously directing one's attention to alter his or her state of consciousness
- Produces physiological effects such as decreased heart rate, blood pressure, and respiratory rate; decreased anxiety; and increased alpha brain waves.

Reflexology
- Stimulates the body's natural healing power through massaging the feet, hands, and ears
- Alleviates tension by cleaning crystalline deposits under the skin that may interfere with the natural flow of the body's energy
- Body parts mapped out on the soles and sides of the feet, hands, and ears
- Disorders related to the represented body parts relieved by application of pressure
- Used for back pain, migraines, infertility, sleep disorders, digestive disorders, and stress-related conditions.

Macrobiotics

- Use of a balanced diet in attempt to live in harmony with nature
- Foods classified as yin (cold and wet) and yang (hot and dry)
- Goal to keep the yin and yang in balance.

Case Study

You are an existential therapist in session with Bill, who has anxiety and states, "No one really understands me or cares about me. That is why I have low self-esteem and feel 'less than.' That is why I act the way I do." He has been self-medicating with alcohol and illicit drugs.

- Using an existential style, how would you respond to Bill's statement?
- What existential tenet does your response display?
- According to existential theory, how do you view Bill's anxiety?

Review Questions

1. Group therapy is beneficial because it

    a. Increases social skills

    b. Is cost-effective

    c. Enables participants to acquire the curative factors

    d. All of the above

2. You are using Beck's cognitive–behavioral therapy and know that this will help the client

    a. Recognize and change his or her automatic thoughts

    b. See reality as you see it

    c. Change his or her reality by changing his or her environment

    d. Recognize and accept that automatic thoughts suggest delusional thinking

3. Homeostasis in a family refers to

    a. Choices a family makes to keep the peace

    b. Balance or stability that the family returns to despite its dysfunction

    c. Need for change and balance in a family

    d. Calm in a family that returns after a crisis

4. In an attempt to bring the client toward the goal he or she is working on, you ask the client, "If a miracle were to happen tonight while you slept, and you awoke in the morning and the problem no longer existed, how would you know, and what would be different?" This technique is used in which type of therapy?

   a. Behavioral therapy

   b. Solution-focused therapy

   c. Adlerian therapy

   d. Existential therapy

References and Resources

Brown, J., & Christensen, D. (1999). *Family therapy: Theory and practice* (2nd ed.). Pacific Grove, CA: Brooks/Cole.

Corey, G. (2005). *Theory and practice of counseling and psychotherapy* (7th ed.). Belmont, CA: Thompson, Brooks/Cole.

Corey, M., & Corey, G. (2006). *Groups: Process and practice* (7th ed.). Pacific Grove, CA: Thompson, Brooks/Cole.

Goldenberg, I., & Goldenberg, H. (2004). *Family therapy: An overview* (6th ed.). Stamford, CT: Wadsworth.

Hawks, J., & Moyad, M. (2003). CAM: Definition and classification overview. *Urologic Nursing, 23*(3), 221–223.

Kazdin, A. E., & Weisz, J. R. (2003). *Evidence-based psychotherapies for children and adolescents*. New York: Guilford Press.

Long, L., Huntley, A., & Ernst, E. (2001). Which complementary and alternative therapies benefit which conditions? A survey of the opinions of 223 professional organizations. *Complementary Therapy in Medicine, 9*(3), 178–185.

Nichols, N. P., & Schwartz, R. C. (2003). *Family therapy: Concepts and methods* (6th ed.). Boston: Allyn & Bacon.

Sadock, B., & Sadock, V. (2007). *Kaplan and Sadock's synopsis of psychiatry* (10th ed.). New York: Lippincott Williams & Wilkins.

Sholevar, G. P., Schwoeri, L. D. (Eds). (2003). *Textbook of family and couples therapy: Clinical applications*. Arlington, VA: American Psychiatric Publishing, Inc.

Yalom, I. (2005). *Theory and practice of group psychotherapy* (5th ed.). New York: Basic Books.

Notes:

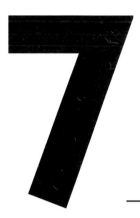

Mood Disorders

This chapter reviews the mood disorders encountered by psychiatric–mental health nurse practitioners (PMHNPs). These are the most common of all psychiatric illnesses and can manifest initially as physical health states. Often only after extensive, unnecessary assessment and diagnostic evaluation is the client's problem correctly identified as a mood disorder.

It has become increasingly common for mood disorders to be treated in primary care settings, and often clients first present in such settings because of the high degree of somatic symptomatology that accompanies these disorders. Many studies have indicated that mood disorders are not well identified or treated in primary care settings if a psychiatric care provider is not involved.

Depression is a very common, very normal human emotion. PMHNPs caring for clients who present for evaluation of depression must distinguish between normal levels of depression and pathological levels that are symptomatic of an underlying brain-based illness. Pathological levels of depression require treatment and generally will not fully abate without therapeutic intervention. Untreated depression predisposes individuals to other serious health problems, so pathological levels of depression should not go untreated.

Depression as a Common Emotional State

- Depression, one of the most common human emotions, exists on a continuum ranging from the absence of depression at one end to pathological levels that produce significant symptoms of psychiatric disorder at the other.
- Cultural differences affect behavioral manifestations of depression.
- Depression can be a normal, healthy reaction to life stressors that motivates an individual to deal with events and emotions.
- Depression can be pathological if
    - It is disproportionate to events and sustained over a significant time period.
    - It significantly impairs normal social functioning (e.g., occupational, social, school, relational functioning).
    - It significantly impairs normal somatic functioning (e.g., loss of appetite, altered sleep, altered self-care activities, altered sexual functioning).
    - It is apparently unrelated to any identifiable event or situation in an individual's life.

Major Depressive Disorder (MDD)

Description
- One of the most common psychiatric disorders; represents the primary unipolar affective disorder
- A complex brain-based illness with a primary characteristic of a persistent disturbance in mood
- Represents an excessive or distorted degree of sadness and manifests with behavioral, affective, cognitive, and somatic symptoms
- May have known precipitating event, situation, or concern but often occurs without any precipitating stressor identified
- Significantly interferes with daily functioning and goal attainment
- Has complex genetic, biochemical, and environmental etiological factors.

Etiology
- Multiple theories of the etiology of depression range from psychological to neurobiological.
- Theories are categorized as psychodynamic and biological.

Psychodynamic Theories

Object Loss Theory (Ronald Fairbairn, 1889–1964; D. W. Winnicott, 1896–1971; Harry Guntrip, 1901–1975)
- This theory assumes that early psychological developmental issues lay the foundation for depressive responses in later life; that the accomplishment of the first stage of development in which the child is able to form relationships is normal; and that during the second stage of development, the child experiences traumatic separation from significant objects of attachment (usually maternal object).
- Loss may be related to maternal death, illness, or emotional lack of availability and is unexpected and overwhelming.
- Depth of loss produces constellation of responses dominated by separation anxiety, grief, mourning, and despair.
- This critical object loss event predisposes the child to respond in similar ways to any future losses or significant separation.

Aggression-Turned-Inward Theory (Sigmund Freud, 1856–1939)
- This theory assumes that early psychological developmental issues lay the foundation for depressive responses in later life; that the accomplishment of the first stage of development in which the child is able to form relationships is normal; and that during the second stage of development, the child experiences loss of significant mothering individual.
- The loss can be real or imagined and is unexpected and overwhelming.
- The loss may be related to maternal death, illness, or emotional lack of availability or to the birth of a new sibling and the child's perception of losing undivided, individualized attention from the mother. The child's initial reaction is anger; however, the child feels unsafe to express this anger openly and directly. This may relate to the child's fearing further loss if he or she responds with anger or his or her subjective perception that anger is unacceptable.

- The child uses defense mechanisms to deal with conflict created by desire for the love object but co-occurring with anger for the love object.
- Instead of anger being expressed outward at the maternal figure, it turns inward because it is more acceptable and safer to be angry at oneself than at the mother.
- Anger at oneself is rationalized as the child assumes that loss of the mother was related to something bad that he or she did rather than to the caregiver's actions.
- Excessive guilt becomes a manifestation of the process of dealing with aggression experienced with the loss of the mother's attention.
- A similar emotional reaction (e.g., low self-esteem, excessive guilt, inability to cope with anger, self-destructive impulses) occurs as an adult whenever a loss is experienced.

Cognitive Theory (Aaron Beck, 1921–)
- This theory represents a cognitive diathesis–stress model in which developmental experiences sensitize an individual to respond to stressful life events in a depressed manner.
- This theory assumes that individuals with a tendency to be depressed think about the world differently than nondepressed individuals and that depressed individuals are more negative and believe that bad things are going to happen to them because of their own personal shortcomings and inadequacies.
- This thinking promotes low self-esteem and beliefs that the individual deserves to have bad things happen to him or her and promotes pessimistic perceptions about the world at large and about the individual's future. It also globalizes the negativity to all events, situations, and people in the person's life.
- When confronted by stressful events, these individuals tend to appraise them and the potential consequences in a negative, hopeless manner and therefore are more depressed than individuals with different cognitive styles.

Learned Helplessness-Hopelessness Theory (M. Seligman, 1942–)
- This theory is a modified aspect of cognitive theory, which assumes that an individual becomes depressed related to perceptions of lack of control over life events and experiences. These perceptions are learned over time, especially as the individual perceives others seeing him or her as inadequate.
- Perceptions of lack of control lead to the individual not adapting or coping.
- The individual's behavior becomes passive and nonreactive because of self-perceptions of personal characteristics of being helpless, hopeless, and powerless.

Biological Theories
Genetic Predisposition
- There is a clear genetic predisposition to depressive disorders; one assumption is a polygenic single nucleotide polymorphism (SNP) disorder.
- Having a depressed parent is the single strongest predictor of depression. Children of depressed parents are 3 times more likely to experience MDD in their lifetime than the general population and have a 40% chance of having a depressive episode before age 18 years.
- The earlier the age of onset of MDD and the more severe the symptoms, the more likely it is that a person has a strong genetic load for depression.

Endocrine Dysfunction

- MDD has symptoms that suggest endocrine abnormalities as part of the etiologic picture.
- Neurovegetative symptoms commonly seen in MDD (e.g., sleep disturbances, appetite disturbances, libido disturbances, lethargy, anhedonia) are related to functions of the hypothalamus and pituitary and the hormones they secrete.
- A high incidence of postpartum mood disturbances is suggestive of endocrine dysfunction.
- Deregulation of *hypothalamic–pituitary–adrenal axis* (HPA, which controls the physiological response to stress and is composed of interconnective feedback pathways between the hypothalamus, pituitary gland, and the adrenal glands) is another theory of endocrine basis of MDD. In this theory, MDD is presumed to be, at least in part, a result of an abnormal stress response related to HPA dysregulation.
  - The HPA functions in response to stress.
  - The hypothalamus releases corticotropin-releasing hormone (CRH), which then stimulates the pituitary to release adrenocorticotropin hormone (ACTH). This then stimulates the adrenals to release cortisol.
  - Hyperactivity of the HPA axis has been demonstrated to be present in individuals with MDD, and who have possible elevated cortisol levels.
  - Elevated cortisol levels over time damage the central nervous system (CNS) by altering neurotransmission and electrical signal conduction.
  - Evidence supports that cortisol over time can cause changes in size and function of brain tissue.
- HPA dysregulation is the rational and scientific basis for the dexamethasone suppression test (DST), a screening test for depression, which has proved to be too nonspecific and is not commonly used in clinical practice.

Abnormalities of Neurotransmitter Function

- All of the following are possible neurotransmitter function abnormalities causing depression:
  - Deregulation of one or more biogenic amine neurotransmitters: dopamine, serotonin, norepinephrine
  - Low levels of endogenous catecholamines in specific areas of the brain
    - Serotonin levels were shown to be low in postmortem studies on individuals who commit suicide and in individuals with MDD.
  - Low levels of precursor tryptophan
  - Low levels of serotonin metabolite 5HTIAA
  - Receptor sensitivity for neurotransmitters set unusually high in specific areas of the brain
    - A stronger neurotransmitter receptor cascade is required to induce neuronal activity.
  - Low density of receptor sites in specific areas of the brain
  - Hypometabolism in specific areas of the brain regulating mood, appetite, and cognition
  - Complexity of brain functions imply that the etiology of complex disorders like MDD involves the relative balance of available neurotransmitters and not just a low level of one neurotransmitter.

Structural Brain Changes

- Neuroimaging has demonstrated consistent abnormalities in certain structures of the brain in individuals with chronic and severe depression.
  - Hypovolemic hippocampus
  - Hypovolemic prefrontal cortex–limbic striatal regions.
- MDD is a common comorbidity in individuals who have experienced brain damage, including damage from stroke and trauma.

Chronobiological Theory

- Desynchronization of the circadian rhythms produces the symptom constellation collectively called MDD.
- Circadian rhythms control biological processes that are frequent problems in depressed individuals:
  - Interrupted sleep–rest cycle
  - REM abnormalities
  - Frequent waking
  - More intensified dreaming
  - Diurnal variations to circadian-related behaviors
  - Decreased arousal and energy levels
  - Decreased activity patterns
  - Increased cortisol secretion
  - Increased emotional reactivity.

Incidence and Demographics

- MDD is a common illness, with approximately 5% of the U.S. population ages 18 and older in a given year having the disorder. This represents 9.9 million American adults.
- MDD is the leading cause of disability in the U.S. and is the most common psychiatric illness seen in primary care practices; however, only 50% of people with MDD ever receive treatment.
- MDD can occur at any age; however, the average age of onset is mid-20s.
- During reproductive years, the lifetime risk for MDD varies with gender—25% for women, 12% for men; the risk is equal for the genders before puberty and after menopause.
- MDD is a greater source of morbidity for women than any other illness.
- MDD is associated with high mortality; 15% of people with MDD will commit suicide. People with MDD have 4 times greater risk of premature death than the normal control population.
- The disease course is variable and can involve isolated episodes separated by many years, clusters of episodes, or a severe episode with some remission of symptoms but with chronic symptoms persisting over time.
- If left untreated, an episode of symptoms of MDD usually lasts 4 months or longer.
- MDD tends to be a chronic, recurrent illness.
- One year after initial diagnosis of MDD, symptoms often persist.
  - 40% of clients have significant enough symptoms to meet full *DSM-IV* (American Psychiatric Association, 2000a) criteria for MDD.
  - 20% of clients do not meet full *DSM-IV* criteria but still have significant symptom level that impairs functioning.
  - 40% have no symptoms.

- The number of prior episodes predict likelihood of future episodes (Judd, Paulus, & Schettler, 2000).
  - There is approximately a 60% risk of a second episode in individuals with first episode MDD.
  - There is approximately a 70% risk of a third episode after the second.
  - There is approximately a 90% risk of a fourth episode after the third.

Risk Factors
- Genetic loading
  - Family history, especially first-degree relative
- Prior episode of MDD
- Female gender
- Postpartum period
- Medical comorbidity
- Single marital status
- Significant environmental stressors, especially multiple losses.

Prevention and Screening
- Provide at-risk family education
- Provide community education to help reduce stigma, to convey signs and symptoms of illness, and to emphasize the treatment potential for control of symptoms
- Provide significant screening efforts to help recognize, intervene, and initiate treatment early
- Provide health care provider education to facilitate early recognition and effective treatment
- Significant and protracted prodromal symptom period usually noted before full onset of illness.

Assessment
History–Assess for the Following:
- Detailed history of present illness, including time frame, progression, and any associated symptoms
- Social history, including present living situation; marital status; occupation; spirituality; education; and alcohol, tobacco, or illicit drug use
- Medication use, including prescription, over-the-counter, alternative, supplements, and home remedies
- Recent medical illness or surgery
- Initial and periodic functional history and assessment
- Validation of history with family member
  - *Initial Presentation*—Often manifests as vague somatic complaints.
    - Bodily aches, pains
    - Headaches
    - Muscle pains
    - Lack of energy
    - Gastrointestinal problems.
  - When mood is presenting complaint, client word choice is often vague or indirect.
    - Individual may describe mood as *depressed, discouraged, sad, "blue," "blah,"* or *"down in the dumps."*

- Irritable mood is a frequent subjective state validated by significant individual in client's life.
- Characteristic low energy is seen, so assess for individual activity intolerance without other apparent cause.
- Anhedonia is almost always present to some degree.
- Sleep disturbance is almost always present.
  - Typically problems occur with middle or terminal insomnia.
  - Hypersomnia can be present.
  - Diurnal variations can be present.
- A prodromal episode consisting of a high level of subjective anxiety and mild depressive symptoms often develops over days to weeks before onset of a full episode.
- Women often report symptoms occurring in fixed pattern around several days before onset of menses, so assess menstrual history.
- Psychotic features can be present, so always assess for their presence.
- Assess for client's symptoms according to *diagnostic criteria for MDD:*
  - Anhedonia or a depressed mood, or both
  - Depressed mood most of the day, nearly every day, as indicated by subjective reports or observations of others
    - In children, irritable mood.
  - Marked anhedonia in all or almost all activities of daily living
  - At least three or more significant symptoms present during the same 2-week period that represent a change in previous functioning
  - Significant, unintentional weight loss or gain of more than 5% of body weight, with increased appetite and usually a concurrent craving for specific foods, such as carbohydrates or sweets
  - Hypersomnia or insomnia nearly every day
  - Psychomotor agitation or retardation
  - Fatigue or loss of energy
  - Self-deprecating comments or thoughts
  - Feelings of worthlessness or excessive or inappropriate guilt nearly every day
  - Decreased concentration and memory
  - Recurrent morbid thoughts or suicidal ideation
  - Symptoms that begin within 2 months of significant loss such as death of a loved one and do not persist beyond 2 months are generally considered bereavement and not MDD.

Physical Exam Findings
- There are no specific physical findings.
- Individuals with certain other disorders (e.g., diabetes, myocardial infarction, carcinomas, stroke) have a statistically significant increased risk for MDD.
  - Prognosis for treatment of other disorders is poor if MDD is not recognized and effectively treated.
- Clients with MDD often have trouble participating with assessments related to the cognitive problems of the disorder.
  - Impaired ability to report chronological timeline of illness
  - Poor decision making

- Slowed thought processes
- Requires focus assessment.
- Clients with MDD often have psychomotor findings.
  - Agitation
  - Retardation.

Mental Status Exam Findings

Appearance
- Unkempt
- Tired looking
- Clothing showing little attention or care about how the individual looks
- Dark-colored, loose-fitting clothing
- Significant weight change from baseline.

Speech
- Underproductive
- Blocking
- Slowed response times
- Monotonal intonation.

Affect
- Constricted or blunted
- Sad
- Anxious
- Irritable.

Mood
- Sad
- Depressed
- Hopeless
- Helpless
- Guilty and worried
- Anxious
- Irritable.

Thought Process
- Usually organized but may be disorganized if psychosis present
- Slowing
- Distractible
- Rumination.

Thought Content
- Morbid preoccupation
- Suicidal ideation exists on continuum of severity
- Thoughts that others would be better off if individual was "gone"
- Transient recurrent thoughts of suicide
- Nonspecific thoughts of active action to commit suicide

- Specific plan for committing suicide
- Specific plan with timeline for completion
- Specific plan with acquisition of the means to carry out plan
  - Suicidal motivation differs for different clients.
- Despair
- Desire to give up struggle
- Attempt to end significant emotional pain
- Lack of any visible options for dealing with stressors
- Anger and frustration with poor impulse control
  - Research evidence supports that it is not possible to predict accurately whether or when an individual will attempt suicide (see Table 7–1 for review of suicide assessment).
  - Suicide risk especially high for individuals with certain symptoms or history:
    - Presence of psychotic symptoms
    - History of past attempts
    - History of first-degree relative who committed suicide
    - Concurrent substance abuse or dependency
    - Current serious health problem (see below for clinical management of suicidality).

Table 7–1. Assessing for Suicidal Behavior

- Past history for suicide attempts or completed suicide in client or family
- Negativity and morbidity
- Suicidal ideation currently
- Plan and intent for suicide action
- Means and access to commit suicide
- Perceived social supports
- Lethality of intended suicide action
  - **High Lethality:** Jumping significant height, gun, hanging
  - **Moderate Lethality:** Overdose of toxic agents (e.g., aspirin, sleeping pills)
  - **Low Lethality:** Superficial wrist cutting, breath holding
- Ability to contract for safety
- Impulsivity
- Substance abuse/dependence
- History of psychiatric disorder

Cognition
- Usually impaired.

Orientation
- Individual is usually oriented to person, place, and time unless psychosis present.

Memory
- Usually impaired recent and short-term memory.

Concentration
- Usually significantly impaired.

Abstraction
- Abstract ability on proverb testing usually intact
- If concrete, assess for other psychotic findings.

Judgment
- Impaired for self-welfare.

Diagnostic and Laboratory Findings

- Do CBC, chemistry profile, thyroid function tests, or B_{12} level to rule out metabolic causes or unidentified conditions.
- Do drug toxicity screening, if indicated by history.
- The more severe the depression, the more likely laboratory abnormalities are present.
- No specific lab findings specific to MDD exist; however, research has found that individuals with depression seem to have the following abnormal lab findings:
  - Elevated glucocorticoid levels
  - Increased urinary free cortisol levels
  - Decreased hormonal levels
  - Decreased thyroid-stimulating hormone levels
  - Decreased growth hormone levels.

- Before establishing MDD diagnosis, obtain baseline lab studies to rule out other differential diagnosis:
  - Thyroid panel
  - CBC with differential
  - Electrolyte panel
  - Drug screen.

- Polysomnographic testing abnormalities include
  - Sleep continuity disturbances (e.g., prolonged latency)
  - Reduced non-rapid eye movement (NREM) Stages 3–4 (i.e., slow-wave sleep)
  - Decreased rapid eye movement (REM) latency
  - Increased phasic REM activity
  - Increased duration of early REM.

Differential Diagnosis
Endocrine Disorders
- Hypothyroidism
- Diabetes
- Hyperaldosteronism
- Cushing's/Addison's disease.

Neurological Disorders

- Stroke
- Epilepsy
- Dementia
- Huntington's disease
- Sleep apnea
- Wilson's disease
- Neoplasms
- Head trauma
- Multiple sclerosis
- Parkinson's disease.

Cardiac Disorders

- Myocardial infarction
- Congestive heart failure
- Hypertension.

Infectious and Inflammatory States

- Mononucleosis
- AIDS
- Pneumonia: Viral and bacterial
- Systemic lupus erythematosus
- Temporal arteritis
- Tuberculosis.

Nutritional Disorders

- Pernicious anemia
- Pellagra.

Other Disorders

- Fibromyalgia
- Chronic fatigue syndrome
- Bereavement or grief reaction
- Electrolyte imbalance
- Uremia and other renal conditions.

Psychiatric Disorders

- Anxiety disorders
- Eating disorders
- Bipolar affective disorder
- Substance dependence–related disorders.

Medications With Altered Mood States as Side Effects

- Steroids
- Estrogen compounds
- Antihypertensive agents
- Anti-Parkinson's agents
- Anti-neoplastic agents
- Sulphanamides
- Tetracycline
- Analgesics
- Opiates
- Antibacterial/antifungal agents
- Ampicillin
- Cycloserine
- Metronidazole
- Streptomycin
- Nonsteroidal anti-inflammatory drugs (NSAIDs)
- Indomethacin
- Ibuprofen
- Beta blockers.

Clinical Management

- The top goal in the acute phase of MDD is ensuring client safety.
- A general consideration is to rule out or treat any conditions that may contribute to depression and cognitive impairment.
- Assess for the acuity level of client presentation.
  - Reasons for brief hospitalization during acute episodes of MDD
    - To ensure client safety
    - To initiate medication change
    - To restabilize on medication
    - To monitor suicidality
    - To ensure client compliance with treatment to reach stabilization.
  - Clinical management during nonacute episodes occurs most often in community settings.
    - Obtain baseline labs before initiation of treatment.
      - Pharmacological clinical management
      - Nonpharmacological clinical management (counseling).

Pharmacological Management

- Inform client that therapeutic effect may take at least 4–6 weeks.
- Once started, continue antidepressants for a minimum of 8–12 months.
  - If client has more than one prior episode of MDD, consider longer term use.
- Not all symptoms of MDD will respond to pharmacological interventions.
- Identify clear, measurable target symptoms and educate the client about these symptoms (see Table 7–2).
- Research has found that the most effective intervention is a combination of medication and counseling.

Table 7–2. Target Symptoms of Antidepressant Treatment

- Depressed mood
- Sleep–rest disturbances
- Anxiety
- Irritability
- Impaired concentration
- Impaired memory
- Appetite disturbance
- Agitation
- Anhedonia

Classes of Antidepressants

Selective Serotonin Reuptake Inhibitors (SSRIs)

- Action primarily to increase serotonin levels in CNS by inhibiting their reuptake
- See Table 7–3 for examples.

Tricyclic Antidepressants (TCAs)
- Elevate serotonin and norepinephrine levels primarily by inhibiting their reuptake
- See Table 7–4 for examples.

Monoamine Oxidase Inhibitors (MAOIs)
- Elevate serotonin and norepinephrine levels primarily by inhibiting MAO, the enzyme that destroys neurotransmitters
- See Table 7–5 for examples.

Serotonin Norepinephrine Reuptake Inhibitors (SNRIs)
- Inhibit dual reuptake
- Action very selective on neurotransmitters
- Elevate serotonin and norepinephrine levels by inhibiting their reuptake
- See Table 7–6 for examples.

Norepinephrine Dopamine Reuptake Inhibitors (NDRIs)
- Inhibit dual reuptake
- Action very selective on neurotransmitters
- Elevate dopamine and norepinephrine levels by inhibiting their reuptake
- See Table 7–6 for examples.

Serotonin Agonist and Reuptake Inhibitors (SARIs)
- Dual action
- Agonist of serotonin 5HT-2 receptors
- Action very selective on neurotransmitters
- Elevate serotonin levels by inhibiting serotonin reuptake
- See Table 7–6 for examples.

  - The various antidepressants differ markedly in characteristics such as
    - Cost
    - Side-effect profile
    - Safety in overdose
    - Safety in clients with other disorders
    - Drug–drug interactions
    - Cytochrome P450 liver effects.

  - To achieve best control of symptoms, match client's symptom profile to the pharmacodynamic and pharmacokinetic properties of specific antidepressant agents.

SSRIs

- Serious side effects typically few
- The most common side effects of SSRIs are
  - GI upset
  - Sexual dysfunction
  - Nervousness

- Headache
- Dry mouth.

- Much safer in overdose than TCAs
- Also effective for panic disorder, obsessive–compulsive disorder, bulimia, generalized anxiety disorder, social phobia, posttraumatic stress disorder, and premenstrual dysphoric disorder.

Table 7–3. Selective Serotonin Reuptake Inhibitors

Drug	Brand Name	Dosage Forms/ Daily Dosage	Side Effects	Comments
Citalopram (SSRI)	Celexa	Tablet/20–60 mg/d	Sedation Sexual dysfunction Agitation Yawning GI disturbances Weight gain	
Escitalo-pram (SSRI)	Lexapro	Tablet/10–20 mg/d	Somnolence Headache Sexual dysfunction GI disturbances	
Fluoxetine (SSRI)	Prozac	Capsule/Tablet/ Liquid	Insomnia Headache GI disturbances Sexual dysfunction	• Long half-life
Fluvoxa-mine (SSRI)	Luvox	Tablet, 100–300 mg/d	Sedation Sexual dysfunction Agitation GI disturbances	• Black box warning for liver toxicity
Paroxetine (SSRI)	Paxil/CR Pexeva	Tablet/Liquid, 20–60 mg/d	Headache GI disturbances Sexual dysfunction	• Teratogenic effect possible • Significant discontinuation syndrome
Sertraline (SSRI)	Zoloft	Tablet, 50–200 mg/d	Sexual dysfunction GI disturbances Somnolence Headache	• Teratogenic effect possible • Significant discontinuation syndrome

TCAs

- Considered second-line drugs for treating MDD (see Table 7–4)
- Dirty side-effect profile promotes poor patient compliance
  - *Anticholinergic:* Dry mouth, blurred vision, constipation, memory problems (from muscarinic receptor blockade)
  - *Antiadrenergic:* Orthostatic hypotension (from alpha 1 receptor blockade)
  - *Antihistaminergic:* Sedation and weight gain (from histamine receptor blockade)
  - EKG changes and cardiac dysrythmias
  - Unsafe in many co-occurring disorders (e.g., cardiac disease)
  - Known to induce hypomania in certain patients.
- Can have well-identified serum blood levels that assist in dosing strategies to reach symptom control
- Are inexpensive and available in generic forms
- Slow down the gut, so are good for individuals with significant GI problems
- Avoid abrupt withdrawal due to significant abstinence syndrome
- Avoid prescribing to suicidal individuals; **lethal dose is 1,000 mg or more (a week's supply of an average dose)**
- ✓ **Remember not to prescribe TCAs with MAOIs. This can cause a lethal reaction.**
- Use caution if individual is taking both a TCA and an SSRI, as the SSRI can possibly elevate TCA concentrations in the bloodstream. Monitor TCA levels.

Table 7–4. Tricyclic Antidepressants

Drug	Brand Name/ Manufacturer	Dosage Forms/ Daily Dosage	Comments
Amitriptyline	Elavil	Tablet/IM 50–300 mg/d	• Also used for chronic pain, insomnia, sciatica, fibromyalgia, trigeminal neuralgia, and diabetic neuropathy
Clomipramine	Anafranil	Capsule/100–250 mg/d	• Approved for obsessive–compulsive disorder; 250 mg/d maximum due to increased seizure risk
Desipramine	Norpramin	Tablet, Capsule/ 100–300 mg/d	• Also used for attention-deficit/ hyperactivity disorder
Doxepin	Sinequan	Capsule, Liquid/ 100–300 mg/d	• Also used for insomnia
Imipramine	Tofranil	Tablet, Capsule/ IM 100–300 mg/d	• Also used for enuresis and separation anxiety
Nortriptyline	Pamelor	Capsule, Liquid/ 50–150 mg/d	• Also used for enuresis and attention-deficit/hyperactivity disorder
Protriptyline	Vivactil	Tablet, 15–60 mg/d	
Trimipramine	Surmontil	Capsule, 100–300 mg/d	

MAOIs

- Normally are never first- or second-line agents for MDD because of dangerous food and drug interactions (see Tables 7–5 and 7–7).
  - *Hypertensive crisis* occurs when MAOIs are taken in conjunction with foods containing *tyramine,* a dietary precursor to norepinephrine.
  - Tyramine exerts strong vasopressor effect (i.e., stimulates the release of catecholamines, epinephrine, and norepinephrine, which can increase blood pressure and heart rate) when MAO is inhibited.
  - Hypertensive crisis is life threatening and irreversible until more MAO is produced by the body.
    - Hypertensive crisis and possible death also may occur when MAOIs are taken in conjunction with certain medications:
      - Meperidine
      - SSRIs
      - Decongestants
      - TCAs
      - Atypical antipsychotics
      - St. John's wort
      - L-Trytophan
      - Ritalin
      - Asthma medications.

  - *Symptoms of Hypertensive Crisis*
    - Sudden, explosive-like headache, usually in occipital region
    - Elevated blood pressure
    - Facial flushing
    - Palpitations
    - Pupillary dilation
    - Diaphoresis
    - Fever.

  - *Treatment of Hypertensive Crisis*
    - Hold the MAOI.
    - Give phentolamine (binds with norepinephrine receptor sites, blocks norepinephrine).
    - Stabilize fever.
    - Reevaluate the individual's diet and adherence, and reiterate medication guidelines as necessary.

  - Individuals on MAOIs must be on a *tyramine-free diet* and must avoid many medications, including most over-the-counter cold and allergy preparations.
  - There is little safety in overdose.
  - Dirty side-effect profile and stringent dietary restrictions promote poor client compliance.

  - *Clinically Significant Side Effects of MAOIs Include*
    - Insomnia
    - Hypertension crisis
    - Weight gain
    - Anticholinergic side effects
    - Light-headedness and dizziness
    - Sexual dysfunction.

- MAOIs are unsafe in many co-occurring disorders
- MAOIs are inexpensive, and most come in generic form.

Table 7–5. Monoamine Oxidase Inhibitors

Drug	Brand Name/ Manufacturer	Dosage Forms/ Daily Dosage	Comments
Isocarboxazid Phenelzine Tranylcypromine	Marplan Nardil Parnate	Tablet/100–60 mg/d Tablet/45–90 mg/d Tablet/20–50 mg/d	• Also used for panic disorder, phobic disorders, selective mutism • *Caution:* High tyramine diet; sympathomimetic agents. • Divided dosing: bid and qid
Selegiline	EMSAM	Transdermal patch/ 6–12 mg/d	No dietary restrictions with 6 mg dosage

Other Antidepressants

- Other antidepressants used in the treatment of MDD are SNRIs (Effexor and Cymbalta) and NDRIs (Wellbutrin) (see Table 7–6).

Table 7–6. Other Antidepressant Agents

Drug	Brand Name/ Manufacturer	Dosage Forms/ Daily Dosage	Side Effects	Comments
Bupropion (NDRI)	Wellbutrin	Tablet/150–450 mg/d	Headache Nervousness Tremors Tachycardia Insomnia Decreased appetite	• Contraindicated if patient has seizures, eating disorder SR offers bid dosing; XL offers once daily dosing • Can increase energy level • Also used for attention-deficit/ hyperactivity disorder and smoking cessation
Bupropion SR/XL	Wellbutrin SR	Sustained release/ 150–400 mg/d Extended release/ 150–450 mg/d		• Caution with caffeine and in individuals with panic disorder

Continued on the next page

Table 7–6. Continued

Drug	Brand Name/ Manufacturer	Dosage Forms/ Daily Dosage	Side Effects	Comments
Mirtazapine	Remeron	Tablet/15–45 mg/d	Sedation Weight gain Increased cholesterol	• Inverse relationship between dosage and sedation
Nefazodone (SARI)	Serzone	Tablet/ 300–600 mg/d	Headache Drowsiness GI disturbances	• **Must** monitor LFTs • Can cause liver failure • Safer in overdose than TCAs • qhs or bid dosing • Potent P450 3A4 inhibitor
Trazodone (SARI)	Desyrel	Tablet/ 200–600 mg/d	Sedation Nausea Headache	• Safer in overdose than TCAs • Priapism possible • Not well tolerated at antidepressant dosage due to sedation • Most commonly used as hypnotic at 50–200 mg/hs • May potentially prolong QTc interval
Venlafaxine (SNRI)	Effexor, Effexor XR	Capsule (XR), Tablet/75–375 mg/d XR 75–225 mg/d GI disturbances	Diaphoresis Headache Dizziness	• Can raise BP • Potent inhibitor of CYP450 system • qd for XR capsules • bid–tid dosing for tablets • Safer in overdose than TCAs • Has *significant* discontinuation syndrome if stopped abruptly
Duloxetine (SNRI)	Cymbalta	Capsule/ 30–120 mg/d	Dizziness Headache GI disturbances	• Once-daily dosing • Can possibly elevate BP • Can possibly elevate liver function tests • Has *significant* discontinuation syndrome if stopped abruptly

Table 7–7. Tyramine-Free Dietary Considerations

Category of Food	Specific Foods to Avoid
Cheese	Aged cheeses such as blue, Brie, Camembert, and Roquefort
Meat	Smoked, aged, and cured meats such as sausages, pastrami, and salami
Fish	Smoked, aged, and cured fish such as pickled herring and salted fish
Beverages	Any aged and fermented beverages such as wine, chianti, aged liquors, whiskey, beer, and alcohol-free beers; caffeine
Other	Bean curd, soy bean paste, sauerkraut, soy sauce, miso soup, yeast extract, chocolate, MSG, nuts, and bananas

- Psychotic features can be present with MDD.
  - Should routinely assess for the presence of psychotic symptoms during periods of symptom exacerbation
  - Are usually mood congruent
  - Can be managed with short-term use of antipsychotic medications (see Chapter 9).

- Common comorbidities with MDD are medical comorbidities (as noted earlier in chapter) as well as psychiatric comorbidities such as panic disorder, obsessive–compulsive disorder, and substance abuse/dependence.
- Altered appetite and sleep–rest patterns predispose clients with MDD to decreased overall health status.
- Increased mortality exists in individuals with MDD.

Nonpharmacological Clinical Management

Electroconvulsive Therapy (ECT)
- Grand mal seizure induced in anesthetized individual
- Usual course 6–12 treatments
  - *Mechanism of action*
    - *Neurotransmitter theory*—Increases dopamine, serotonin, and norepinephrine
    - *Neuroendocrine theory*—Releases hormones such as prolactin, thyroid-stimulating hormone, pituitary hormones, endorphins, and adrenocorticotropic hormone
    - *Anticonvulsant theory*—Exerts an anticonvulsant effect, which then produces an antidepressant effect.

  - *Situations in which ECT is used*
    - Client preference
    - Need for rapid response due to severity of illness
    - Risk of other treatment outweighs risk of ECT
    - Treatment resistance.
  - *Contraindications*
    - Cardiac disease
    - Compromised pulmonary status
    - History of brain injury or brain tumor
    - Anesthesia medical complications.

- *Adverse effects*
  - Possible cardiovascular effects
  - Systemic effects (e.g., headaches, anorexia, muscle aches, drowsiness)
  - Cognitive effects (e.g., memory disturbance and confusion)

Transcranial Magnetic Stimulation (TMS)
Vagal Nerve Stimulation (VNS)
Phototherapy

Individual Therapy

- Cognitive–Behavioral Therapy (CBT)
  - Modify perceptions
  - Decrease negativity
  - Increase sense of internal control
  - Enhance coping skills
  - Modify environmental factors contributing to illness.

- Brief Therapy (Solution-Focused Therapy)
  - Focus on precipitant stressor
  - Cope with immediate impact of MDD on personal life
  - Modify contributory environmental factors.

- Group Therapy
  - Improve decision making
  - Improve socialization skills
  - Improve assessment of individual strengths
  - Gain new coping skills.

- Family Therapy
  - Enhance family coping
  - Improve knowledge base
  - Plan for relapse
  - Gain insight into effects of MDD on family unit
  - Undertake psychoeducation for family members about the illness state of MDD.

- Clinical Management of Suicidality
  - Pay significant attention to positive assessments for suicidality
  - Always assume client is serious when he or she vocalizes suicidal thoughts
  - Identify current stressors that may be contributing to crisis
  - Generally do not manage in community setting during acute suicidal ideation periods unless client is able to make "no-harm" agreement
  - Consider hospitalization
  - Consider mobilizing available social resources.
  - *Risk factors for suicide*
    - Ages 45 or older if male
    - Ages 55 or older if female
    - Divorced/single/separated
    - White
    - Living alone
    - Psychiatric disorder
    - Physical illness
    - Substance abuse
    - Previous suicide attempt
    - Family history of suicide
    - Recent loss
    - Male gender.

Life Span Considerations: Children

- Core symptoms of MDD are the same for children. However, some symptoms are more pronounced in children:
    - Irritability
    - Somatic complaints
    - Social withdrawal.
- Some core symptoms are less common in children before onset of puberty:
    - Psychosis
    - Motor retardation
    - Hypersomnia
    - Increased appetite.
- MDD often has a strong separation anxiety component in children.
- Children usually do not respond well to tricyclics; however, they do respond well to SSRIs.
- Monitor closely for suicidal behavior, agitation, and aggression in children taking antidepressants.

Life Span Considerations: Older Adults

- Individuals with MDD admitted to a long-term-care facility have significantly shorter life spans than normal control population.
    - 65% are more likely to die within the first year in a long-term care facility.
- Cognition and memory symptoms of MDD in the elderly population often are confused with dementia-related symptoms (pseudodementia).
- In dementia, there is usually a premorbid history of slowly declining cognition.
- In MDD, cognitive changes have a relatively acute onset and are significant when compared to premorbid functioning.
- It is important to complete a *functional assessment* for elderly individuals.
    - Determines the degree to which the individual's abilities and performance match the demands of his or her life
    - Determines the impact of illness on the overall functioning
        - *Skill deficit*—Inability to perform a functional skill despite the physical ability, as in dementia
        - *Performance deficit*—Ability to perform a functional skill but lacks the motivation to do so, as in depression
    - *Reasons for Performing Functional Assessment*
        - To correctly diagnose (i.e., to differentiate depression from dementia)
        - To track client improvement or decompensation
        - To help families set realistic expectations.
    - *Components of Functional Assessment*
        - *Activities of daily living (ADLs)*—Basic self-care skills, such as bathing, dressing, eating, and toileting
        - *Instrumental activities of daily living (IADLs)*—Complex activities needed for independent functioning, such as shopping, cooking, driving, and housekeeping
        - *Executive functioning*—Judgment and planning; ability to maintain calendar, manage money and appointments, and prioritize activities.

- The degree of change over time and the speed of change are better observed with objective recording and when the assessment is measured at intervals such as every 6 months.

Follow-up

- *Follow-up Care Practices for the PMHNP to Consider*
  - Include in client teaching the risks, benefits, and potential side effects of medication treatment.
  - Continuously monitor client's response to medication; the treatment goal is complete remission of symptoms.
  - Teach clients the symptoms of depression and that it is a chronic illness; establish a relapse plan for all clients.
  - Assess for suicidality during every client contact.
  - Assess for the presence of psychotic symptoms during every client contact.
  - Assess and manage client for side effects of treatment, including sexual side effects, in an attempt to increase medication compliance.
  - Observe all clients treated with antidepressants for development of *serotonin syndrome* (overstimulation of serotonin receptors usually caused from drug–drug interactions).

- *Drug Combinations That May Cause Serotonin Syndrome*
  - SSRIs and MAOIs
  - Drug and herbal interactions
  - SSRIs and St. John's wort.

- *Symptoms of Serotonin Syndrome*
  - Autonomic instability
  - Restlessness
  - Agitation
  - Myoclonis
  - Hyperreflexia
  - Hyperthermia
  - Diaphoresis
  - Altered sensorium
  - Tremor
  - Chills
  - Diarrhea and cramps
  - Ataxia
  - Headache
  - Insomnia.

  - ✓ Remember to monitor for adverse effects over time.
    - Some SSRIs are known to increase blood glucose and contribute to hyperlipidemia, and others may elevate liver function tests.
  - ✓ Discontinue SSRIs slowly to prevent *discontinuation syndrome*.

- *Symptoms of Discontinuation Syndrome*
  - Flu-like symptoms
  - Fatigue and lethargy
  - Myalgia
  - Decreased concentration
  - Nausea/vomiting
  - Impaired memory

- Shock-like sensations
- Irritability
- Anxiety
- Insomnia
- Crying without provocation
- Dizziness and vertigo.

- *Risk Factors for Discontinuation Syndrome*
  - Medications with short half-life
  - Abrupt discontinuation
  - Noncompliant, irregular use pattern
  - High dose range
  - Long-term treatment
  - Prior history of discontinuation syndrome
    - Discontinue TCAs slowly.
      - Clients can get *cholinergic rebound syndrome:*
        - Nausea
        - GI upset
        - Diaphoresis
        - Myalgias, especially of neck muscles.

- *Expected Course of MDD*
  - Evidence indicates the best treatment outcomes if medications are used in conjunction with appropriate therapy.
  - Evidence indicates that clients should take an antidepressant agent for at least 12 months after remission of symptoms.
  - Clients who have had two or more episodes of MDD usually require lifelong medication.

Dysthymic Disorder

Description
- A disorder similar to MDD but with less acute symptoms; with a more protracted, chronic disease course; and without any manifestations of psychotic symptoms
- Less discrete episodes of illness than MDD
- Symptoms often go undetected and therefore untreated for years
- Vegetative symptoms (e.g., sleep, appetite, weight changes) much less common in dysthymic disorder than in MDD.

Etiology
- Similar to MDD.

Incidence and Demographics
- 6% of people in the U.S. will develop dysthmic disorder in their lifetime
- Affects 5.4% of the U.S. population ages 18 or older, or 10.9 million Americans.
- Individuals with dysthymia have an increased risk for developing MDD; 15%–25% of individuals diagnosed with dysthymic disorder will have a lifetime episode of MDD.

- In individuals with the onset of symptoms before age 21, there is a 75% likelihood that they will have a lifetime episode of MDD.
- Women are 2–3 times more likely to develop dysthymic disorder than men.
- Symptoms can be described as one of two types:
  - *Early Onset*
    - Dysthymic symptoms occur before age 21
    - Usually type with most symptoms
    - Most at risk for onset of MDD.
  - *Late Onset*
    - Dysthymic symptoms occur at or after age 21.

Risk Factors
- Genetic loading
- A first-degree relative with MDD
- A first-degree relative with dysthymic disorder
- Female gender.

Prevention and Screening
- At-risk family education
- Community education
- Stigma reduction
- Signs and symptoms of illness
- Treatment potential for control of symptoms
- Early recognition, intervention, and initiation of treatment
- Because of chronic nature of disorder, symptoms become part of client's day-to-day existence and often go unreported unless solicited by direct questioning
- Aggressive screening procedure required.

Assessment
History—Assess for the Following:
- Chronically depressed mood that occurs for most of the day, more days than not, for at least 2 years
- Prominent presence of low self-esteem, self-criticism, and a perception of general incompetence compared to others.

Other Common Symptoms
- Low energy and fatigue
- Poor concentration
- Difficulty with decision making
- Feelings of hopelessness
- Feelings of inadequacy
- Mild anhedonia
- Social withdrawal
- Brooding about past issues
- Subjective irritability or anger
- Decreased productivity and activity.

Less Common Symptoms
- Alteration in appetite
- Alteration in sleep–rest patterns.

Physical Exam Findings
- Similar to MDD.

Mental Status Exam Findings
- Similar to MDD
- Usually no vegetative findings
- Mood described as *sad, "down for all of my life."*

Diagnostic and Laboratory Findings
- Nonspecific.
- Polysomnographic findings are similar to those found in MDD.

Differential Diagnosis
- Similar to MDD.

Clinical Management
Pharmacological Management
- Because of increased risk for development of MDD, dysthymia is usually treated with antidepressant medications in a manner similar to MDD.

Nonpharmacological Management
- Similar to MDD
- Often good clinical outcomes with just nonpharmacological treatment if client is willing.

Common Comorbidities
- Dysthymic disorder is often superimposed on MDD.
- The subjective worsening of symptoms or onset of new symptoms such as vegetative ones often brings individual into treatment.
- When dysthymia precedes MDD, clinical management is more complex and outcomes can be less positive.
- Dysthymic disorder is associated with personality disorders:
  - Borderline
  - Histrionic
  - Narcissistic
  - Avoidant
  - Dependent.

Life Span Considerations
- Similar to MDD
- In children, prevalence rates of dysthymia equal for boys and girls
- Associated with several childhood disorders:
  - Attention-deficit/hyperactivity disorder

- Conduct disorder
- Anxiety disorders
- Learning disorders
- Mental retardation.

- Period of symptoms required for diagnosis only 1 year for children, compared with 2 years for adults
- In children, the mood is usually described as *irritable* rather than *sad*, but may report both irritability and sadness
- Low self-esteem, poor social skills, and pessimism.

Follow-up
- Similar to MDD.

Bipolar (BP) Disorder

Description
- Complex brain-based illness with a primary characteristic of disturbance in mood
- Mood disturbance often of both polarities:
  - Depressive
  - Expansive or manic.

- One of three patterns of symptoms present:
  - Single-polarity symptom only
  - Manic symptoms only
  - Cyclic symptom patterns of alternating polarity—Manic symptoms alternating with depressive symptoms, mixed-polarity symptoms at the same time

- Represents an excessive or distorted degree of sadness or elation, or both
- Manifests with behavioral, affective, cognitive, and somatic symptoms
- May have precipitating event, situation, or concern, but often occurs without any precipitating stressor identified
- Has complex genetic, biochemical, and environmental etiological factors.

Etiology
- Multiple theories ranging from psychological to neurobiological
- Probable multifactorial etiological profile
  - *Biological Theories*
    - Neurotransmitter deregulation.
    - Gamma-aminobutyric (GABA) deregulation.
    - Increased noradrenergic activity.
    - Voltage-gated ion channel abnormalities.
    - Abnormalities lead to abnormal balances of intracellular and extracellular levels of neurotransmitters, which then cause subsequent disruption of electric signal transmission in brain regions.
    - *Kindling*—Process of neuronal membrane threshold sensitivity dysfunction
    - Long-lasting, epileptogenic changes induced by daily subthreshold brain stimulation.

- Brain becomes overly sensitive to electrical stimuli.
- Neuronal misfiring occurs.
- Process becomes automatic; neuronal firing occurs even without stimuli.

Incidence and Demographics

- Less common than MDD
- 0.7% of general population at risk
- Affects 2.3 million American adults; 1.2% of the U.S. adult population older than age 18
- Mean age of onset early 20s
- Common in adolescent years.

Risk Factors

- Genetic loading
- Family history of first-order relative having MDD or BP disorder
- 24% increased risk if relative has BP disorder Type I (see below)
- 5% increased risk if relative has BP disorder Type II (see below)
- 25% increased risk if relative has MDD
- For BP disorder Type II, similar to MDD.

Prevention and Screening

- At-risk family education
- Community education
  - Stigma reduction
  - Signs and symptoms of illness
  - Treatment potential for control of symptoms.
- Early recognition, intervention, and initiation of treatment
  - Significant and protracted prodromal symptom period usually noted before full onset of illness
  - Usually mild manifestations of criteria symptoms before full clinical syndrome apparent
  - The longer time period between onset of symptoms and diagnosis, the more difficult to interrupt cyclicity of illness.

Assessment

History—Assess for the Following:

- Detailed history of present illness, including time frame, progression, and any associated symptoms
- Social history, including present living situation; marital status; occupation; education; and alcohol, tobacco, or illicit drug use
- Medication use, including prescription, over-the-counter, alternative, supplements, and home remedies
- Initial and periodic functional history and assessment
- Validate history with family member.

Diagnostic Criteria

- Period of abnormally or persistently elevated, expansive, or irritable mood, lasting for at least 1 week

- Mood episode has rapid development and escalation of symptoms over a few days
- Often precipitated by significant environmental stressor
- Mood disturbance may result in brief psychotic symptoms
- Manic episodes last days to several months
- Briefer duration and ending more abruptly than major depressive episodes
- In 60% of individuals, a major depressive episode immediately precedes or follows the manic episode
- Persistence of other suggestive symptoms:
  - Decreased need for sleep
  - Feels rested after 3 hours sleep on average
  - Usually a marked difference from normal baseline sleep pattern
  - Inflated self-esteem
  - Grandiosity
  - Increased goal-directed activities
  - Excessive involvement in pleasurable activities with a high potential for painful consequences
  - Unrestrained buying sprees
  - Sexual indiscretions
  - Unsound business ventures
  - Excessive substance use or abuse.

- Recurrent shifts in polarity
  - Major depressive episode shifting to a manic episode
  - Manic episode shifting to a major depressive episode.

- Expansive or elated mood symptoms
  - Manic
    - Symptoms as described above.
  - Hypomanic
    - Similar to mania
    - Briefer in duration
    - Episode not as severe as mania
    - Does not require hospitalization
    - Does not cause significant functional impairment.

Two Common Types

Type I
- Clinical history characterized by occurrence of one or more manic or mixed episodes.

Type II
- Clinical history characterized by occurrence of one or more major depressive episodes accompanied by at least one manic or hypomanic episode.

  ✓ Remember that, in a small subset of individuals with BP disorder, the recurrent shifts in polarity can occur more frequently—*rapid cycling*.

    - Occurrence of four or more mood episodes during previous 12 months
    - Mood episodes either major depressive or manic
    - Other than occurring more frequently, mood episodes same as non–rapid cycling episodes

- 20% of individuals with BP disorder have rapid cycling
- Most rapid cyclers are women (90%).

✓ Identifying rapid cycling is important.
✓ Antidepressants may accelerate rapid cycling.
✓ Individuals with rapid cycling have poorer prognosis.

Physical Exam Findings
- Nonspecific
- Clinical findings consistent with thyroid dysfunction.

Mental Status Exam Findings
Appearance
- Psychomotor restlessness or agitation
- Frequent change of dress
- Prone to light-colored, often sexualized dress
- Dramatic or flamboyant dress usually out of character for person when compared to nonsymptomatic periods.

Speech
- Rapid
- Loud
- Pressured
- Difficult to interrupt
- Joking, irreverent, amusing
- Word clanging in severely ill clients.

Affect
- Labile
- Irritable
- Overly theatrical and dramatic.

Mood
- Euphoric
- Cheerful
- High
- Expansive
- Irritable.

Thought Process
- Thoughts racing
- Flight of ideas
- Thoughts disorganized and incoherent in severely ill clients.

Thought Content
- Inflated self-esteem
- Indiscriminate enthusiasm

- Inflated sense of abilities bordering on delusional
- Increased sexual content.

Orientation
- Fully oriented.

Memory
- Impaired short term
- Impaired recall.

Concentration
- Highly distractible.

Abstraction
- Generally abstractive
- Can be concrete on proverb testing during psychotic episodes.

Judgment
- Poor
- Prone to imprudent behavioral choice with potential for negative consequences.

Insight
- Individual usually does not recognize that he or she is ill.
- Resists treatment options.

Diagnostic and Laboratory Findings
- CBC, chemistry profile, thyroid function tests, and B_{12} level to rule out metabolic causes or unidentified conditions
- Drug toxicity screening if indicated by history
- Laboratory findings
  - Abnormalities in neurotransmitter metabolite levels: serotonin, dopamine, and GABA
  - Abnormalities in pharmacological provocation tests; increased cortisol secretion.
- Polysomnographic findings are similar to those found in MDD.

Differential Diagnosis
- If first onset of manic symptoms occurs after age 40, most likely symptoms are caused by another medical condition.
- Many medical conditions mimic manic symptoms:
  - Endocrine disorders
  - Hyperthyroidism
  - Intoxication or withdrawal from illicit drug use:
    - Amphetamines
    - Cocaine
    - Hallucinogens
    - Opiates.

- Medications:
  - Captopril
  - Cimetidine
  - Corticosteroids
  - Cyclosporine
  - Disulfiram
  - Hydralazine
  - Isoniazid.
- Mania can be precipitated by treatments used for MDD or other unipolar mood disorders:
  - Antidepressants
  - ECT
  - Light therapy.

Clinical Management

- Rule out or treat any conditions that may contribute to current symptom manifestation.
- Assess and identify client's level of acuity.
- Determine severity of illness.
- Determine duration of illness.
- Ascertain history of response to treatment.
- During acute manic episodes or significant depressive episodes, client may require brief hospitalization.
  - To ensure client safety
  - To ensure client compliance with treatment to reach stabilization
  - To rapidly stabilize on medication.
- Clinical management during non-acute episodes occurs most often in community settings.

Pharmacological Management

- Pharmacological management should never entail the use of an antidepressant agent if a mood stabilizing agent is not in place.
  - Especially important in clients who are rapid cycling
  - Well known to precipitate manic polarity shift
  - Can worsen the kindling process.

Mood Stabilizing Agents

- Commonly used pharmacological agents
  - *Lithium Carbonate*
    - Gold standard for treating manic episodes
    - Action largely unknown
    - Long history of use; drug profile well established
    - Evidence exists showing some effectiveness on depressive symptoms as well as on manic symptoms
    - Has many clinically significant side effects; clients on this drug require careful monitoring (see Table 7–8)
    - Narrow therapeutic window

- Therapeutic effect and potential for adverse side effects monitored by use of serum lithium level
  - Drawn as trough level
  - 12 hours post-dose
  - Therapeutic serum range 0.5–1.2 mEq/L
  - Greater than 1.2 mEq/L increases risk for toxic side effects.
  - Need baseline labs before initiation of lithium to ensure safety and efficacy
    - Thyroid panel
    - Serum creatinine
    - Blood urea nitrogen (BUN)
    - Urinalysis
    - CBC
    - EKG for clients older than age 50.
- Rapid-cycling clients seldom respond to lithium.

- *Anticonvulsant Mood Stabilizing Agents*
  - Anticonvulsant medication (see Table 7–9)
  - Often considered first-line agents and almost always first-line agents for rapid-cycling clients
  - Action reduces kindling
  - Response to treatment with lithium or anticonvulsant medications 1–2 weeks.

Table 7–8. Clinically Significant Side Effects of Lithium

Organ System Affected	Clinical Finding
Endocrine	Weight gain
	Impaired thyroid functioning
Central nervous system	Fine hand tremors
	Fatigue
	Fasciculations
	Mental cloudiness
	Headaches
	Coarse hand tremors with toxicity
	Nystagmus
Dermatological	Maculopapular rash
	Pruritis
	Acne
GI	GI upset
	Diarrhea
	Vomiting
	Cramps
	Anorexia
Renal	Polyuria with related polydipsia
	Diabetes insipidus
	Edema
	Microscopic tubular changes

Table 7–8, Continued

Organ System Affected	Clinical Finding
Cardiac	T-wave inversions Dysrhythmias
Hematological	Leukocytosis

Table 7–9. Drugs for Mood Disorders: Mood Disorders/Anticonvulsants

Drug	Brand Name	Daily Dosage	Therapeutic Plasma Level	Side Effects	Comments
Lithium carbonate	Eskalith Lithobid	1,200–2,400 mg/d (acute) 900–1,200 mg/d (maintenance)	0.8–1.2 mEq/L 0.6–1.2 mEq/L	• *Common* Nausea, fine hand tremors, increased urination and thirst • *Toxicity* Slurred speech, confusion, severe GI effect	• Established standard treatment for bipolar disorder • Risk of hypothyroidism • Avoid in pregnancy, especially 1st trimester
Carba-mazepine	Tegretol	10–20 mg/kg/d	6–12 mcg/ml	• *Rare* Agranulocytosis, aplastic anemia • *Common* Nausea, dizziness, sedation, headache, dry mouth, constipation, skin rash	• Hepatic enzyme inducer • Monitor LFTs • Alternative to lithium or valproic acid • Avoid in pregnancy, especially in 1st trimester
Valproic Acid, Divalproex Sodium	Depakene, Depakote	15–40 mg/kg/d	50–125 mcg/mL	• *Common* Nausea, diarrhea, abdominal cramps, sedation, tremor • *Rare* Increased liver enzymes	• Depakote minimizes GI effects • More effective than lithium for rapid cycling and mixed bipolar • Loading dose: 20 mg/kg • Avoid in pregnancy, especially 1st trimester

Continued on the next page

Table 7–9. Continued

Drug	Brand Name	Daily Dosage	Therapeutic Plasma Level	Side Effects	Comments
Lamotri-gene	Lamictal	25–600 mg/d	Blood monitoring not necessary	• *Common* Dizziness, ataxia, somnolence, diplopia, nausea, headache, hepatotoxicity *Rare:* Life-threatening rashes, leukopenia	• Helps in depressive phase of bipolar affective disorder • Monitor for blood dyscrasia • Titrate dosages slowly
Topira-mate	Topamax	400–1,200 mg/d	Blood monitoring not necessary	• *Common* Somnolence, fatigue, altered cognition, paresthesias • *Rare* Kidney stones, glaucoma	• Monitor for glaucoma • Monitor for renal stones • Can cause weight loss • Decreases efficacy of birth control agents and digoxin
Oxcar-bazepine	Trileptal	300–2,400 mg/d	Blood monitoring not necessary	• *Common* Sedation, dizziness, headache, fatigue, GI distress, abnormal vision, weight gain • *Rare* Hyponatremia	• May cause hyponatremia • Monitor sodium levels • May decrease efficacy of birth control pills
Carba-mazepine ER	Equetro	200–1,600 mg/d	Blood monitoring not necessary	• *Common* Dizziness, sedation, headache • *Rare* Transient decrease in platelets and white blood cells	• No need to obtain blood levels as with Tegretol
Levetira-cetam	Keppra	250–3,000 mg/d	Blood monitoring not necessary	• *Common* Sedation, dizziness • *Rare* Anemia	• Monitor for leukopenia

Table 7–9. Continued

Drug	Brand Name	Daily Dosage	Therapeutic Plasma Level	Side Effects	Comments
Zonisamide	Zonegran	100–600 mg/d	Blood monitoring not necessary	• *Common* Sedation, dizziness, ataxia, headache, GI distress • *Rare* Kidney stones, elevated serum creatinine and blood urea nitrogen, anemia, Steven Johnson's syndrome, agranulocytosis	• Contraindicated with sulfonamide allergy • May potentially cause weight loss

Nonpharmacological Management

- Somatic treatments
  - Treatment as previously discussed for MDD episodes.
- Therapies
  - Treatment as previously discussed for MDD episodes.
- During acute phase of manic episode:
  - Monitor and help client meet nutritional needs.
  - Help client meet sleep–rest needs.
  - Monitor safety.
- During less acute periods:
  - CBT
  - Behavioral therapies
  - Interpersonal therapies
  - Supportive groups
  - Milieu therapy
    - Provides for structure and safety needs
    - Provides socialization and interpersonal support
    - Encourages independency.
- Client and family education
  - Explain underlying pathology of illness.
  - Discuss signs and symptoms.
  - Help identify strategies for living with illness.
  - Help understand and make decisions regarding care options.
- Relapse prevention plan
- Overall health promotion.

Common Comorbidities
- Hypothyroidism
- Substance abuse.

General Health Considerations
- High-risk activities from manic behavior
  - Sexual
    - Client education for sexually transmitted diseases (STDs)
    - Assessment and monitoring for STDs.
  - Financial/legal
    - Client access to community resources
    - Nutritional counseling.
- Client health education.

Life Span Considerations
- Adolescent manic episodes present differently than adult episodes.
  - More psychotic features
  - Often associated with antisocial behavior
  - Often associated with substance abuse
  - Prodromal period of significant behavioral problems
    - School truancy
    - Failing grades.

Follow-up
- Clients initially should be seen weekly to titrate medications and monitor serum blood levels of pharmacological agents.
- Treatment duration and success rates vary with individual characteristics and motivation.
- Clients should be taught symptoms of mania and depression and that the disorders are chronic illnesses.
- Relapse is common and frequently occurs.
- Relapse plans need to be developed.
- Client teaching should include risk, benefits, and potential side effects of medication treatment.
  - Pharmacological agents for BP disorder, especially lithium, are teratogenic.
  - Women of child-bearing years need effective contraceptive care while on BP disorder treatment medication.
- Routine use of lab tests to monitor for therapeutic serum levels of anticonvulsants and lithium is needed.
  - Routine evaluation of CBC, renal function, and thyroid function for clients taking lithium long term is needed.
- Assessment for suicidality should occur during every client contact.
- All clients should be observed for development of adverse effects of pharmacological treatment.
- Standardized rating scales are needed to monitor clinical status, establish baseline functioning, and monitor disorder course over time.

- Young Mania Rating Scale (YMRS; Young, Biggs, Ziegler, & Meyer, 1978)
- Mood Disorder Questionnaire (MDQ; Hirschfeld, Holzer, Calabrese, Weissman, Reed, Davies, et al., 2003).

Cyclothymic Disorder

Description
- Chronic, fluctuating mood disorder whose symptoms are similar to but less severe than BP disorder
- Numerous periods of hypomanic and dysthymic symptoms.

Etiology
- Similar to BP disorder.

Incidence and Demographics
- Lifetime prevalence .4%–1%
- Insidious onset
- Chronic course
- Begins early in life
- 15%–50% of individuals with cyclothymic disorder subsequently develop BP disorder.

Risk Factors
- Genetic loading
- Family history
- BP disorder Type I
- Substance abuse.

Prevention and Screening
- At-risk family education
- Community education
  - Stigma reduction
  - Signs and symptoms of illness
  - Treatment potential for control of symptoms.
- Early recognition, intervention, and initiation of treatment
  - Significant and protracted prodromal symptom period usually noted before full onset of illness
  - The longer the time period between onset of symptoms and diagnosis, the more difficult to interrupt cyclicity of illness.

Assessment
History–Assess for the Following:
- Fluctuating mood episodes
- Individuals can function well during hypomanic episodes
- May experience clinically significant distress or impaired function related to cyclicity
- Unpredictable mood changes

- Often regarded by others as *temperamental, moody, unpredictable, inconsistent, and unreliable.*
- No psychotic episodes.

Physical Exam Findings
- Similar to MDD and BP disorder.

Mental Status Exam Findings
- Similar to MDD and BP disorder but with less severity of symptoms.

Diagnostic and Laboratory Findings
- Similar to MDD and BP disorder.

Differential Diagnosis
Nonpsychiatric
- Similar to MDD and BP disorder.

Psychiatric
- BP disorder
- Dysthymia
- Substance abuse.

Clinical Management
Pharmacological Management
- Similar to MDD and BP disorder
- Because of increased risk for development of BP disorder, commonly treated with medication.

Nonpharmacological Management
- Similar to MDD and BP disorder.

Life Span Considerations
- Usually begins in adolescence
- Onset in later life usually suggests general medical condition such as multiple sclerosis.

Follow-up
- Similar to MDD and BP disorder.

Case Study

Mary, a 35-year-old homemaker and mother of two children, accompanied by her husband presents to her primary care provider with complaints of lack of energy and inability to sleep, both of which are getting progressively worse. The symptoms are affecting her ability to take care of her children and the household. Her husband reports that she often has crying spells, is not eating well, and cannot seem to concentrate. When questioned further,

her husband said that she has mentioned not wanting to live, but he thought that she was just having a bad day.

Past Medical History
- Seasonal allergies and stress-induced asthma
- No significant surgical history, except for a tonsillectomy as a child
- Normal pregnancies and deliveries
- No chronic health problems identified.

Family History
- Significant for grandmother and father, who had "breakdowns."
- Father had alcoholism.

Social History
Mary is a homemaker and has two children, ages 8 and 10. She and her husband moved to the area 6 months ago. She does not smoke or use drugs but drinks socially. She has an MA in English and plans to go back to school to get her teaching certificate when her children begin high school.

Mental Status Exam
Mary appears clean but somewhat disheveled. Her hair is not combed or washed. She appears very tired. She avoids eye contact, talks very softly, and is slow to respond to questions. She hardly moves during the interview. Her affect is constricted and sad. She says has no energy, and her mood is "very sad." She does not hear voices or have hallucinations. Her thoughts are appropriate and organized. She does admit to having episodic thoughts of suicide and has a vague plan to ingest an overdose of aspirin, acetaminophen, and alcohol when the children are with their father but has no clear timeline or planned intent. She is unable to do serial number testing and shows impaired short-term memory. She exhibits a few problems with immediate recall. She has difficulty concentrating but no difficulty with abstractions. She is oriented times three, and shows good judgment and insight. She has above-average intelligence.

Current Medications
Mary takes Zyrtec for allergies and is now on OrthoTri-Cyclen contraceptive pills.

Labs
- Platelets 230/mm
- White blood cells 6,000/mm
- Hematocrit 33%, hemoglobin 8.0
- NA 140, K^+ 4.0, Cl 101, CO_2 26, BUN 15, creatinine 0.9, glucose 102
- TSH 1.1, T3 179, T4 1.3.

There are several issues to consider in planning care for Mary:
- What is the most probable diagnosis?
- What further assessment is needed?
- What target symptoms does Mary display that are consistent with the probable diagnosis?
- What medications would be considered?

- If Mary had psychotic features with her depression, how would this change the treatment plan?
- How would the plan differ if Mary had a heart condition and was taking no other medications?

Review Questions

1. Mrs. Thomas has been diagnosed with MDD and is placed on Serzone 20 mg for her depression. For the PMHNP to effectively monitor this client's use of the medication, which of the following actions should be part of ongoing care?

   a. Use of a standardized rating scale of depression

   b. Monitoring for potential abuse of medication

   c. Monitoring of renal functioning

   d. Monitoring for potential cardiac side effects

2. A 23-year-old female in brought into the ER after attempting suicide by cutting her wrists. Which nursing action by the PMHNP would be of highest priority initially?

   a. Assess her coping behaviors

   b. Assess her current level of suicidality

   c. Take her vital signs

   d. Assess her health history

3. The TCA class of medications can be characterized by all of the following properties except

   a. Safety in overdose

   b. Inexpensive cost of medications

   c. Significant side effect concerns

   d. Long half-life

4. For the PMHNP to provide a client with an adequate trial on an antidepressant medication, what time period of continuous medication use is required?

   a. 6 weeks of continuous medication use

   b. 6 months of continuous medication use

   c. 3 weeks of continuous medication use

   d. 10 weeks of continuous medication use

References and Resources

Agency for Health Care Policy and Research. (1993). *Depression in primary care treatment of major depression* (Clinical Practice Guideline 5, AHCPR Publication No. 93-0551). Rockville, MD: U.S. Department of Health and Human Services.

American Psychiatric Association. (1998). *Practice parameters for the assessment and treatment of children and adolescents with bipolar disorder.* Washington, DC: Author.

American Psychiatric Association. (2000a). *Diagnostic and statistical manual of mental disorders* (4th ed., text rev.). Washington, DC: Author.

American Psychiatric Association. (2000b). *Practice guidelines for the treatment of patients with major depressive disorder.* Washington, DC: Author.

Beck, A. (1979). *Cognitive therapy of depression.* New York: Guilford Press.

Beck, A. T., Ward, C. H., Mendelson, M., Mock, J., & Erbaugh, J. (1961). An inventory for measuring depression. *Archives of General Psychiatry, 4,* 561–571.

Beydoun, A. (2001). Innovative treatment strategies with anticonvulsants: A focus on bipolar disorder. *Primary Psychiatry, 8*(6), 49–52.

Birmaher, B., Brent, D. A., & Benson, R. S. (1998). Summary of the practice parameters for the assessment and treatment of children and adolescents with depressive disorders. *Journal of the American Academy of Child and Adolescent Psychiatry, 37,* 1234–1238.

Freidrich, M. (1999). Lithium: Proving its mettle for 50 years. *Journal of the American Medical Association, 281,* 2271–2275.

George, M. S., Wassermann, E. M., Williams, W. A., Callahan, A., Ketter, T. A., Basser, P., et al. (1995). Daily repetitive transcranial magnetic stimulation (rTMS) improves mood in depression. *Neuroreport, 6,* 1853–1856.

Ghaemi, S. N. (2001). Bipolar disorder and antidepressants: An ongoing controversy. *Primary Psychiatry, 6*(2), 28–34.

Giles, D. E., Kupfer, D. J., Rush, A. J., & Roffwarg, H. P. (1998). Controlled comparison of electrophysiological sleep in families of probands with unipolar depression. *American Journal of Psychiatry, 155,* 192–196.

Gloaguen, V., Cottraux, J., Cucherat, M., & Blackburn, I. M. (1998). A meta-analysis of the effects of cognitive therapy in depressed patients. *Journal of Affective Disorders, 49*(1), 59–62.

Green, J. (2001). Helping patients understand depression and its treatment. *Primary Psychiatry, 8*(11), 49–53.

Hirschfeld, R., Holzer, C., Calabrese, J., Weissman, M., Reed, M., Davies, M., et al. (2003). Validity of the mood disorder questionnaire: A general population study. *American Journal of Psychiatry, 160,* 178–180.

Hoyert, D. L., Kochanek, K. D., & Murphy, S. L. (1998). *Deaths: Final data for 1997* (National Vital Statistics Report, DHHS Publication No. PHS-99-1120). Hyattsville, MD: National Center for Health Statistics.

Judd, L., Paulus, M., Schettler, P., Hagop, S., Endicott, A., Leon, A., et al. (2007). Does incomplete recovery from first lifetime major depressive episode herald a chronic course of illness? *American Journal of Psychiatry, 157,* 1501–1504.

Kimrell, T., Little, R., & Dunn, T. (1999). Frequency dependence of antidepressant response to left prefrontal repetitive transcranial magnetic stimulation (rTMS) as a function of baseline cerebral glucose metabolism. *Biological Psychiatry, 46,* 1603–1613.

Klein, D. N., Schwartz, J. E., & Rose S. (2000). Five-year course and outcome of dysthymic disorder: A prospective, naturalistic follow-up study. *American Journal of Psychiatry, 157,* 931–939.

Lowe-Ponsford, F. L., & Nutt, D. J. (2001). Pathophysiology of depression. *Primary Psychiatry, 8*(11), 43–48.

McBride, A., & Austin, J. (1996). *Psychiatric mental health nursing: Integrating the behavioral and biological sciences.* Philadelphia: W. B. Saunders.

McQuade, R., & Young, A. (2000). Future therapeutic targets in mood disorders: The glucocorticoid receptor. *British Journal of Psychiatry, 177,* 390–395.

Monroe, S. M., Rohde, P., & Seeley, J. R. (1999). Life events and depression in adolescence: Relationship loss as a prospective risk factor for first onset of major depressive disorder. *Journal of Abnormal Psychology, 108,* 606–614.

Ornstein, S., Stuart, G., & Jenkins, R. (2000). Depression diagnosis and antidepressant use in primary care practices. *Journal of Family Practice, 49*(1), 68–71.

Saeed, M. (2001). Assessment and management of the suicidal patient in the managed care era. *Primary Psychiatry, 8*(6), 38–45.

Shaffer, D., & Craft, L. (1999). Methods of adolescent suicide prevention. *Journal of Clinical Psychiatry, 60*(Suppl. 2), 70–74.

Spencer, T., Biederman, J., & Wilens, T. (1999). Attention-deficit/hyperactivity disorder and comorbidity. *Pediatric Clinics of North America, 46,* 915–927.

Stuart, G. W., & Laraia, M. (2004). *Principles and practice of psychiatric nursing* (8th ed.). St. Louis, MO: Mosby.

Young, R. C., Biggs, J. T., Ziegler, V. E., & Meyer, D. A. (1978). A rating scale for mania: Reliability, Validity, and sensitivity. *British Journal of Psychiatry, 133,* 429–435.

Notes:

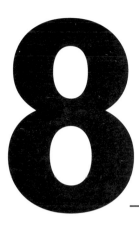

Anxiety Disorders

This chapter reviews anxiety disorders encountered by psychiatric–mental health nurse practitioners (PMHNPs). These, some of the most common of all psychiatric illnesses, can manifest initially as physical health states. Often only after extensive, unnecessary assessment and diagnostic evaluation is a client's problem correctly identified as an anxiety disorder. It has become increasingly common for these disorders to be treated in primary care settings, and often clients first present in such settings because of the high degree of somatic symptomatology.

Anxiety is a very common and normal human emotion. PMHNPs caring for clients who present for evaluation of anxiety must be able to distinguish between normal levels of anxiety and pathological levels that are symptomatic of an underlying brain-based illness. Pathological levels of anxiety require treatment and generally will not fully abate without therapeutic intervention. Untreated high levels of anxiety predispose individuals to other serious health problems; therefore, pathological levels of anxiety should not go untreated (Narrow, Rae, & Regier, 1998).

Normal Emotion of Anxiety

- Anxiety is one of the most common human emotions.
- Cultural differences can affect behavioral manifestations of anxiety.
- Anxiety exists on a continuum ranging from the absence of anxiety at one end to pathological levels that produce significant symptoms of psychiatric disorder at the other (see Table 8–1).
- Anxiety can be a normal, healthy reaction to life stressors that motivates an individual to deal with events and emotions.
- Anxiety can be pathological if it is disproportionate to events, if it is sustained over a significant time frame, if it significantly impairs functioning, or if it is apparently unrelated to any identifiable event or situation in an individual's life.
- High pathological levels of anxiety interfere with perceptions, memory, judgment, and motor responses.
- The role of the PMHNP in assessing anxiety is to separate normal vs. pathological levels of anxiety, to intervene to lower the level of anxiety, and to improve overall functioning.

Table 8–1. Assessing Levels of Anxiety

Level of Anxiety	Definition	Physiological Signs/Symptoms	Psychological Signs/Symptoms
Level I. Mild	Normative level experienced by all; functions to motivate	Vital signs normal, pupils constricted, minimal increase in muscle tone	Perceptual field broadened, heightened awareness of environment
Level II. Moderate	Normative level experienced by most in response to significant stressors	Vital signs normal, mild increased heart rate, moderate increase in muscle tone	Subjective feeling of tension or worry, narrowed perceptions
Level III. Severe	Pathological level	Autonomic nervous system triggered, flight-or-fight response, pupils dilated, vital signs increased, diaphoresis, muscles rigid, hearing decreased, pain threshold increased, urinary frequency, diarrhea	Perceptual field greatly narrowed, difficulty with problem solving, distorted perception of time, selective inattention, dissociative sensations, automatic behavior
Level IV. Panic	Pathological level	Severe symptoms markedly increased; patient is pale, hypotensive, has poor eye–hand coordination, muscle pains, marked decrease in hearing, dizziness, shortness of breath	Scattered perceptions, unable to attend to environmental stimuli, illogical thinking, may exhibit hallucinations or delusions

Anxiety Disorders

Description

- Anxiety disorders are the most common group of psychiatric disorders and are characterized by the degree of anxiety experienced by the client, the duration and severity of the anxiety, and the typical behavioral manifestation of anxiety observed in the client. Anxiety ranges from acute states to chronic disorders and is accompanied by multiple somatic complaints.
- Individuals most often present first in primary care settings with nonspecific physical complaints.
  - Often confused with cardiac and respiratory disorders, so careful differential diagnostic assessment is essential.
- Frequent comorbidity exists with substance abuse, depression, and eating disorders.
- Symptoms significantly impair functioning and occur more days than not for a period of at least 6 months, with the individual reporting little or no volitional control over the symptoms.

- Nine specific anxiety disorders are identified in the *DSM-IV-TR* (American Psychiatric Association, 2000) and are described in more detail in this chapter.

Etiology

- Multiple theories range from psychological to neurobiological; however, more likely there is a multifactorial etiological profile.

Psychodynamic Theory

- This theory is based on the work of Sigmund Freud (1856–1939), who believed that anxiety initially occurs in response to the stimulation of birth and need of the infant to adapt to the changed environment.
- Subsequent anxiety results from intrapsychic conflict.
- The process of unconscious repression of sexual drive is at the core of much of the conflict.
- Conflict exists between instinctual needs of the *id* and the *superego* (*conscience*); anxiety signals the individual of the need to deal with the id–superego conflict.
- Conflict is unconscious, but anxiety is consciously perceived.
- Conflict entails fear of punishment and of doing wrong.
- Defense mechanisms are unconsciously used by the individual to deal with the conflict.
- The behavioral manifestations of anxiety disorders stem from the pathological overuse of defense mechanisms.

Interpersonal Theory

- This theory is based on the work of Harry Stack Sullivan (1892–1949), who believed that humans are goal directed toward attainment of satisfaction and security needs.
- Satisfaction and security needs are normally met in interpersonal interactions.
- Anxiety arises when an individual's needs are unmet.
- Anxiety is first experienced in an infant's interactions with his or her mother.
- Subsequent anxiety arises because of interpersonal conflict.
- Conflict occurs when an individual perceives his or her needs will not be met because of rejection, feelings of inferiority, or inability to engage with significant others.
- Sense of self becomes based on the individual's perception of how others view him or her.

Neurobiological Theory

- Pathological levels of anxiety result from neurobiological deficits in normal brain functioning.
- Deficits are genetically mediated by and involve predominantly the limbic system, midline brain stem area, and sections of the cortex.
- Deficits predispose the individual to abnormal stress responses, with hyperactivity of autonomic nervous system causing symptoms such as increased heart rate and blood pressure, diaphoresis, papillary dilation, tremors, and increased respiratory rate.
- Problems with the hypothalamic pituitary adrenal (HPA) axis:
  - Threat is perceived, and amygdala signals the hypothalamus to secrete corticotropin-releasing hormone (CRH).
  - The amygdala also activates the sympathetic nervous system to start the fight-or-flight response.

- The pituitary is stimulated to release adrenocorticotropic hormone (ACTH).
- The adrenal glands are then stimulated to release cortisol, which shuts off the alarm system and restores the body to homeostasis.
- In anxiety disorders, the amygdala may not be able to shut off the response (overactive amygdala), or there may not be enough cortisol to stop the fight-or-flight response.
- Neurobiological deficits result in low levels of the neurotransmitter GABA (gamma-aminobutyric acid), the chemical responsible for inhibitory responses of neurons, and in high levels of norepinephrine, the chemical associated with the fight-or-flight response.
- Neurotransmitters involved in suppressing the HPA axis are serotonin and GABA.

Incidence and Demographics

- Anxiety disorders are common disorders experienced by 18.1% of the general U.S. population.
- Except for obsessive–compulsive disorder (OCD) and social phobia, anxiety disorders are more common in girls and women than in boys and men.
- Most anxiety disorders manifest in adolescence and early adulthood (Narrow, Rae, & Regier, 1998).

Risk Factors

- Genetic loading (National Institute of Mental Health, Genetics Workgroup, 1998)
  - A first-degree relative of an individual with panic disorder is up to eight times more likely than the general population to develop panic disorder.
  - If a first-degree relative of an individual developed panic disorder before age 20, that individual is up to 20 times more likely than the general population to develop panic disorder.
- Limited range of coping skills.

Prevention and Screening

- At-risk family education
- Community education
  - Stigma reduction
  - Signs and symptoms of illness
  - Treatment potential for control of symptoms.

- Early recognition, intervention, and initiation of treatment
  - Teach at-risk individuals to recognize and manage anxiety levels.
  - Help at-risk individuals reduce anxiety through improved coping activities.

Assessment

History–Assess for the Following:

- Detailed history of present illness, including time frame and progression, any associated symptoms.
- Social history, including present living situation; marital status; occupation; education; and alcohol, tobacco, or illicit drug use.
- Medication use, including prescription, over-the-counter, alternative, supplements, and home remedies.

- Validate history with family member.
- Initial presentation and periodic functional history and assessment
- Individuals are usually more troubled by and complain more often of physical symptoms and may initially not identify anxiety as a concern.
- Question the client regarding subjective sensations of being nervous, tense, worried, anxious, or stressed out.
- Identify current environmental stressors as experienced by the client.
- Determine if anxiety is normative or pathological.
- Assess for common indicators of *pathological* levels of anxiety indicative of underlying anxiety disorder:
    - Anxiety is perceived as out of the control of the individual.
    - Anxiety does not respond, even momentarily, to conscious suppression.
    - More pervasive anxiety overlaps into all spheres of functioning.
    - Anxiety is pronounced, distressing, and of long duration.
    - Anxiety is unlinked and not seen as caused by life events.
    - Anxiety is accompanied by somatic complaints, which is more uncommon in normal anxiety levels.
    - Anxiety interferes with social, occupational, and recreational activities and with activities of daily living.
- Determine the level of the client's anxiety using the four-point scale of mild to panic levels (1 = mild to 4 = panic; see Table 8–1).
- Use standardized rating scales such as the Hamilton Rating Scale for Anxiety (HAM-A; Hamilton, 1959) for establishing and monitoring the client's anxiety level over time.
- Assess general level of health and presence of concomitant illnesses.
- Assess for *dysfunctional and self-medicating strategies in anxious clients:*
    - Substance use or abuse
    - Increased caffeine use
    - Increased nicotine use.

- Assess for *psychological symptoms of anxiety:*
    - Fear of dying, losing one's mind, or a sense of unreality
    - Belief that he or she is very ill, with no findings to support this belief
    - Narrowed perceptions
    - Limited eye contact
    - Thought content exhibiting increased worry.

Physical Exam Findings
- Anxiety manifests in many physical ways:
    - Pupillary dilation
    - Tachycardia
    - Increased muscle tone
    - Headaches
    - Hypertension
    - Motor restlessness
    - Diaphoresis
    - Palpitations, often with tightness of chest
    - GI problems
    - Dizziness or light-headedness.

Mental Status Exam Findings

Appearance

- Psychomotor restlessness
- Fidgeting
- Tremors
- Inability to sit still
- Hand-wringing.

Speech

- Overproductive
- Rapid
- Distractible speech patterns
- Thought blocking.

Affect

- Anxious
- Worried.

Mood

- Tense
- Nervous
- Worried.

Thought Process

- Overall organized
- Goal directed
- Redirectable.

Thought Content

- Thematic for worry
- Mild perseveration on topics of concern.

Orientation

- Usually fully oriented.

Memory

- Impaired short-term and immediate memory
- Forgetful.

Concentration

- Inattentive
- Decreased concentration.

Abstraction

- Abstract on proverbs and similarities.

Judgment
- Poor judgment for self-welfare.

Insight
- Limited insight.

Diagnostic and Laboratory Findings
- Obtain baseline labs such as CBC, chemistry profile, thyroid function tests, and B_{12} level to rule out metabolic causes or unidentified conditions.
- Obtain drug toxicity screening if indicated by history.
- In some cases, clients may have labs reflecting compensated respiratory alkalosis:
  - Decreased carbon dioxide levels
  - Decreased bicarbonate levels
  - Normal pH.

Differential Diagnosis
- Many medical conditions can cause worry, fear, and normal levels of anxiety (see Table 8–2).
- Ensure that client symptoms meet criteria for anxiety disorders.

Table 8–2. Medical Conditions That May Mimic Anxiety Disorders

General Category of Disorder	Specific Illness
Cardiovascular	Congestive heart failure
	Mitral valve prolapse
	Myocardial infarct
	Arrhythmia, especially tachycardic arrhythmia
	Pulmonary embolism
	Coronary artery disease
Respiratory	Asthma
	Chronic obstructive pulmonary disorder
	Pneumonia
Endocrine	Hyperthyroidism
	Hyperparathyroidism
	Cushing's disease
Neurological	Seizure disorder
	Transient ischemic attack
	Cerebral vascular accident
	Encephalitis
	Central nervous system (CNS) neoplasm
Metabolic	Hypoglycemia
	Vitamin B deficiency
	Porphyria
Substance Abuse or Dependency	Intoxication with CNS stimulants (e.g., cocaine, amphetamines, caffeine)
	Withdrawal from CNS depressants (e.g., alcohol, marijuana)

General Clinical Management

- Rule out or treat any conditions that may contribute to pathological levels of anxiety.

Pharmacological Management

- Most of the medications known to improve symptoms of anxiety act on the GABA system.

- Selective serotonin reuptake inhibitors (SSRIs)
  - Considered *first-line agents* for chronic anxiety disorders
  - Action on serotonin system and indirectly on GABA system
  - Carry no risk of dependency
  - Cannot be used prn
  - Clean side-effect profile
  - Take time to reach symptom control (usually 3–4 weeks)
  - Best when combined with psychotherapy.

- Benzodiazepines (BNZs)
  - Potentiate the effect of GABA
  - Rapid onset of action
  - Can be used prn
  - Limit to lowest possible dose and short-term use if possible, as long-term use may lead to tolerance, dependence, memory impairment, and depression
  - Use should be limited to period of excessive symptoms, period of high stress, or in unremitting symptoms
  - Contraindicated in clients with history of substance dependence
  - Effective but carry high risk for addiction
  - BNZs with *longer half-lives* require less frequent dosing, have less severe withdrawal, and have less rebound anxiety:
    - Klonopin (clonazepam)
    - Valium (diazepam).

- BNZs with *shorter half-lives* require more frequent dosing, have more severe withdrawal, and have more rebound anxiety:
  - Xanax (alprazolam)
  - Ativan (lorazepam).

- *Advantages of BNZs with short half-lives:*
  - Less daytime sedation
  - Less drug accumulation
  - Quick onset of action
  - Useful for treatment of insomnia.

- *Disadvantages of BNZs with short half-lives:*
  - Increased risk of addiction.

- Tricyclics (TCAs)
  - Effective but have dirty side-effect profiles
  - Side effects often affect compliance.

- Non-BNZ anxiolytics (see Table 8–3)
  - Buspar (buspirone)
    - Must be taken regularly, not as prn

- • Gabitril (tiagabine)
- • Neurontin (gabapentin)
- • Usually adjunctive use with other pharmacological agent.
- • Life span considerations
  - • In children, alpha-agonists are often used for anxiety.
  - • Catapres (clonidine, .003–.01 mg/kg/d)
  - • Tenex (guanfacine, .015–.05 mg/kg/d).

Table 8–3. Non-Benzodiazepine Anxiolytics for Adults

Generic	Brand	Dosage Range	Side Effects	Comments
Buspirone	BuSpar	20–60 mg/d	Dizziness, insomnia, tremors, akathisia, stomach upset, dry mouth	Helpful adjunct for anxiety
Tiagabine	Gabitril	4–56 mg/d	Dizziness, somnolence, stomach upset, tremors, dry mouth	Helpful adjunct for anxiety
Gabapentin	Neurontin	300–3,600 mg/d	Ataxia, decreased coordination, sedation, disequilibrium	Used for anxiety, neuropathic pain, fibromyalgia, and as an anti-craving medication

Nonpharmacological Management

- • Behavioral therapy
  - • Systematic desensitization
  - • Exposure therapy
  - • Relaxation therapies
  - • Biofeedback.
- • Cognitive–behavioral therapy (CBT)
- • Interpersonal therapies
- • Community self-help groups
- • Alternative therapies as adjunctive treatments.

Comorbidities

- • Anemia
- • Cardiac disorders, especially in clients with dysrhythmias
- • Endocrine disorders
  - • Cushing's disease
  - • Hyperthyroidism
  - • Hypoglycemia.
- • Pulmonary conditions
  - • Chronic obstructive pulmonary disorder

- • Asthma
- • Pulmonary embolism
- • Pneumothorax.
- Adverse medication reactions
  - • Caffeine
  - • Nicotine
  - • Anticholinergics
  - • Antihistamines
  - • Antipsychotics
  - • Steroids
  - • Bronchodilators
  - • Anesthetics.
- Mood disorders
- Substance abuse–related disorders.

General Health Considerations

- Chronic anxiety is wearing on the body; therefore, assess for effects on the cardiovascular system.
- Perform a general assessment for a healthy lifestyle.

Follow-up

General Considerations

- Clients should initially be seen weekly or biweekly to titrate medications.
- Client teaching should include risk, benefits, and potential side effects of medication treatment.
  - • If the client is taking BNZs, monitor for potential dependence.
  - • If the client is taking SSRIs, monitor for common side effects and adverse effects.
- Clients should be taught symptoms of anxiety and the fact that disorders are chronic illnesses; a relapse plan should be established for all clients.
- Assessment for suicidality should occur during symptom exacerbation periods.
- Because of frequent comorbidity with major depressive disorder, assess frequently for depression levels using standardized rating scales (see below).
- Medication should be combined with therapy to reach maximum control of symptoms.
- Clients may need encouragement to continue treatment, especially after initial symptom relief occurs.

Standardized Rating Scales for Anxiety Disorders

- Zung Self-rating Anxiety Scale (Zung, 1971)
- Hamilton Rating Scale for Anxiety (HAM–A; Hamilton, 1959)
- Yale-Brown Obsessive-Compulsive Scale (Y–BOCS; Goodman et al., 1989).

Panic Disorder

Description

- Panic disorder is experienced as discrete episodes or attacks with sudden onset of intense apprehension, fearfulness, or terror, often associated with sense of impending doom.

- May be diagnosed with or without agoraphobia.
- Attacks occur without warning and in the absence of any real danger.
- Attacks build to a peak of intensity within a short, self-limiting time, usually within 10 minutes of onset.
- Panic disorder is more common in women than in men.

Assessment

History–Assess for the Following:

- Assess for *diagnostic criteria* of panic disorder:
  - Discrete episode in which client experiences 4 or more of the following symptoms, having a sudden onset, and peaking within 10 minute of onset:
    - Paresthesias
    - Chills or hot flushing
    - Fear of losing control or of going crazy
    - Fear of dying
    - Shortness of breath or smothering sensation
    - Palpitations, pounding, or accelerated heart rate
    - Chest pain, tightness, or discomfort
    - Sweating
    - Trembling or shaking
    - Nausea or abdominal distress.

- After first attack, persistent concern over having another attack, worry over the consequences of initial attack, or a significant behavioral change related to attack
- With high somatic sensations, clients often sensitive to new somatic experiences or perceptions
- Often intolerant of or concerned with common side effects of medication treatments
- Discouraged or ashamed about "failure" to control emotions and over concern about dying when no other pathology identified
  - In two-thirds of cases, major depression occurs first, followed by panic disorder symptoms.
  - In one-third of cases, panic disorder symptoms precede major depression symptoms.

Three Characteristic Types

- Client presentation is defined by relationship between onset of attack and presence or absence of triggers for attacks.

  - Type 1: Uncued
    - No associated internal or external trigger
    - Experienced as spontaneous or "out of the blue" attack
    - May over time become cued or situationally cued (see below) or may, less commonly, remain uncued
    - NOTE: Recurrent, unexpected, uncued attacks are required for initial fulfillment of *DSM-IV-TR* diagnostic criteria for panic disorder. If initial onset is *not* this type, consider an alternative diagnosis (e.g., phobia, posttraumatic stress disorder [PTSD], generalized anxiety disorder [GAD]; see below).

- Type 2: Cued
  - Occurs immediately and invariably on exposure to or in anticipation of a situational cue or trigger.
- Type 3: Situationally Cued
  - Similar to cued but is not immediate and not invariably cued to trigger.

Type Determined by Assessment of

- Client's focus of anxiety
- Type and number of attacks
- Number of situations avoided by client
- Level of anxiety experienced between panic attacks.

Physical Exam Findings

- Nonspecific, especially when client not experiencing panic attack
- Nonspecific cardiac-related complaints during panic episodes often bring client into treatment:
  - Chest pain
  - Numbness
  - Shortness of breath.

Mental Status Exam Findings

- General findings of anxiety as described earlier
- Findings very pronounced during panic episodes and less pronounced during nonpanic periods
- High level of anticipatory anxiety between panic episodes.

Diagnostic and Laboratory Findings

- None specific.

Differential Diagnosis

- Rule out general medical conditions known to produce similar symptoms, including
  - Hyperthyroidism
  - Hyperparathyroidism
  - Pheochromocytosis
  - Vestibular dysfunction
  - Seizure disorders
  - Cardiac arrhythmias such as supraventricular tachycardia (SVT)
  - Use of CNS stimulants, including
    - Cocaine
    - Amphetamines
    - Caffeine.
- Panic attacks with another anxiety disorder such as PTSD or phobias
- Separation anxiety disorder
- Avoidance behavior in delusional disorder
- Consider general medical disorder if
  - First episode panic attack symptoms occur after age 45

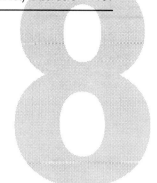

- Panic symptoms are atypical, such as
  - Vertigo
  - Loss of consciousness
  - Incontinence
  - Headache
  - Slurred speech
  - Amnesic pattern after attacks.
- Differentiated from other anxiety conditions by
  - Sudden onset of attack
  - Discrete, self-limiting nature of symptoms
  - Paroxysmal symptom profile
  - Level III–IV anxiety symptoms with somatic symptoms that are experienced as distressing and severe by the client.

Clinical Management
- Follow guidelines of general clinical management of anxiety disorders.

Pharmacological Management
- SSRIs
- BNZs, usually used for short-term symptom control
- Buspar effective as an adjunct to an antidepressant
- Other non-BNZ anxiolytic meds used as adjuncts.

Nonpharmacological Management
- CBT
- Individual or group therapy
- Exposure therapy
- Relaxation therapies.

Common Comorbidities
- Frequent with major depressive disorder
- Estimated between 10% and 65%, depending on source:
  - Social phobia
  - OCD
  - Substance abuse.

Agoraphobia

Description
- Agoraphobia is characterized by avoidance of places or situations from which escape may be difficult or embarrassing or in which help may not be available in the event of perceived need, such as a panic attack.
- The anxiety usually leads to avoidant behavior that impairs an individual's ability to travel, to work, or to carry out responsibilities of daily living.

- Differential diagnosis is assisted by the awareness that individuals with agoraphobia feel better and report less significant concerns with anxiety when accompanied by a trusted companion.
- Agoraphobia is not an independently coded *DSM-IV-TR* diagnosis and is always diagnosed in relationship to presence or absence of panic disorder.
- Agoraphobia most commonly occurs in conjunction with panic disorder and is labeled as *panic disorder with agoraphobia.*
- For clients to be diagnosed *panic disorder with agoraphobia,* they must meet the criteria for panic disorder and must experience agoraphobic anxiety about being in places or situations from which escape might be difficult or in which help may not be available in the event of a panic attack.
- If agoraphobia experienced *without panic disorder,* the anxiety disorder is labeled *agoraphobia without history of panic disorder.*

Assessment
History–Assess for the Following:
- Clinical presentation meets *diagnostic criteria* for agoraphobia:
  - Presence of agoraphobic anxiety related to fear of developing panic-like symptoms
  - Never met criteria for panic disorder
  - Avoidant behavior as a result of the agoraphobic anxiety.

Physical Exam Findings
- Nonspecific for agoraphobia.

Mental Status Exam Findings
- Consistent with finding for anxiety
- Thought content consistent with criteria for agoraphobia.

Diagnostic and Laboratory Findings
- Nonspecific for agoraphobia.

Clinical Management
- Follow guidelines of general clinical management of anxiety disorders.

Pharmacological Management
- SSRIs
- BNZs for short-term use.

Nonpharmacological Management
- CBT
- Supportive group therapy
- Desensitization therapy.

Common Comorbidities
- Panic disorder.

Specific Phobias (Simple Phobias)

Description
- In specific phobias there is a clinically significant level of marked and persistent fear that is clearly observable and is, by client perception, clearly related to specific objects or situations.
- In adults, but not in children, there exists the conscious recognition that the fear is excessive or unreasonable.
- In children, the degree of insight to the unreasonable nature of the fear increases as age increases.

Risk Factors
- Traumatic past exposure
  - Having been bitten by dog, having choked on food, and so forth.
- Observation of another's trauma
  - Seeing others having been bitten by dog, seeing others having choked on food, and so forth.
- Excessive informational transmission
  - Repeated graphic parental warnings of dangers of certain events or situations.
- Genetic loading
  - Having family member with specific phobia
  - Blood-injection-injury subtype most familial
  - Subtype aggregation patterns noted within families; for example, if an individual's first-degree relative has animal subtype, the risk is highest for him or her to develop animal subtype.

Assessment
History–Assess for the Following:
- The content of phobias, which can vary with culture, ethnicity, and age
  - Children manifest fear and anxiety as crying, freezing, tantrums, or excessive clinging behavior.
  - Children normatively express a transient fear of animals and other natural objects.
  - Phobic diagnosis should occur only when accompanied by significant functional impairment, such as full avoidance of school related to fear of encountering a spider.
- Exposure to the specific feared object or situation, which immediately provokes the onset of clinically significant levels of anxiety
  - This anxiety may fit the criteria for cued panic attack.
  - The level of anxiety is directly related to how physically close the object or situation is to the person and the degree to which escape from the object or situation is possible.
- Individual engages in avoidant behavior to prevent reaction to object or situation or endures object or situation with dread.
  - Avoidant behavior is distressful and has implications for social, recreational, or occupational or school functioning.

Assess for Subtypes

- There are five common subtypes: situational, natural environment, blood injection injury, animal, and other.
- An individual can experience more than one subtype at a time.
- A phobia to one object or situation in a subclass predisposes an individual to another phobia within the same subclass (e.g., fear of rats increases the risk for fear of spiders).
  1. **Situational Type:** Cued by specific situations; examples include driving, enclosed spaces, tunnels or bridges, and flying.
     - Most common adult form
     - In elderly people, fear of closed-in situations most common
     - Bimodal peak of onset
       - First peak, childhood
       - Second peak, mid-20s.

  2. **Natural Environment Type:** Fear cued by objects in the natural environment; examples include storms, lightning, water, and heights.
     - Second most common adult form
     - Onset usually during childhood.

  3. **Blood-Injection-Injury Type:** Cued by seeing blood or an injury or by receiving an injection or other invasive medical procedure.
  - Third most common adult form
  - Highly familiar subtype
  - Strong vasovagal component that can produce other somatic sensations
    - May exacerbate underlying cardiac or respiratory disorders
    - Person often presents with fainting as chief complaint
    - Experiences paroxysmal tachycardia and hypertension followed by deceleration of heart rate and drop in blood pressure
    - Clinical presentation and disease natural history similar to panic disorder with agoraphobia.

  4. **Animal Type:** Fear cued by animals or insects; examples include rats, snakes, and spiders.
     - Fourth most common adult form
     - Onset usually during childhood.

  5. **Other Type:** Fear cued by range of other stimuli; examples include fear of choking, vomiting, and fear of a specific illness.
     - In children, often manifests as fear of loud sounds or costumed characters.

Differential Diagnosis

- Avoidance behavior in PTSD, OCD, separation anxiety disorder, or psychotic disorders.

Physical Exam Findings

- Nonspecific.

Mental Status Exam Findings

- Consistent with finding for anxiety
- Thought content consistent with criteria for phobia.

Diagnostic and Laboratory Findings
- Nonspecific.

Clinical Management
- Follow guidelines of general clinical management of anxiety disorders.

Pharmacological Management
- SSRIs
- TCAs
- Short-term use of BNZs.

Nonpharmacological Management
- CBT
- Biofeedback
- Desensitization therapy.

Social Anxiety (Phobia) Disorder

Description
- Social anxiety disorder is a marked and persistent fear of social or performance situations in which embarrassment may occur.
- Anxiety levels often are sufficient to fit criteria for a situationally bound panic attack.
- The disorder has an estimated 3%–13% prevalence rate among the U.S. population.
- Rates are equal for the genders.

Assessment
History–Assess for the Following:
- Some degree of social anxiety is common and normative in adolescence.
- Social phobia should be diagnosed only if symptoms persist for longer than 6 months.
- Onset is in the mid-teens, often following stressful or humiliating experience, and tends to remit with age.
- Differential diagnosis is assisted by awareness that individuals with social phobia do *not* feel better or experience decreased anxiety when accompanied by a trusted companion.

Common Descriptive Features
- Hypersensitivity to criticism
- Negative self-evaluations
- Sensitivity to rejection
- Low self-esteem
- Inferiority feelings
- Lack of assertiveness
- Protracted anticipatory anxiety may occur days or weeks before the feared social situation

- Levels of subjective distress and impaired functioning can be significant and have been associated with suicidal ideation.

Physical Exam Findings
- Sweating
- Tremors
- Palpitations
- Muscle tension
- Diarrhea
- Blushing.

Mental Status Exam Findings
- Consistent for anxiety
- Thought content consistent with criteria for social anxiety.

Diagnostic and Laboratory Findings
- Nonspecific.

Clinical Management
- Follow guidelines of general clinical management of anxiety disorders.

Pharmacological Management
- SSRIs
- BNZs, for short-term use
- Beta blockers
  - Used for discrete-episode relief
  - *Example:* Before having to attend a scheduled social function.

Nonpharmacological Management
- CBT
- Exposure therapy
- Relaxation therapy.

Obsessive–Compulsive Disorder (OCD)

Description
- OCD is the presence of anxiety-provoking obsessions or compulsions that function to reduce the individual's subjective anxiety level.

Obsession
- Defined as recurrent and persistent thought, impulse, or images that are experienced and that cause anxiety and distress
- Experienced as intrusive and inappropriate
- Ego-dystonic experience in which an individual feels the content of obsession is alien to his or her belief structure and not the kind of common thought, impulse, or image he or she usually experiences.

Compulsion
- Defined as repetitive behaviors or mental actions such that an individual feels driven to perform in response to an obsession.

Incidence and Demographics
- Rates are equal in men and women.
- Onset is most common during adolescence or early adulthood.
  - Age of onset is earlier in men (usually age 15) than women (usually age 20).

Risk Factors
- Genetic loading
  - Familial transmission pattern
    - Disease rates higher in individuals with a first-degree relative who has OCD than in the general population.
    - Rates are also higher in individuals with a first-degree relative who has Tourette's syndrome than in the general population.

Assessment
History—Assess for the Following:
- Diagnostic criteria
  - Presence of *either* obsessions *or* compulsions
  - The individual recognizing that the obsession or compulsion is excessive or unreasonable
  - The obsession or compulsion is causing marked distress, is time-consuming, or interferes with normal daily activity.

- Common obsessions include
  - Repeated thoughts about contamination, dirt, or germs
  - Repeated doubts, such as having hit someone with a car or having left an oven on, without evidence
  - Need to have things in a specific order, with marked distress when that order is disturbed
  - Aggressive or horrific impulses
  - Sexual imagery.
- Obsessions usually do not involve real-world worries such as concern over finances.
- An individual recognizes that the thought, impulse, or images are a product of his or her own mind.
- An individual attempts to ignore or suppress thoughts, impulse, or images or to override them with other thoughts or actions.
- Individuals often avoid situations in which content of obsession may be encountered (e.g., avoiding public restrooms to avoid contamination).

- Common compulsions include
  - Repetitive actions, usually behavioral, and often called *rituals*
  - Level III anxiety levels
  - Common behaviors include
    - Hand washing
    - Excessive cleaning

- Checking to see, for example, if the lights are turned off, the stove is turned off, or the doors are locked
- Ordering behaviors.

- Common mental actions include
  - Counting
  - Silently repeating words
  - Praying.

- Behaviors or mental acts are not experienced as pleasurable and are intended to prevent or reduce distress and subjective anxiety.
- If the individual resists the compulsion, anxiety and subjective tension usually increase.
- Some individuals believe the compulsion can prevent some dreaded event or situation that is experienced as an obsession, such as sexual or horrific images.

Differential Diagnosis
- Body dysmorphic disorder
- Eating disorders
- Trichotillomania
- Hypochondriasis
- Obsessive–compulsive personality disorder
- Tic or stereotypic movement disorder.

Physical Exam Findings
- Nonspecific
- Dermatitis often present related to excessive hand washing or overuse of caustic cleaning agents.
- Hypochondriasis and somatic fixation common.

Mental Status Exam Findings
- Consistent with finding for anxiety
- Thought content dominated by obsessions
- Behavioral manifestations of rituals may be noted.

Diagnostic and Laboratory Findings
- Nonspecific.

Common Comorbidities
- Major depression
- Eating disorders
- Other anxiety disorders.

Clinical Management
- Follow guidelines of general clinical management of anxiety disorders.

Pharmacological Management
- SSRIs
- TCAs.

Nonpharmacological Management
- CBT
- Behavioral therapies.

Life Span Considerations

Children
- Common in childhood, usually with prepubertal onset
- More common in boys than girls
- Washing, checking, and ordering the most common behavioral manifestations
- Common comorbidities in children:
  - Learning disorders
  - Disruptive behavioral disorders
  - Tourette's syndrome.
- Associated in children with Group A beta-hemolytic streptococcal infections (e.g., scarlet fever, strep throat).

Older Adults
- More obsessions than compulsions usually present
- Obsessive content characteristically about dying
- Compulsions characteristically about washing and cleaning.

Posttraumatic Stress Disorder (PTSD)

Description
- PTSD is the reexperiencing of an extremely traumatic event accompanied by symptoms of increased arousal and avoidance of stimuli associated with the trauma.
- The traumatic event can be experienced directly or witnessed.

- Common *experienced* trauma includes
  - Military combat
  - Violent personal assault such as robbery or rape
  - Kidnapping or hostage situation
  - Terrorist attack
  - Torture
  - Prolonged sexual abuse
  - Natural or human-made disasters.

- Common *witnessed* trauma includes
  - Observing the death of or significant injury to another
  - Unexpectedly witnessing any of the above traumas
  - Learning of the sudden or unexpected death of or significant injury to a family member or close friend.

- A relationship exists between the individual's physical proximity to the traumatic event and the likelihood of symptom onset.

Risk Factors

*   Genetic loading
    *   Assumed to have strong genetic etiological component and tends to run in families
    *   Experienced trauma or witnessed trauma
    *   History of major depression in first-degree relative related to increased risk of developing PTSD.

Assessment

History–Assess for the Following:

*   Symptoms cannot predate exposure to trauma.
*   Presenting symptoms and history can be delineated as one of *three subtypes:*
    *   *Acute*—Duration of symptoms less than 3 months
    *   *Chronic*—Symptoms lasting 3 months or longer
    *   *Delayed onset*—At least 6 months between traumatic event and the onset of symptoms.

*   *Diagnostic Criteria (symptoms for 1 month or longer)*
    *   Exposure to a traumatic event
        *   The individual experienced, witnessed, or was confronted with an event involving actual or threatened death or serious injury, *and* the individual's response involved intense fear, helplessness, or horror.

    *   The traumatic event is persistently reexperienced in one or more of the following:
        *   One or more reexperiencing symptoms
            *   Recurrent and intrusive distressing recollection of the event, including images, thoughts, and perceptions
                *   May be experienced as flashbacks
                *   Rare cases involve dissociative states lasting hours to days.

        *   Recurrent distressing dreams about the event
        *   Acting or feeling as if the traumatic event were recurring
        *   Intense psychological distress at exposure to cues that symbolize or resemble aspects of the traumatic event
        *   Physiological reactivity on exposure to cues that symbolize or resemble aspects of the traumatic event.

        *   Three or more avoidance symptoms
            *   Persistent avoidance of stimuli associated with the traumatic event and numbing of responsiveness
            *   Efforts to avoid talking about or thinking about traumatic event
            *   Avoidance of activities, places, or people that arouse recollections of traumatic event
            *   Inability to recall important aspects of event
            *   Marked decreased interest or participation in activities
            *   Feelings of detachment or estrangement from others
            *   Restricted range of affect
            *   Sense of foreboding and of shortened future, or premature death, or no expectation for success or happiness.

- Two or more increased arousal symptoms
  - Persistent symptoms of increased arousal
    - Difficulty falling asleep
    - Irritability or outburst of anger
    - Difficulty concentrating
    - Hypervigilance
    - Exaggerated startle response.
  - Symptoms causing significant distress or impairment in the ability to carry out activities of daily functioning
  - Symptoms usually occur within 3 months of trauma
  - Duration of symptoms highly variable
    - Symptoms remitting within 3 months in one-half of cases
    - Common waxing and waning of symptoms related to internal and external cues that resemble the trauma.

Differential Diagnosis
- Adjustment disorder
- Brief psychotic disorder
- Acute stress disorder
- Intrusive thoughts in OCD.

Physical Exam Findings
- Nonspecific
- Increased rates of somatic complaints
- Insomnia frequently chief complaint on presentation for evaluation
- Distractibility in motor tasks
- Measurable increased autonomic functioning
  - Tachycardia
  - Diaphoresis
  - Increased respiratory rates
  - Pupilary dilation
  - Increased startle response.

Mental Status Exam Findings
- Consistent with finding for anxiety
- Thought content consistent with criteria for PTSD and often dominated by traumatic experience
- May demonstrate some psychotic findings during flashback episodes.

Diagnostic and Laboratory Findings
- Nonspecific.

Clinical Management
- Follow guidelines of general clinical management of anxiety disorders.

Pharmacological Management
- SSRIs
- TCAs

- BNZs
- Antipsychotics during episodes of flashbacks.

Nonpharmacological Management
- CBT
- Supportive group therapy
- Relaxation therapies
- Eye movement desensitization and reprocessing.

Common Comorbidities
- Major depression
- Dysthymia
- Substance abuse or dependence.

Life Span Considerations
- Can occur at any age, including childhood.

Children
- Expression of fear and horror occurs in disorganized or agitated behavior.
- Repetitive play behaviors show themes or aspects of trauma.
- Frightening dreams, but without recognized content, are common.

Generalized Anxiety Disorder (GAD)

Description
- In GAD, excessive worry, apprehension, or anxiety about events or activities occurs more days than not for a period of at least 6 months.
  - The individual finds it hard to control the anxiety.
  - No clear link exists for the anxiety to life events or stressors.
  - Worry and anxiety interfere with activities of daily living.
  - The nature and focus of worry shift frequently.
  - A pattern of waxing and waning of symptoms exists.
- Symptoms worsen as life events stress the individual.

Incidence and Demographics
- Onset usually by age 20
- More frequent in women than in men
  - Two-thirds of patients are female.

Risk Factors
- Genetic loading, with familial pattern of transmission.

Assessment

History–Assess for the Following:

- In GAD, anxiety and worry are out of proportion to the actual likelihood or impact of the feared event.
  - Individuals report subjective distress caused by the constant worry but do not always describe the worry as excessive.
- Excessive anxiety and worry last for more days than not for at least 6 months.
- The individual finds it difficult to control anxiety.

Differential Diagnosis

- PTSD
- Adjustment disorder with anxiety
- Obsessions in OCD
- Anxiety associated with another disorder such as hypochondriasis or social phobia.

Physical Exam Findings

- Nonspecific
- Associated with other health states
  - Irritable bowel syndrome
  - Migraine and other headache disorders.
- Physical signs of anxiety include
  - Muscle tension
  - Generalized muscle ache and soreness
  - Tremors
  - Twitching
  - Subjective complaints of shakiness
  - Shortness of breath
  - Autonomic hyperarousal signs
  - Tachycardia
  - Increased respiratory rates
  - Dizziness
  - Numbness
  - Easily fatigued, often experienced as activity intolerance
  - Muscle tension and increased tone
  - Sleep disturbance.

Mental Status Exam Findings

Appearance

- Psychomotor restlessness.

Mood

- Anxious
- Feeling keyed up or on edge
- Irritability.

Concentration

- Difficulty concentrating.

Thought Content
- Thematic for the anxiety and worry
- Descriptive of the significant distress and impairment in daily functioning caused by GAD.

Diagnostic and Laboratory Findings
- Nonspecific.

Clinical Management
Pharmacological Management
- SSRIs
- Buspar
- BNZs as prn agents.

Nonpharmacological Management
- Good candidates for therapy as single-treatment modality
- CBT
- Relaxation therapies
- Stress management
- Supportive counseling.

Common Comorbidities
- Mood disorders
- Other anxiety disorders
- Substance-related disorders.

Life Span Considerations
Children
- Anxiety is common in children, but it is important to assess normal vs. pathological levels.
- Anxiety is manifested in excessive worry over competence or quality of performance in school or work, sports, or other activities.
- Common worry often manifests as anxiety over punctuality or natural catastrophes such as earthquakes or war.
- Often accompanied by
  - Overly conforming behavior
  - Perfectionist self-expectations
  - Excessive seeking of approval of others
  - Need for frequent reassurance about performance.

Case Study

John, a 47-year-old teacher, has a long-standing history of GAD. He had been doing well until about 4 weeks ago. At that time he was traveling overseas with his church group, participating in a caring mission in South America. He began to feel more and more depressed and anxious as he saw the "poverty and despair" in developing countries. He started not sleeping and having "bad dreams" whenever he did try to sleep. He is beginning to think he is physically sick, as his anxiety is now beginning to interfere with work, and he is worried that he may need to be in the hospital to find out "what's wrong with me."

One week ago John began to feel overwhelmingly anxious, was convinced he was dying, and had the first of six discrete episodes that he calls "panic attacks." He went to the local ER and was diagnosed with anxiety and given Valium 5 mg #30 to use prn. At first he felt like the Valium was helping, but now he is feeling "like nothing helps." He is increasingly despondent, sure he is dying and that no one will believe him, and has contemplated suicide. He says he would not do it but is bothered by thinking about suicide. He is having increased tremors with anxiety, headaches, and nausea, which the ER diagnosed as anxiety reaction. His wife agrees that all of his symptoms are anxiety, but she reports that he is sure he is dying of cancer and no one will tell him the truth.

Mental Status Exam Findings
- Appearance: Well nourished, well dressed
- Motor: Some motor restlessness
- Speech: Some slowing and underproduction
- Affect: Anxious
- Mood: Depressed
- Thought process/content: Thematic for fear of becoming sicker and dying early; some vague suicidality without intent or plan; denies delusions or hallucinations
- Abstractive on proverbs
- Memory: Impaired
- Concentration: Impaired.

Social History
- Married and has three children
- Works as high school gym teacher
- Overweight at 280 lbs., with sedentary lifestyle
- Smokes two packs of cigarettes a day
- Does not drink alcohol for religious reasons
- Wife very concerned and supportive.

Past Psychiatric History
- Hospitalized in 1998 for "nerves"
- At that time started on Paxil 20 mg/d
- After 3 months, dose raised to 40 mg/d; has been doing well until recently
- Has had no significant exacerbation of symptoms since initial treatment.

Past Medical History
- History of seizure disorder since childhood; well controlled with meds
- Recent exposure to tuberculosis during international travel.

Current Medications
- Paxil 40 mg/d
- Valium 5 mg po prn q 4 hrs.
- Isoniazid for prophylaxis treatment for 6 months.

Labs
- All labs within normal limits.

Screening Tools
- Beck Anxiety Inventory (BAI): Severe score range.

There are many issues to consider in planning care for John:
- What is the most likely diagnosis?
- How will you separate comorbidity from complications of current diagnosis?
- What medication adjustments would you make?
- How will you address the family issues?
- How often will you plan to see the client?

Review Questions

1. The psychodynamic theory of anxiety states that the etiology of anxiety is

    a. Conflict between the id and the superego
    b. Conflict between the ego and the id
    c. Interpersonal conflict between significant others
    d. Perceived disapproval from significant others

2. The interpersonal theory of anxiety states that the etiology of anxiety is

    a. Conflict between the id and the superego
    b. Conflict between the ego and the id
    c. Distortions in perceived interpersonal relationships with significant others
    d. Perceived disapproval from significant others

3. Mr. Zimms is admitted to the hospital with a diagnosis of OCD. He exhibits high use of defense mechanisms; has automatic behavior, physical discomfort, and feelings of dread and horror; and is trembling and ritualistically washing his hands. You would assess his level of anxiety as

    a. Mild
    b. Moderate
    c. Severe
    d. Panic

4. Which of the following levels of anxiety is considered normal and useful in motivating a person to action?

    a. Mild
    b. Moderate
    c. Severe
    d. Panic

References and Resources

American Nurses Association. (2000). *Scope and standards of psychiatric–mental health clinical nursing practice.* Washington, DC: Author.

American Psychiatric Association. (2000). *Diagnostic and statistical manual of mental disorders* (4th ed., text rev.). Washington, DC: Author.

Bremner, J. D. (2002). Neuroimaging studies in post-traumatic stress disorder. *Current Psychiatric Reports, 4,* 254–263.

Christensen, D. D. (2001). The challenge of obsessive–compulsive hoarding. *Primary Psychiatry, 6* (2), 79–84.

Davidson, J. R. (2000). Trauma: The impact of post-traumatic stress disorder. *Journal of Psychopharmacology, 14* (Suppl. 1), 5–12.

Gold, P. W., & Chrousos, G. (1998). The endocrinology of melancholic and atypical depression: Relation to neurocircuitry and somatic consequences. *Proceedings of the Association of American Physicians, 111* (1), 22–34.

Goodman, W. K., Price, L. H., Rasmussen, S. A., Mazure, C., Fleischmann, R. L., Hill, S. A., et al. (1989). The Yale–Brown obsessive-compulsive scale I: Development, use, and reliability. *Archives of General Psychiatry, 46,* 1006–1011.

Gould, E., Reeves, A. J., & Fallah, M. (1999). Hippocampal neurogenesis in adult Old World primates. *Proceedings of the National Academy of Sciences USA, 96,* 5263–5267.

Guess, K. (2006). Posttraumatic stress disorder: Early detection is key. *The Nurse Practitioner, 31* (3), 1–8.

Hamilton, M. (1959). The assessment of anxiety states by rating. *British Journal of Medical Psychology, 32* (1), 50–55.

Hembree, E. (2002). Psychosocial treatment of post-traumatic stress disorder. *Primary Psychiatry, 9* (2), 49–52.

Margolin, G., & Gordis, E. B. (2000). The effects of family and community violence on children. *Annual Review of Psychology, 51,* 445–479.

Mathew, J. (2002). Future pharmacotherapy for post-traumatic stress disorder: Prevention and treatment. *Psychiatric Clinics of North America, 25,* 427–441.

Meredith, P. V., & Horan, N. M. (2000). *Adult primary care.* Philadelphia: W. B. Saunders.

Narrow, W. E., Rae, D. S., & Regier, D. A. (1998). *NIMH epidemiology note: Prevalence of anxiety disorders. One-year prevalence best estimates calculated from ECA and NCS data.* Washington, DC: National Institute of Mental Health.

National Institute of Mental Health, Genetics Workgroup. (1998). *Genetics and mental disorders* (NIH Publication No. 98-4268). Rockville, MD: Author.

Regier, D. A., Rae, D. S., & Narrow, W. E. (1998). Prevalence of anxiety disorders and their comorbidity with mood and addictive disorders. *British Journal of Psychiatry* (Suppl. 34), 24–28.

Stuart, G. W., & Laraia, M. (2001). *Principles and practice of psychiatric nursing.* St. Louis, MO: Mosby.

Turner, S. (1999). Place of pharmacotherapy in PTSD. *The Lancet, 354,* 1404–1407.

Yehuda, R. (1999). Biological factors associated with susceptibility to posttraumatic stress disorder. *Canadian Journal of Psychiatry, 44*(1), 34–39.

Yehuda, R. (2000). Biology of posttraumatic stress disorder. *Journal of Clinical Psychiatry, 61*(Suppl. 7), 14–21.

Zung, W. W. K. (1971). A rating instrument for anxiety disorders. *Psychometrics, 12,* 371–379.

Notes:

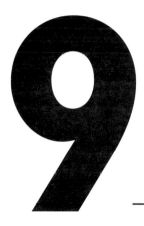

Schizophrenia and Other Psychotic Disorders

This chapter describes a category of illnesses that represents some of the most debilitating of the psychiatric disorders. Schizophrenia, the prototypic disease of this category of illnesses, is a multifaceted disorder that gravely affects an individual's ability to function in many spheres of daily life. It is the psychotic illness that has been most heavily researched in the past few years and the one we know the most about.

The other illness states that make up this category of disorders will be presented after the in-depth discussion of schizophrenia. Almost all of the information provided for schizophrenia and for the clinical management of this disorder will pertain to the other psychotic disorders presented in this chapter.

General Description of Psychotic Disorders

- These brain-based psychiatric disorders are grouped together because of similarity in frequent psychotic symptoms, but each has somewhat different etiologies.
- Psychotic disorders are one of the most debilitating classes of psychiatric disorders, as determined by the degree of functional impairment and financial burden of this chronic illness.
- *Psychotic* implies inability to test reality.
  - Manifests in symptoms such as (see Table 9–1)
    - Hallucinations
    - Delusions
    - Disorganized thinking and speech
    - Referential thinking
    - Frequent illusional perceptions.
- Psychotic disorders are generally known to have a strong genetic component.

Schizophrenia

Description
- Schizophrenia causes significant disturbance in many areas of functioning:
  - Cognition

- Perception
- Emotionality
- Behavior
- Movement
- Socialization.

Etiology

- Multiple theories exist, ranging from psychological to neurobiological.
- A probable multifactorial etiological profile exists.

Biological Theory

- Implicates three areas of biological functioning: genetics, neurodevelopment, and neurobiological defects

    - Genetics
        - Studies of twins have identified schizophrenia as having a strong genetic etiological component.
        - Incidence increases from 1% risk of illness in general population to
            - 50% risk in monozygotic twin of a person with schizophrenia
            - 15% risk in dizygotic twin of a person with schizophrenia
            - 40% risk in children if both parents have schizophrenia.

    - No one specific gene has yet been identified.
    - A polygenic single nucleotide polymorphism (SNP) defect is believed to exist.
    - Chromosomes 5, 6, 8, 11, 18, 19, and 22 have been implicated (Gershon & Badner, 2001).

Table 9–1. Symptoms of Psychosis

Clinical Manifestation	Definition	Type
Hallucinations	False sensory experience without a stimuli being present	(Arranged in order of commonality) Auditory Visual Tactile Olfactory Gustatory NOTE: *Hypnopompic** and *Hypnogogic*** are considered normative and do not fall under the true definition of hallucinations.
Delusions	A false belief firmly maintained despite evidence to the contrary	Persecutory Religious Grandiosity Somatic Referential Jealousy Erotomanic

Table 9–1. Continued

Clinical Manifestation	Definition	Type
Disorganized thinking (often referred to as *formal thought disturbance* or *disorder*)	Problems with information organization and interpretation that are best assessed in the speech patterns of patients	Loose association Derailment Tangentiality Word salad
Disorganized behavior	Unusual behavior ranging from childlike silliness to anger. Is a symptom of schizophrenia.	Silliness Unpredictable anger Difficulties with activities of daily living Disheveled Odd or unusual dress Inappropriate sexual activity Stereotypic motor activities
Referential thinking and delusions of control	Belief that events, actions, or situations in the environment hold special significance or meaning	Thought insertion Thought withdrawal Thought control Thought broadcasting
Illusional perceptions	Misperception of actual environmental stimuli	Auditory Visual Tactile Olfactory Gustatory

*Hypnopompic hallucination—A false perception that occurs when one is waking up.
**Hypnogogic hallucination—A false perception that occurs when one is falling asleep. Not considered pathological.

- Neurodevelopment
    - Genetic defects are believed to cause abnormal neuronal cell development, connection, organization, and migration.
    - These include inadequate synapse formation, excessive pruning of synapses, and excitotoxic death of neurons.
    - Intrauterine insults may contribute to etiological picture:
        - Prenatal exposure to toxins, including viral agents
        - Oxygenation deprivation
        - Maternal malnutrition, substance use, or other illness.
- Neurobiological Defect
    - Several abnormal brain structures have been identified in individuals with schizophrenia:
        - Enlarged ventricles
        - Smaller frontal and temporal lobes
        - Cortical atrophy

- Decreased cerebral blood flow
- Hippocampal reduction (Lencz, Bilder, & Cornblatt, 2001).
- Abnormalities lead to suspected impaired neuronal communication:
  - Suspected alterations in chemical neuronal signal transmission
    - Excess dopamine in mesolimbic pathway
    - Decreased dopamine in the mesocortical pathway
    - Excess glutamate
    - Decreased gamma-aminobutyric acid (GABA)
    - Decreased serotonin.

Incidence and Demographics

- Schizophrenia affects approximately 1%–1.5% of the U.S. population.
- Geographic and historical variations in incidence give insight into etiological factors:
  - Higher rates in urban-born individuals
  - Higher rates in first-born individuals
  - Higher rates in individuals with lower socioeconomic status.
- Schizophrenia is equally prevalent in men and women.
  - *Men*—Onset ages 18–25 years
    - Tend to have more negative symptoms than women
    - Tend to have poorer prognosis, more hospitalizations, and less responsiveness to medications than women.
  - *Women*—Onset ages 25–35 years
    - Usually have less premorbid dysfunction than men
    - Usually experience more dysphoria than men
    - Tend to have paranoid delusions and more hallucinations than men.
- Age of onset has pathophysiological and prognostic significance
  - *Characteristics of Earlier Age of Onset*
    - Tend to be men
    - Have poorer premorbid functioning
    - Have more evidence of structural brain abnormalities
    - Have more prominent negative symptoms
    - Have more cognitive impairment
    - Have poorer prognosis.
  - *Characteristics of Later Age of Onset*
    - Tend to be women
    - Have less evidence of structural abnormalities
    - Have less cognitive impairment
    - Have better prognosis.

Possible Risk Factors

- Genetic loading
  - First-order relative with schizophrenia.
- Prenatal exposure to flu or virus
- Prenatal malnutrition
- Obstetrical complications
- Central nervous system (CNS) infection in early childhood.

Prevention and Screening

- At-risk family education
- Community education
  - Stigma reduction
  - Signs and symptoms of illness
  - Treatment potential for control of symptoms.

- Early recognition, intervention, and initiation of treatment
  - Significant and protracted prodromal symptom period usually noted before full onset of illness
  - Usually mild manifestations of criteria symptoms:
    - Odd or unusual beliefs but not to delusional proportion
    - Feel unliked or picked on but not to delusional proportion
    - Odd speech patterns but not illogical
      - Digressions
      - Tangentiality.

  - Overly concrete or abstractive
  - Odd behavior but not disorganized
    - Collects odd or worthless items
    - Mumbles to self
    - Isolates self and avoids interaction with others.

Assessment

History—Assess for the Following:

- There exists no single pathognomonic symptom of schizophrenia but rather a constellation of clustered symptoms.
- Schizophrenia is a disease of information processing.
- The clusters of symptoms are behavioral and cognitive.
- The illness is associated with marked social or occupational functioning.
- Prominent dysfunction exists in many spheres of daily living.

Interpersonal Relationships

- 60%–70% of clients do not marry.

Social or Occupational Functioning

- "Downdrift" functionality is noted over time.
  - Go less far in school than unaffected siblings
  - Have difficulty holding jobs
  - Are underemployed relative to intellectual capacity.

Self-Care Deficits

- Poor hygiene
- Poor money management
- Limited ability for independent living.

Characteristic symptom clusters for the illness (see Table 9–2) include
- Positive symptom cluster
- Negative symptom cluster
- Associated symptoms.

Table 9–2. Positive and Negative Symptom Clusters of Schizophrenia

Symptom Cluster	Explanation	Clinical Manifestations
Positive symptoms	• Symptoms that respond positively to and that can be controlled by typical antipsychotic medications • Reflect excesses or distortions of normal brain functioning • Caused by increased dopamine in the mesolimbic pathway	Hallucinations Delusions Referential thinking Disorganized behavior Hostility Grandiosity Mania Suspiciousness
Negative symptoms	• Symptoms less responsive to typical antipsychotic medications but may respond to and be controlled by atypical antipsychotic medications • Represent a decrease or loss of normal functioning • Caused by decreased dopamine in the mesocortical pathway	Affective flattening Alogia or poverty of speech Avolition Apathy Abstract-thinking problems Anhedonia Attention deficits
Associated symptoms	• Symptoms not required to be present to diagnose condition but often are present and a focus of treatment	Inappropriate affect Dysphoric mood Depersonalization Derealization High anxiety

DSM-IV-TR (American Psychiatric Association, 2000)
Diagnostic Criteria for Schizophrenia
- Two or more of the following frequently are present during a 1-month period (only one if delusions are bizarre or hallucinations consist of a voice that is running commentary or two or more voices conversing with each other):
  - *Delusions*—Bizarre and unorganized type; examples include delusions that manifest as loss of control over mind or body:
    - Thought withdrawal
    - Thought insertion.

  - *Hallucinations*—Bizarre and unorganized type; examples include hallucinations that are improbable or readily apparent as not likely to have occurred

- Disorganized speech
- Grossly disorganized behavior
- Presence of negative symptoms.

- Significant impairment usually is evident by social or occupational dysfunction.
- Duration of symptoms lasts for at least 6 months.

- Complete remission is uncommon.
- The course of illness is variable.
  - Many clients have a fairly stable illness course.
  - Some clients have clear episodic remissions and exacerbation periods.
  - Negative symptoms tend to appear first as the illness develops.
  - Positive symptoms appear to decrease over time, but negative symptoms persist.

Factors Predictive of Good Prognosis

- Good premorbid functioning
- Acute onset
- Later age of onset
- Clear precipitating event
- Married client
- Good support system
- Positive symptoms
- Short interval between treatment and onset of first symptoms
  - The sooner the client is treated, the better the prognosis.
  - The longer the premorbid period is untreated, the worse the prognosis.

- Absence of structural brain abnormalities
- Family history of mood disorders
- No family history of schizophrenia.

Subtypes of Schizophrenia

- Subtypes are defined by predominant patient symptomatology (see Table 9–3).
  - *Disorganized type*—Most severe type
  - *Paranoid type*—Least severe type
  - *Catatonic type*
  - *Undifferentiated type*
  - *Residual type.*

- Subtype identification is of limited clinical value, because illness course, response to treatment, and prognosis appear unrelated to subtype.

Table 9–3. Subtypes of Schizophrenia

Subtype	Characteristic
Paranoid	Prominent delusions or auditory hallucinations Lack of prominence of disorganized speech or behavior
Disorganized	Prominence of disorganized speech, behavior, and flat or inappropriate affect

Continued on the next page

Table 9–3. Continued

Subtype	Characteristic
Catatonic	Prominence of motor symptoms, including immobility as evidenced by catalepsy or stupor, excessive motor movement that is purposeless and not influenced by environmental stimuli, extreme negativity, mutism, oddities of posturing, echolalia,* and echopraxia**
Undifferentiated	Presence of symptoms consistent with schizophrenia but not a prominence of symptoms consistent with any of the other subtypes
Residual	Absence of prominent delusions, hallucinations, disorganized speech, and disorganized or catatonic behavior, and the continued presence of disturbance as indicated by presence of negative symptoms

Echolalia—Repetition of the last-heard words of other individuals.
**Echopraxia*—Imitation of observed behavior or movements.

Physical Exam Findings
- Abnormal smooth pursuit eye movement
- Abnormal saccadic eye movement
- Poor eye–hand coordination
    - Client identified as "clumsy" or "awkward."

- Presence of neurological nonlocalizing "soft signs"
    - *Astereognosis*—Loss of ability to judge the form of an object by touch
    - Twitches, tics, or rapid eye blinking
    - *Dysdiadochokinesia*—Impairment of the ability to perform rapidly alternating movements
    - Impaired fine-motor movement
    - Left–right confusion
    - Mirroring.

- Presence of neurological localizing "hard signs"
    - Weakness
    - Decreased reflexes.

- Other abnormalities that may be noted:
    - Highly arched palate
    - Narrow or wide-set eyes
    - Subtle malformations of the ears.

Mental Status Exam Findings
Appearance
- Odd
- Unusual
- Peculiar.

Speech
- Bizarre content
- Disorganized
- Tangential
- Loose association.

Affect
- Blunted
- Flat
- Inappropriate.

Mood
- Blandness
- Impoverished.

Thought Process
- Psychotic
  - Hallucination
  - Delusion
  - Referential
  - Thought control, insertion, or withdrawal.

Thought Content
- Thematically matched to psychotic content
- May be impoverished.

Cognition
- Illogical
- Disorganized.

Orientation
- Usually intact.

Memory
- Impaired short term.

Concentration
- Impaired during acute episodes.

Abstraction
- Concrete on formal testing.

Judgment
- Impaired for self-welfare.

Diagnostic and Laboratory Findings
- No specific diagnostic lab findings exist.

Abnormalities Noted in Structural Studies
- Enlargement of lateral ventricles
- Widened cortical sulci
- Diffuse decrease in volume of white and gray matter
- Decreased volume of temporal lobe
- Hypovolume in hippocampus, amygdala, and thalamus (Lencz, Bilder, & Cornblatt, 2001).

Abnormalities Noted in Functional Studies
- Hypofrontality
- Decreased cerebral blood flow and metabolism
- Diffuse hypometabolic action in cortical–subcortical circuitry.

Differential Diagnosis
Nonpsychiatric Disorders
- Epilepsy
- CNS neoplasm
- AIDS
- Acute intermittent porphyria
- B_{12} deficiency
- Heavy-metal poisoning
- Huntington's disease
- Neurosyphilis
- Systemic lupus erythematosus
- Wernicke–Korsakoff syndrome
- Wilson's disease.

Psychiatric Disorders
- Bipolar affective disorder
- Substance-induced psychotic disorder
  - Amphetamines
  - Hallucinogens
  - Alcoholic hallucinosis
  - Barbiturate withdrawal
  - Cocaine
  - PCP.

- Mood disorders with psychotic features (see Chapter 7)
- Schizoaffective disorder (see below)
- Schizophreniform disorder (see below)
- Brief psychotic disorder (see below)
- Delusional disorder (see below)
- Schizotypal personality disorder (see Chapter 12)
- Schizoid personality disorder (see Chapter 12)
- Paranoid personality disorder (see Chapter 12).

Clinical Management
- Assess for acuity level.
  - During acute psychotic episodes, client may require brief hospitalization to
    - Ensure client safety
    - Rapidly stabilize client's symptom level in a controlled environment
    - Monitor client adherence with treatment to reach stabilization.

- Clinical management during nonacute episodes occurs most often in community settings.

Pharmacological Management
- Pharmacological therapy is the primary treatment modality.
- *Atypical antipsychotics* (second generation; see Table 9–4)
  - Primary first-line treatment agents
  - First introduced in the 1990s
  - Have less significant neurological side effects
  - Effectively treat positive *and* negative symptoms
  - Function as serotonin–dopamine antagonists
    - D_2 and 5HT2a blockade.

  - Expensive; no generic forms at present
  - Have less clinically significant side effects
  - Can cause extrapyramidal side effects (EPS; see five common types in Table 9–5) but is much less significant an issue than with typical antipsychotics
    - Not known to produce tardive dyskinesia (TD; see below).

  - Improved compliance
  - *Mode of Action:* Positive symptoms are decreased by the blockade of dopamine in the mesolimbic pathway. Serotonin inhibits dopamine. Negative symptoms are decreased when serotonin dopamine antagonists (SDAs) block serotonin; therefore, dopamine increases in the mesocortical pathway.
  - *Dopamine Pathways:* These explain both the therapeutic effects *and* the side effects of the atypical antipsychotics.
    - *Mesolimbic Pathway*—SDAs block dopamine in this pathway, causing decreased positive symptoms.
    - *Mesocortical Pathway*—SDAs increase dopamine in this pathway, causing decreased negative symptoms.
    - *Nigrostriatal Pathway*—Dopamine has a reciprocal relationship with acetylcholine (ACh). When serotonin is blocked by the SDA, dopamine increases; therefore, ACh decreases, which causes decreased EPS (EPS is caused by increased ACh).
    - *Tuberoinfundibular Pathway*—Dopamine inhibits prolactin. The blockade of dopamine by SDAs causes prolactin to increase, causing galactorrhea.
      - Hyperprolactinemia associated with the antipsychotics may cause sexual problems, galactorrhea, amenorrhea, and bone demineralization in postmenopausal women not on estrogen.

Table 9–4. Atypical (Second-Generation) Antipsychotics

Drug	Brand Name	Dosage Forms/ Daily Dosage	Side Effects	Comments
Clozapine	Clozaril	Tablet/25–900 mg/d	*Common:* Tachycardia, drowsiness, dizziness, sialorrhea, weight gain, hyperlipidemia *Rare:* Agranulocytosis, myocarditis, neuroleptic malignant syndrome	• Only drug for treatment-resistant schizophrenia • White blood count (WBC) monitoring required due to risk of agranulocytosis • During first 6 months: weekly; during second 6 months: every 2 weeks; then monthly if WBC/ANC normal • Monitor for myocarditis • Dose-related seizure risk • Significant weight gain and risk of diabetes • No prolactin elevation
Quetiapine	Seroquel	Tablet/50–800 mg/d	*Common:* Sedation and hypotension, weight gain *Rare:* Cataract formation	• Less weight gain than with Clozaril or Zyprexa • Transient and asymptomatic elevated LFTs • Monitor for cataract development • Divided doses: bid or tid • No prolactin elevation
Olanzapine	Zyprexa	Tablet/5–20 mg/d	Sedation, weight gain, hyperlipidemia, elevated glucose, elevated LFTs, mild prolactin elevation	• Significant weight gain • Monitor BMI, waist circumference • Monitor serum lipids • Monitor blood sugar
Risperidone	Risperdal, Risperdal Consta	Tablet, Liquid, Injectable/2–6 mg/d	Hypotension, galactorrhea nausea, insomnia	• Doses >6 mg associated with a higher incidence of extrapyramidal symptoms • Less weight gain than with Clozaril or Zyprexa • Greatest prolactin elevation among atypical psychotics

Table 9–4. Continued

Drug	Brand Name	Dosage Forms/ Daily Dosage	Side Effects	Comments
Ziprasidone	Geodon	Tablets, Injectable/ 40–160 mg/d	*Common:* Hypotension, sedation, dizziness *Rare:* Prolongation of QTc interval	• Requires QTc monitoring • Avoid coadministration with other drugs known to prolong QTc • Taking with food increases absorption twofold • Weight gain uncommon • Use extreme caution when administering with patients at risk for hypokalemia, hypomagnesemia, after myocardial infarction, or with congestive heart failure
Paliperidone	Invega	Tablets/3–12 mg/d	Orthostatic hypotension, hyperprolactinemia, GI upset, dizziness, headache	• Extended-release risperidone
Aripiprizole	Abilify	Tablets/5–30 mg/d	Headache, agitation, anxiety, insomnia, somnolence, akathisia, GI problems	• Is a partial agonist of D_2 receptors • Weight gain, elevated lipids, and blood glucose not problematic • Akathisia usually dissipates and is alleviated by short-term benzodiazepine

- Typical antipsychotics (first generation; see Table 9–6)
- Cross-classified as neuroleptics because of significant side effects
- First introduced in the 1950s
- Useful for treating positive symptoms by blocking dopamine in the mesolimbic pathway
- Can make negative symptoms worse by blocking dopamine in the mesocortical pathway
- Therapeutic effect related primarily to D_2 receptor blockade
- Inexpensive
- Can be used as sustained-released injectable agents
    - Decanoate long-acting injectable dose forms of typical antipsychotics:
        - Prolixin-D
        - Haldol-D.

- *High potency*—Have a greater risk of EPS but less risk of sedation and anticholinergic symptoms
- *Low potency*—Have a greater risk of sedation and anticholinergic side effects but less risk of EPS
- Caffeine and nicotine cause diminished antipsychotic effect; dose may need to be higher
- Because of multiple clinically significant side effects, are not considered first-line treatment agents
  - Side effects leading to poor compliance
  - High client teaching needs
  - Significant safety issues
  - EPS most common side effect.
    - Caused by D_2 receptor antagonism (when dopamine receptors are blocked, ACh increases, which causes EPS; a reciprocal relationship exists between ACh and dopamine).
    - Treated by use of anti-Parkinsonian drugs (cross-classified; see Table 9–7)
      - Anticholinergics
      - Antihistamines
      - Dopamine agonists
      - Benzodiazepines (BNZs).

- Tardive dyskinesia (TD)
  - TD is a potentially irreversible movement disorder that may occur in individuals who are treated for more than 1 year with typical antipsychotics.
  - Symptoms consist of abnormal, involuntary movements such as lip smacking, chewing, tongue protrusion, or twisting movements of the trunk or limbs.
  - Perioral movements are most common.
  - First-line treatment involves prevention and use of atypical antipsychotics.
  - Clients on typical antipsychotics should have routine abnormal involuntary muscle movement screening (see AIMS below) every 3–6 months.
  - If abnormal movements are noted, consider reducing the dosage or switching to an atypical antipsychotic.
  - Risk factors include
    - Long-term treatment with neuroleptics
    - Older age
    - Female gender
    - Presence of mood or cognitive disorder.

  - Abnormal Involuntary Movement Scale (AIMS; Guy, 1976)
  - After observing the client, rate symptoms on a scale (0 = none, 1 = minimal, 2 = mild, 3 = moderate, 4 = severe) according to the severity of symptoms.
  - Ensure that client does not have gum in his or her mouth.
  - Assess the following:
    - Gait as client is walking into the assessment area
    - Client's profile
    - Sitting in chair with feet on floor
    - Sitting in chair with hands hanging
    - Arms outstretched in front
    - Touching thumb to each finger
    - Opening mouth and protruding tongue
    - Flexing and extending arms.

- If symptoms are evident, ascertain client's awareness of them and if the symptoms are interfering with daily functioning.

- Neuroleptic malignant syndrome (NMS)
  - Rare but potentially life threatening
  - Can occur at any point during treatment
  - Most common with typical but has been reported with atypical antipsychotics
  - Risk factors include
    - Rapid dose escalation
    - Use of high-potency typical antipsychotics
    - Parental administration of antipsychotics.

  - Assess for the following abnormal labs:
    - Elevated creatine phosphokinase (CPK)
    - Elevated white blood cell count (WBC)
    - Elevated liver function tests (LFT).

  - Assess for symptoms known to occur first:
    - Altered sensorium
    - Hyperthermia
    - Hyper-reflexia.

  - Assess for symptoms of autonomic instability:
    - Hypotension
    - Extreme muscular rigidity
    - Hyperthermia
    - Tachycardia
    - Diaphoresis
    - Tachypnea
    - Coma and potentially death.

  - Treatment
    - Immediate medical intervention
    - Discontinuation of antipsychotic medications
    - Supportive therapies
    - Administration of Dantrium (dantrolene) or Parlodel (bromocriptine).

Table 9–5. Extrapyramidal Side Effects (EPS)

Side Effect	Definition
Akathisia	Motor restlessness; inability to remain still; rocking, pacing, or constant motion of unilateral limb; also can manifest as a subjective sense of restlessness without objective finding *Note:* Often mistaken for increasing anxiety
Akinesia	Absence of movement, difficulty initiating motion, subjective feeling of lack of motivation to move *Note:* Often mistaken for laziness or lack of interest

Continued on the next page

Table 9–5. Continued

Dystonia	Muscle spasm; spasticity of muscle group, especially back or neck muscles; subjectively painful but generally not clinically significant except as it affects adherence *Note:* Often mistaken for agitation or unusual, stereotypic movements characteristic of schizophrenia
Pseudo Parkinson's	Presence of symptoms of Parkinson's disorder produced by D_2 blockade; includes shuffling gait, motor slowing, mask-like facial expression, pill rolling, tremors, and muscle rigidity *Note:* Mask-like facial expression often confused as affective blunting or flattening
Tardive dyskinesia	Involuntary abnormal muscle movement of the mouth, tongue, face, and jaw that may progress to limbs; can be irreversible; can occur as an acute process at initiation of medications or as a chronic condition at any point in treatment

Table 9–6. Typical Antipsychotics

Drug	Brand Name	Dosage Forms/ Daily Dosage	Side Effects	Comments
Chlorpro-mazine	Thorazine	Tablet, SR, Liquid/ 50–2,000 mg/d	*High:* Sedation, hypotension *Moderate:* EPS, anticholinergic	Allergic dermatitis Photosensitivity EKG changes
Mesori-dazine	Serentil	Tablet, liquid, injection/100–400 mg/d	*High:* Anticholinergic, sedation, hypotension *Low:* EPS	EKG changes
Thioridazine	Mellaril	Tablet, Liquid/ 50–800 mg/d	*High:* Anticholinergic, sedation, hypotension, prolonged QT interval *Low:* EPS	QTc monitoring Irreversible retinal pigmentation at doses >800 mg/d Decreased libido Retrograde ejaculation
Fluphena-zine	Permitil Prolixin	Tablet, Liquid, Injection/2–40 mg/d, 12.5–75 mg/IM every 2 weeks (decanoate)	*Very high:* EPS *Low:* Anticholinergic, sedation, hypotension	
Perphen-azine	Trilafon	Tablet, Liquid, Injection/8–64 mg/d	*High:* EPS *Low:* Anticholinergic, sedation, hypotension	

Table 9–6. Continued

Drug	Brand Name	Dosage Forms/ Daily Dosage	Side Effects	Comments
Trifluo-perazine	Stelazine	Tablet, Injection/ 5–80 mg/d	*High:* EPS *Low:* Anticholinergic, sedation, hypotension	
Haldo-peridol	Haldol	Tablet, Liquid, Injection/2–40 mg/d, 50–300 mg IM, every month (decanoate)	*Very high:* EPS *High:* Anticholinergic, sedation *Low:* Hypotension	In elderly people, monitor for oculogyric crisis and pneumonia
Loxapine	Loxitane	Capsule, Liquid/ 20–250 mg/d	*High:* EPS *Moderate:* Sedation, hypotension *Low:* Anticholinergic	
Molindone	Moban	Tablet, Liquid/ 50–225 mg/d	*High:* EPS *Low:* Anticholinergic, hypotension *Very low:* Sedation	Little or no weight gain
Thiothixene	Navane	Capsule, Liquid, Injection/5–60 mg/d	*High:* EPS *Low:* Anticholinergic, Sedation, hypotension	

Table 9–7. Medications Used to Treat EPS Symptoms

Effective Drug and Cross-Classification	Akinesia	Akathisia	Dystonia	Pseudo-Parkinson's	Tardive Dyskinesia
Cogentin (benztropine): *Anticholinergic*	X	X	X	X	• Best treatment strategy is prevention through careful monitoring.
Kemadrin (procyclidine): *Anticholinergic*	X	X	X	X	• If present, treat by reducing current dose, or change client to atypical agent.
Artane (trihexyphenidyl): *Anticholinergic*	X	X	X	X	
Benadryl (diphenhydramine): *Antihistamine*	X		X	X	

Continued on the next page

Table 9–7. Continued

Effective Drug and Cross-Classification	Akinesia	Akathisia	Dystonia	Pseudo-Parkinson's	Tardive Dyskinesia
Symmetrel (amantadine): *Dopamine agonist*	X			X	
Inderal (propranolol): *Beta blocker*		X			
Catapres (clonidine): *Alpha 2 agonist*		X			
Klonopin (clonazepam): *Benzodiazepine*		X	X		
Ativan (lorazepam): *Benzodiazepine*		X	X		

- Other common side effects related to effects on receptors other than dopamine:
    - Alpha adrenergic blockade
        - Cardiovascular side effects
        - Orthostatic hypotension.
    - Muscarinic cholinergic blockade
        - Dry mouth
        - Blurred vision
        - Constipation
        - Urinary retention.
    - Endocrine side effects
        - Weight gain
        - Increased prolactin levels.
    - Neurological side effects
        - Lowering of seizure threshold.
    - Other side effects
        - Photosensitivity
        - Agranulocytosis.

Management

Pharmacological Management

- Most clients will require lifelong medication.
- Adjunctive medications may be used to achieve full symptom control
  - Antidepressants
  - Anxiolytics
  - Anticonvulsants.

Nonpharmacological Management

- Individual Therapy
  - Usually supportive rather than insight oriented
    - Focuses on establishing reality testing
    - Builds daily-life skills
    - Assists client in establishing and meeting life goals.
  - Cognitive-behavioral therapy (CBT) for management of hallucinations and delusions.

- Group Therapy
  - Focuses on problem solving
  - Focuses on education
    - Medication groups
    - Life-skills groups.
  - Proactive crisis-management planning to deal with potential relapse needs
    - Identify symptom triggers
    - Identify symptoms that indicate relapse
    - Identify past pattern of relapse to help predict future relapses
    - Identify self-care interventions
    - Identify point at which professional intervention is required
    - Identify support network of family and friends
    - Identify other resources to be mobilized when symptom level increases.

- Milieu Therapy
  - Provides for structure and safety needs
  - Provides socialization and interpersonal support
  - Encourages independency.

- Client and Family Education
  - Explain underlying pathology of illness
  - Discuss signs and symptoms
  - Assist in identifying strategies for living with illness
  - Assist in understanding and making decisions about care options
  - Develop relapse prevention plan
  - Promote overall health.

Common Comorbidities

- Rates of substance abuse and dependency are high.
  - 20%–40% comorbidity

- Nicotine dependence is especially high.
  - 80%–90% comorbidity
  - Tend to use cigarettes with highest nicotine content.
- Other common psychiatric comorbidities are anxiety disorders (see Chapter 8), especially panic disorder and obsessive–compulsive disorder.

General Health Considerations

- Schizophrenia is significantly associated with shorter-than-expected life span when compared to the general population.
  - Reasons are unclear but may include overall general lack of routine health care and high levels of comorbidity (see below).

Suicide

- Suicide rates are high; assess for suicidal ideations at every visit.
- 10% commit suicide.
- 20%–40% attempt suicide.
- Known risk factors for suicide include
  - Male gender
  - Ages 45 or younger
  - Presence of depressive symptoms
  - Hopelessness
  - Unemployed
  - Noncompliance
  - Recent hospitalization
  - Post-psychotic period
  - Comorbid substance abuse.

General Medical Illnesses

- Clients need access to ongoing primary care.
- Monitor client for development of diabetes, hypertension, respiratory illnesses, and cardiac illnesses.
  - Monitor weight gain, lipids, and blood sugar values over time.
  - Provide weight management and nutritional assistance.
  - Use the body mass index (BMI) as the accepted standard for determining if a client's weight places him or her at risk of developing serious health problems.
  - BMI categories
    - *Underweight*—BMI 18.5 or less
    - *Normal weight*—BMI 18.5–24.9
    - *Overweight*—BMI 25.0–29.9
    - *Obese*—BMI 30.0–39.9
    - *Severely obese*—BMI 40 and higher.
  - Risks related to BMI
    - Clients who are overweight to obese as determined by BMI have
      - 2.9 times increased risk for diabetes
      - 2.9 times increased risk for hypertension
      - 2.1 times increased risk of coronary artery disease
      - 3.0 times increased risk for endometrial cancer
      - 2.7 times increased risk for colon cancer.

Life Span Considerations

Children
- Hallucinatory and delusional content less rich, elaborate, and bizarre
- Visual hallucinations more common than auditory.

Older Adults
- More women than men with rare late onset
- Although exhibiting prodromal social isolation, are more often married
- Prognosis usually better; more responsive to medications due to dominance of positive symptom cluster (see below).

Risk Factors
- Postmenopausal states
- Presence of human leukocyte antigen
- Positive family history.

Symptoms
- Predominance of positive symptoms
- High levels of persecutory delusions and hallucinations
- Lower levels of disorganized behavior
- Preservation of social and occupational interest
- Fewer negative symptoms.

Follow-up

Chronic Illness
- Usually requires lifelong treatment
- Case management necessary to coordinate aspects of care.

Relapse Periods
- Develop relapse plan with client and family.

Multiple Health Needs
- Perform frequent assessment of general health status
- Address comorbid nicotine addiction.

Preventive Care
- Monitor routine labs to screen for complications of treatment
  - Blood sugar levels
  - Lipid panels
  - Hematology panels.
- Perform annual eye exam if on typical antipsychotic agent or Seroquel.

Clinical Outcome Measures
- Standardized rating scales include
  - Positive and Negative Syndrome Scale (PANSS; Kay & Fiszbein, 1987)
  - Brief Psychiatric Rating Scale (BPRS; Overall & Gorham, 1962)

- Scale for Assessment of Positive Symptoms (SAPS; Andreason & Olsen, 1982)
- Scale for Assessment of Negative Symptoms (SANS; Andreason, 1982).

Schizophreniform Disorder

Description
- Closely resembles schizophrenia
- Two differences from schizophrenia:
  - Total duration of the illness is at least 1 month but less than 6 months, including prodromal, active illness period, and residual symptom phase
  - Does not require for diagnosis that there be impaired social or occupational functioning, although may be present.

Etiology
- Similar to schizophrenia.

Risk Factors
- Similar to schizophrenia.

Assessment
History–Assess for the Following:
- Two or more of the following frequently present during a 1-month period:
  - Delusions
  - Hallucinations
  - Disorganized speech
  - Grossly disorganized behavior
  - Presence of negative symptoms.

- Duration of symptoms for at least 1 month and for no longer than 6 months
- Almost all information provided for schizophrenia pertains to this disorder, except
  - Occurs much less often than schizophrenia; incidence is 0.03% of general U.S. population
  - Approximately one-third recover completely within 6 months
  - Remaining two-thirds develop schizophrenia or schizoaffective disorder (see below).

Physical Exam Findings
- Similar to schizophrenia.

Mental Status Exam Findings
- Similar to schizophrenia.

Diagnostic and Laboratory Findings
- Similar to schizophrenia.

Clinical Management
- Similar to schizophrenia.

- Assess for acuity level.
- During acute psychotic or affective episodes, client may require brief hospitalization to
  - Ensure client safety
  - Rapidly stabilize client's symptom level in a controlled environment
  - Ensure client compliance with treatment to reach stabilization.
- Clinical management during nonacute episodes occurs most often in community settings.

Pharmacological Management
- Similar to schizophrenia.

Nonpharmacological Management
- Similar to schizophrenia.

Follow-up
- Similar to schizophrenia.

Schizoaffective Disorder

Description
- An uninterrupted period of illness in which the individual experiences psychotic symptoms similar to those seen in schizophrenia as well as mood symptoms similar to major depressive disorder (MDD) or bipolar (BP) disorder (see Chapter 7).
- Presence of schizoaffective disorder increases risk for later development of schizophrenia as a comorbid disorder.

Assessment
History–Assess for the Following:
- Symptoms of schizophrenia—Two or more of the following frequently present during a 1-month period:
  - Delusions
  - Hallucinations
  - Disorganized speech
  - Grossly disorganized behavior
  - Presence of negative symptoms but usually less severe than those in schizophrenia.

- Symptoms of one or more mood disorders (see Chapter 7):
  - Major depressive episode
  - Manic episode
  - Mixed-mood episode.

- Presence of delusions or hallucinations for at least 2 weeks in the absence of prominent mood symptoms.

Subtypes
- Two subtypes differentiated by type of mood-related symptoms:
  - *Depressive*—When predominant mood symptoms are of the depressive type only
  - *Bipolar*—When predominant mood symptoms are manic or mixed type.

Physical Exam Findings
- Similar to schizophrenia.

Mental Status Exam Findings
- Similar to schizophrenia.

Diagnostic and Laboratory Findings
- Similar to schizophrenia.

Clinical Management
Pharmacological Management
- Similar to schizophrenia
- Similar to MDD or BP disorder (see Chapter 7).

Nonpharmacological Management
- Similar to schizophrenia
- Similar to MDD or BP disorder (see Chapter 7).

Follow-up
- Similar to schizophrenia
- Similar to MDD or BP disorder (see Chapter 7).

Delusional Disorder

Description
- Presence of one or more nonbizarre delusions lasting for at least 1 month
- Psychosocial functioning and daily behavior not at all impaired except as they surround content of delusion
- Seldom any other symptoms; in rare cases may have hallucinations or mood disturbances.

Assessment
History–Assess for the Following:
- Presence of delusions
  - Well organized and potentially believable
  - Any unusual behavior is explainable if content of delusion is understood.

- *Subtypes (categorized by thematic content of delusion)*
  - Erotomanic
    - Delusional content focused on false belief that another person is in love with the client
    - Usually focused on idealized or spiritual love and only infrequently has strong sexual content
    - Focus of love usually famous or powerful individual who does not usually know the client
    - In rare cases, individual may know client
    - Leads to obsessive behaviors such as surveillance or stalking.

- Grandiose
  - Delusional content focuses on the client having some great talent, skill, or knowledge
  - May have strong religious component, such as prophecy or deity connections (special connection to God).

- Jealous
  - Delusional content focuses on false belief that client's spouse or partner is being unfaithful with someone else
  - Belief has no connection with realistic evidence
  - Usually seen in men
  - Client may try to control behavior of spouse or partner in an attempt to prevent imagined infidelities.

- Persecutory
  - Delusional content focuses on client's belief that others are out to harm or spy on client
  - Often angry and hostile at perceived persecution.

- Somatic
  - Delusional content focuses on bodily functions and sensations
  - Often belief that a body part is infected, is absent, omits a strange odor, or is misshapen or malformed.

- Mixed
  - No clear predominant theme for the delusional content.

- Related symptoms that can be present but are not required for diagnosis include
  - Depression over protracted problems with thematic content
  - Involvement in legal difficulties related to behaviors based on delusional content
  - Subjection to or requesting unnecessary medical tests or procedures.

Physical Exam Findings
- Nonspecific.

Mental Status Exam Findings
- Normal except for delusions.

Abstraction
- May be concrete on proverbs during delusional episodes.

Thought Process
- Presence of delusions
- Perseveration on topics related to delusion.

Thought Content
- Thematic for type of delusion.

Diagnostic and Laboratory Findings

- Nonspecific.

Clinical Management

Pharmacological Management

- Similar to schizophrenia.

Nonpharmacological Management

- Similar to schizophrenia.

Brief Psychotic Disorder

Description

- Disorder with sudden onset of psychotic symptoms lasting at least 1 day but less than 1 month.

Assessment

History—Assess for the Following:

- Age of onset in adolescence or early adulthood
- Positive-type psychotic symptoms
  - Delusions
  - Hallucinations
  - Grossly disorganized behavior
  - Disorganized speech.

- Can occur with or without identified stressor
- Individual always returns to premorbid level of functioning.

Physical Exam Findings

- Nonspecific.

Mental Status Exam Findings

- Similar to schizophrenia.

Diagnostic and Laboratory Findings

- Nonspecific.

Clinical Management

Pharmacological Management

- Similar to schizophrenia.

Nonpharmacological Management

- Similar to schizophrenia.
- Acute episode requires frequent monitoring for safety needs because of the following:
  - Confusion
  - Rapid shifting in emotions

- Impaired judgment
- Inability to meet nutritional and hygiene needs.

Shared Psychotic Disorder (Folie á Deux)

Description
- Characterized by development of a delusion in a client who has a close relationship with another individual who already has a psychotic disorder with a prominent delusion.

Assessment
History–Assess for the Following:
- Client in close contact with an individual who already has a delusion and
  - That individual usually has schizophrenia.
  - That individual usually is the dominant person in the relationship.
  - That individual gradually imposes his or her delusion on the client.
  - Usually the relationship is long term and very close.

- Aside from the delusional content, the client's behavior otherwise normal.

Physical Exam Findings
- Nonspecific.

Mental Status Exam Findings
- Similar to schizophrenia.

Diagnostic and Laboratory Findings
- Nonspecific.

Clinical Management
Pharmacological Management
- Similar to schizophrenia.

Nonpharmacological Management
- Similar to schizophrenia.

Chronic Disease Course
- Poor prognosis if relationship continues, especially if individual with delusion goes untreated.
- Good prognosis if the client can be separated from individual with the delusion.

Case Study

Jim is a 28-year-old client newly diagnosed with schizophrenia. He initially experienced a psychotic episode while serving in the military and now is living at home with his parents. Jim is still reluctant to accept his diagnosis and continues to believe that he "got bad weed" in the service and that he will be fine once the weed is out of his body. He has not been adherent with treatment, and his parents are threatening to evict him from the house if he does not start accepting treatment.

Jim has a history of juvenile-onset diabetes and has struggled to maintain a diabetic diet and to control his weight. When asked to identify his current goals, Jim will state only that he wishes to find a good wife and settle down to a normal life. There are many issues to consider in planning care with this client.

- What is the top priority for the psychiatric–mental health nurse practitioner (PMHNP)?

- What medications are reasonable to consider for the client at this time?

- What is the relationship between his diabetes and schizophrenia?

- How will his comorbid illness affect care planning?

- What routine ongoing monitoring will he require?

Review Questions

1. The neurotransmitter deregulation theory of the etiology of psychotic disorders such as schizophrenia supports that psychosis is caused, in part, by

    a. An excess of dopamine
    b. A deficiency of dopamine
    c. Poor acetylcholine regulation
    d. Poor synaptic uptake of serotonin receptors

2. The positive–negative model of classifying the symptoms of schizophrenia describes positive symptoms as

    a. Symptoms that positively respond to antipsychotic medication
    b. Symptoms that are less serious to experience
    c. Symptoms that are less socially stigmatizing
    d. Symptoms that positively correlate to drug abuse

3. Mrs. Jay suffers from schizophrenia and is taking Navane 15 mg/d. During her appointment, she complains of feelings of inner restlessness, tremors, drooling, and stiff muscles. The best explanation for these is

    a. Extrapyramidal side effects of Navane
    b. Anticholinergic side effects of Navane
    c. Atypical side effects of Navane
    d. Psychosomatic side effects

4. As part of treatment planning, you place a note on Mrs. Jay's chart about seizure precautions. She notices the note and states that she doesn't understand and that she has no history of seizures. You explain that

   a. It is a clerical error, and you will correct it

   b. Seizures are common in mental illness, and the note is just a precaution

   c. Reactions to psychotropic medications are unpredictable

   d. Typical antipsychotic medications can lower seizure threshold

5. Mrs. Anders, a client with delusional disorder, has been started on Haldol 5 mg po bid, Tylenol 2 tabs po prn, Cogentin 1 mg po prn, and Ativan 2 mg prn for agitation. She is complaining of a sudden painful stiff neck and jaw muscles that started a few hours after she took her medication. These symptoms are most likely related to

   a. Akinesia

   b. Akathisia

   c. Dystonia

   d. Somatic delusions

6. The most appropriate PMHNP action to help relieve Mrs. Anders's pain and stiff muscles is

   a. Switch to an NSAID to control her pain

   b. Increase the Cogentin dose

   c. Teach her relaxation techniques

   d. Work her up for a muscular–skeletal problem

7. After a few weeks, you see Mrs. Anders again. She is refusing to take Haldol because of continued problems with stiff muscles and blurred vision. She tells you that she has not taken her medication for 1 week, and the stiffness and blurred vision are better but still a problem. Mrs. Anders says, "Something else must be seriously wrong with me. I stopped the Haldol, and I'm still not okay." Your best explanation is that Mrs. Anders is

   a. Fixated on her medications

   b. Experiencing an unusual reaction to Haldol

   c. Experiencing a lipophilic reaction to Haldol

   d. Experiencing some problem other than a side effect of Haldol

References and Resources

American Psychiatric Association. (2000). *Diagnostic and statistical manual of mental disorders* (4th ed., text rev.). Washington, DC: Author.

Andreason, N. C. (1982). Negative symptoms in schizophrenia: Definition and reliability. *Archives of General Psychiatry, 39* (7), 784–788.

Andreason, N. C., & Olsen, S. (1982). Negative vs. positive schizophrenia: Definition and validity. *Archives of General Psychiatry, 39* (7), 789–794.

Brzustowicz, L. M., Hodgkinson, K. A., Chow, E.W.C., Honer, W. G., & Bassett, A. S. (2000). Location of a major susceptibility locus for familial schizophrenia on chromosome 1q21-q22. *Science, 288,* 678–682.

Dolder, C. R., Lacro, J., Dunn, L., & Jeste, D. (2002). Antipsychotic medication adherence: Is there a difference between typical and atypical agents? *American Journal of Psychiatry, 159,* 103–108.

Gershon, E. S., & Badner, J. A. (2001). Progress towards discovery of susceptibility genes for bipolar manic–depressive illness and schizophrenia. *CNS Spectrums, 6,* 965–977.

Guy, W. (1976) *ECDEU assessment manual for psychopharmacology* (rev. ed.). Washington, DC: U.S. Department of Health and Human Welfare.

Harkavy-Friedman, J., & Nelson, E. (1997). Management of the suicidal patient with schizophrenia. *Psychiatric Clinics of North America, 20,* 625–629.

Harrop, C. E. (2002). The development of schizophrenia for late-life adolescence. *Current Psychiatric Reports, 4,* 293–298.

Heinssen, R. K., Perkins, R., Appelbaum, P., & Fenton, W. (2001). Informed consent in early psychosis. *Schizophrenia Bulletin, 27,* 571–584.

Heresco-Levy, U., Javitt, D. C., Ermilov, M., Mordel, C., Silipo, G., & Liechtenstein, M. (1999). Efficacy of high-dose glycine in the treatment of enduring negative symptoms of schizophrenia. *Archives of General Psychiatry, 56,* 29–36.

Herz, M., Lamberti, S., Mintz, J., Scott, R., O'Dell, S., McCartan, L., & Nix, G. (2000). A program for relapse prevention in schizophrenia. *Archives of General Psychiatry, 57,* 277–283.

Kay, S. R., & Fiszbein, A. (1987). The positive and negative syndrome scale for schizophrenia. *Schizophrenia Bulletin, 13,* 261–275.

Lencz, T., Bilder, R. M., & Cornblatt, B. (2001). The timing of neurodevelopmental abnormality in schizophrenia: An integrative review of the neuroimaging literature. *CNS Spectrums, 6,* 233–253.

Lewis, D. A., & Lieberman, J. A. (2000). Catching up on schizophrenia: Natural history and neurobiology. *Neuron, 28,* 325–334.

Lindsay, H. (2000). Neurodevelopment of schizophrenia revealed. *Clinical Psychiatric News, 3,* 34–39.

Lyon, E. (1999). A review of the effects of nicotine on schizophrenia and antipsychotic medications. *Psychiatric Services, 50,* 1346–1349.

Mathalon, D. H., Sullivan, E., Lim, K., & Pfefferbaum, A. (2001). Progressive brain volume changes and the clinical course of schizophrenia in men. *Archives of General Psychiatry, 58,* 148–157.

Newcomer, J. W., Haupt, D., Fucetola, R., Melson, A., Schweiser, J., Cooper, B., & Selke, G. (2002). Abnormalities in glucose regulation during antipsychotic treatment of schizophrenia. *Archives of General Psychiatry, 59,* 337–345.

Overall, J. E., & Gorham, D. R. (1962). The brief psychiatric rating scale. *Psychological Reports, 10,* 790–812.

Rector, N. A., & Beck, A. (2002). A clinical review of cognitive therapy for schizophrenia. *Current Psychiatric Reports, 4,* 284–292.

Sable, J. A. (2002). Antipsychotic treatment for late-life schizophrenia. *Current Psychiatric Reports, 4,* 299–306.

Staal, W. G., Hulshoff Pol, H., Schnack, G., van Haren, N. E., Seifert, N., & Kahn, R. (2001). Structural brain abnormalities in chronic schizophrenia at the extremes of the outcome spectrum. *American Journal of Psychiatry, 158,* 1140–1142.

Tamminga, C. (2001). Treating schizophrenia now and developing strategies for the next decade. *CNS Spectrums, 6,* 987–991.

Tandon, R., & Jibson, M. D. (2001). Pharmacologic treatment of schizophrenia: What the future holds. *CNS Spectrums, 6,* 980–986.

Walker, A. (2000). The family and schizophrenia. *Issues in Mental Health Nursing, 21,* 27–31.

Notes:

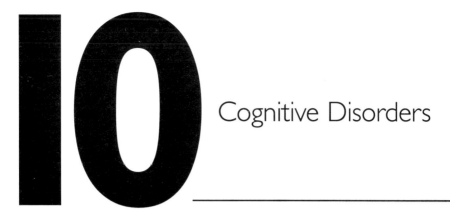

Cognitive Disorders

Cognitive disorders often are thought of as disorders of elderly people. Although most common in this population, cognitive disorders can occur at any age. Very young or very old people with cognitive disorders have multiple health needs. Elderly clients usually have more than one chronic illness, and psychiatric disorders can be accompanied by other comorbidities.

Psychiatric–mental health nurse practitioners (PMHNPs) must approach clients with cognitive disorders by always assessing their needs using a multisystem approach.

Cognitive Disorders

Description
- Cognitive disorders cause a clinically significant deficit in cognition that represents a major change from the individual's previous baseline level of functioning.
- Two common disorders are
  - Delirium
  - Dementia.

Etiology
- Cognitive disorders are a general medical condition, a result of substance use or abuse, a reaction to medications or other ingested agents, or a combination of all of these.

Delirium

Description
- Delirium is a syndrome and not a disease.

- The hallmark symptom is a disturbance of consciousness accompanied by changes in cognition.
- Delirium is not accounted for by other current medical conditions.

Incidence and Demographics
- Common, especially in elderly people
- Often overlooked and mistaken for other conditions
- In individuals with psychiatric disorders, often mistaken for worsening of psychotic symptoms instead of a separate, distinct condition
- Prevalence varies based on age and client setting
  - 0.4% in general U.S. population age 18 or older
  - 1.1% in those age 50 or older
  - 30% in hospitalized clients age 50 or older
  - 60% in elderly clients in skilled-nursing facilities
  - 25% in clients with cancer
  - 40% in hospitalized clients with AIDS
  - 80% in terminal clients nearing death.

Risk Factors
- Age 50 or older
- Multisystem medical illness
  - The more physically ill the client, the higher the risk.

- Substance abuse
- Past episode of delirium.

Prevention and Screening
- At-risk family education
- Community education
  - Stigma reduction
  - Signs and symptoms of illness
  - Treatment potential for control of symptoms.

- Early recognition, intervention, and initiation of treatment
  - Whenever a client's clinical presentation changes rapidly from baseline, consider delirium as one possible differential diagnosis.

Assessment
History–Assess for the Following:
- Key findings
  - Disturbance of consciousness develops over a short time, usually hours to days.
  - This disturbance tends to fluctuate during the course of the day.

- Sleep–wake cycle disturbances
  - Reversal of the sleep–wake cycle is common.
  - Clients are awake at night and sleep during the day.

- Psychomotor agitation
  - The client exhibits purposeless, random actions.

- Illness course may resolve within hours to days.
    - The more quickly the underlying physiological disturbance is recognized and treated, the more rapidly the delirium will resolve.
    - Symptoms may persist for months in an individual when unrecognized.
    - Most symptoms resolve within 3–6 months.

Physical Exam Findings

- Evidence that significant clinical symptoms are a consequence of direct physiological processes, substance use or abuse, or general medical condition
- Usually nonspecific neurological abnormalities
    - Tremors
    - Incoordination
    - Urinary incontinence
    - Myoclonus
    - Nystagmus
    - *Asterixis*—A flapping motion of the wrists
    - Increased muscle tone and reflex.

Mental Status Exam Findings

Appearance

- Unconcerned with appearance
- Disheveled
- Highly inattentive.

Speech

- Impaired
- Disorganized
- Rambling
- Incoherent
- Slurred
- *Dysarthria*—Impaired ability to articulate words
- *Dysnomia*—Impaired ability to name objects
- *Dysgraphia*—Impaired ability to write.

Affect

- Rapid, unpredictable shifts in affective state without known precipitation
    - Lethargic
    - Agitated.

Mood

- Often unable to solicit from patient.

Thought Process

- Disorganized
- Distractible
- Perceptual disturbances
    - Illusions most common
    - Hallucinations less common than illusions but may be present.
- Delusions.

Thought Content
- Often hard to determine
- Hard to engage client in meaningful conversation.

Orientation
- Usually the first symptom to appear
- Usually disoriented to time and place.

Memory
- Grossly impaired.

Concentration
- Grossly impaired.

Abstraction
- Grossly impaired.

Judgment
- Grossly impaired.

Diagnostic and Laboratory Findings
- Findings consistent with underlying physiological etiology
- EEG abnormalities
  - Generalized slowing
  - Generalized increased activity if delirium is related to alcohol withdrawal.

Differential Diagnosis
- Dementia (see below)
- Substance intoxication or withdrawal (see Chapter 11)
- Schizophrenia (see Chapter 9)
- Schizophreniform disorder (see Chapter 9)
- Mood disorders with psychotic features (see Chapter 7).

Clinical Management
- Undertake treatment of underlying condition or disorder.
- Avoid the use of new medications whenever possible, as using them may cloud the diagnostic picture.

Pharmacological Management
- Symptomatic treatment
- Agitation and psychotic symptoms
  - Antipsychotic agents
  - Anxiolytic agents
  - Haldol, Risperdal, and Ativan commonly used.

Nonpharmacological Management
- Monitor for safety needs.

- Determine reality orientation frequently.
- Pay attention to basic needs:
  - Hydration
  - Nutrition.
- Client should be neither sensory deprived nor overstimulated.
- It is helpful to have in the patient's room familiar people; familiar pictures or decorations; a clock or calendar; and regular orientation to person, place, and time.

General Health Considerations
- Delirium is associated with high morbidity, usually from injury.
- High morbidity also results from associated problems related to inactivity
  - Pneumonia
  - Hydration and nutritional deficits.
- Safety concerns exist.

Life Span Considerations
Children
- Especially susceptible
- Related to immature brain development
- Often mistaken for uncooperative behavior
- If a child is not soothed by common methods (e.g., parental presence), delirium is suspected.
  - Most common in febrile states
  - Medications known to affect cognition
    - Especially common with anticholinergic medications.

Older Adults
- Susceptibility related to physiological changes of aging
- Elderly men more prone than elderly women for unknown reasons.

Dementia

Description
- Dementia is a group of disorders characterized by development of multiple cognitive deficits:
  - Impaired executive functioning
  - Impaired global intellect with preservation of level of consciousness
  - Impaired problem solving
  - Impaired organizational skills
  - Altered memory.
- Various forms of dementia share common symptoms but have different underlying pathology.

Dementia of the Alzheimer's Type (DAT)
- Most common type
- Gradual onset and progressive decline without focal neurological deficits
- Hallmark amyloid deposits and neurofibrillary tangles.

Vascular Dementia (VD)
- Second most common type
- Formerly called *multi-infarct dementia*
- Primarily caused by cardiovascular disease and characterized by step-type declines
- Most common in men with preexisting high blood pressure and cardiovascular risk factors
- Hallmarks are carotid bruits, fundoscopic abnormalities, and enlarged cardiac chambers.

Dementia Due to HIV Disease
- Classified as a subcortical dementia
- Parenchymal abnormalities visualized on MRI scan
- HIV-associated neurocognitive disorder or HIV encephalopathy less severe forms
- HIV can cause many psychiatric symptoms
- Manifests by progressive cognitive decline, motor abnormalities, and behavioral abnormalities
- Co-occurring with obsessive–compulsive disorder, posttraumatic stress disorder, generalized anxiety disorder, depression, and mania
- Development of dementia in client with HIV is an indicator of poor prognosis; death usually occurs within 6 months
- Psychotic symptoms usually occur in late-stage infection
- Clinical signs of late-stage HIV-related dementia include cognitive, motor, behavioral, and affective impairment:
  - Global cognitive impairment
  - Mutism
  - Seizures
  - Hallucinations
  - Delusions
  - Apathy
  - Mania.

✓ Remember that protease inhibitors can increase levels of Wellbutrin, benzodiazepines, and selective serotonin reuptake inhibitors (SSRIs). Use caution when prescribing these drugs to individuals taking protease inhibitors.

- Protease inhibitors may induce the metabolism of Depakote and Ativan, thus causing subtherapeutic levels.

Pick's Disease
- Also known as *frontotemporal dementia*
- Neuronal loss, gliosis, and Pick's bodies present
- Personality and behavioral changes in early stage
- Cognitive changes in later stages
- *Kluver–Bucy syndrome*—Hypersexuality, hyperorality, and placidity.

Creutzfeld–Jacob Disease
- Fatal and rapidly progressive disorder
- Occurs mainly in adults middle age or older
- Initially manifests with fatigue, flu-like symptoms, and cognitive impairment
- Later manifests with aphasia, apraxia, emotional lability, depression, mania, psychosis, marked personality changes, and dementia
- Death usually occurs within 6 months.

Huntington's Disease
- Subcortical type of dementia
- Characterized mostly by motor abnormalities (e.g., choreoathetoid movements)
- Psychomotor slowing and difficulty with complex tasks
- Memory, language, and insight usually intact until late stages
- High incidence of depression and psychosis.

Lewy Body Disease
- Caused by lewy inclusion bodies in the cortex
- Presents with hallucinations, Parkinsonian features, and extrapyramidal side effects (EPSs)
- Reacts adversely to antipsychotics.

Etiology
- Multiple theories ranging from psychological to neurobiological
  - Probable multifactorial etiological profile.

- Primary cause mostly unknown
- General medical condition, result of substance use or abuse, reaction to medications or other ingested agents, or combination of all of these
- Diffuse cerebral atrophy and enlarged ventricles in DAT
- Decreased ACh and norepinephrine in DAT
- Genetic loading
- Genes on chromosomes 1, 14, and 21 have been identified in families with history of DAT
- Autosomal dominant trait
- Inherited alleles for apolipoprotein E-4 (APOE4) on chromosome 19 suspected to be related to late-onset dementia.

Incidence and Demographics
- Often misdiagnosed or unrecognized, especially in early stages and in young clients
- Affects 1.6% of individuals in the U.S. age 65 or older
  - 16%–25% in individuals age 85 or older

- DAT the most common
  - Affects an estimated 4 million Americans
  - Duration of illness averages 8–10 years.

Risk Factors
- Age
- Multisystem medical illnesses

- Genetic loading
  - Family history of dementia in first-order relative.

- History of substance use or abuse.

Prevention and Screening
- At-risk family education
- Community education
  - Stigma reduction
  - Signs and symptoms of illness
  - Treatment potential for control of symptoms.

- Early recognition, intervention, and initiation of treatment
  - Allows for ruling out age-related memory changes or unidentified conditions
  - Routine screening not recommended because no definitive treatment exists
  - Cognitive and functional evaluation at least every 3 years for people age 65 or older
  - Baseline and regular cognitive evaluation to monitor cognitive decline and treatment response to medications in individuals diagnosed with dementia.

- Significant and protracted prodromal symptom period usually noted before full onset of illness.

Assessment

History–Assess for the Following:
- Detailed history of present illness, including time frame, progression, and associated symptoms
- Past medical history of hypertension, strokes, head trauma, and psychiatric illness
- Psychiatric history of depression, anxiety, and schizophrenia
- Social history, including present living situation; marital status; occupation; education; and alcohol, tobacco, or illicit drug use
- Medications, including prescription, over-the-counter, alternatives, supplements, and home remedies
- Initial and periodic functional history and assessment
- Validate history with family or caregiver.

Memory Impairment
- Most prominent feature of disorder
- Usually earliest symptom
- Produces multiple deficits in daily functioning
  - Unable to learn new information
  - Forgets past information
  - Loses valuables
  - Forgets daily activities like eating and dressing
  - Becomes easily lost
  - Has other cognitive deficits such as *impaired executive functioning*.

- Instruments for assessing level of impairment
  - Mini-Mental State Examination (MMSE; Crum, Anthony, Bassett, & Folstein, 1993)
  - Short Portable Mental Status Questionnaire (SPMSQ; Pfeiffer, 1975).

- • Blessed Dementia Rating Scale (BDRS; Blessed, Tominson, & Roth, 1968).

- ✓ Remember to always consider visual, sensory, language, physical disabilities, and education when administering mental status tests.

Physical Exam Findings
- • *Amaurosis fugax*—Unilateral transient vision loss, described as "curtain over eye"
- • Unilateral focal–motor weakness
- • Asymmetrical reflexes.

Mental Status Exam Findings
Appearance
- • Apraxia
- • Decreased self-care activities of daily living.

Speech
- • Deterioration of language skills
- • Aphasia
- • Circumlocutory phrases
- • Indefinite object recognition (e.g., calling items "things" and unable to find discrete name)
- • In advanced stages are
  - • Mutism
  - • Echolalia.

Affect
- • Lability.

Mood
- • Difficult to illicit.

Thought Process
- • Agnosia.

Thought Content
- • Difficult to illicit.

Orientation
- • Disoriented to time and place
- • Disoriented to person in late stages of disorder.

Memory
- • Impaired in many dimensions of memory:
  - • Word registration
  - • Recall
  - • Retention
  - • Recognition.

Concentration
*   Distractible.

Abstraction
*   Concrete on proverb testing.

Judgment
*   Grossly impaired for self- and social judgment.

Diagnostic and Laboratory Findings
*   CBC, chemistry profile, thyroid function tests, B_{12} level, and folate level to rule out metabolic causes or unidentified conditions
*   Syphilis drug toxicity screening if indicated by history
*   Alcohol/illicit drug screen if suspected/indicated
*   Urinalysis if urinary tract infection suspected
*   Arterial oxygen or pulse oximetry if hypoxemia suspected
*   CT or MRI not routinely used
*   EEG not useful
*   Neuropsychological testing recommended to complete diagnostic assessment.

Differential Diagnosis
Nonpsychiatric
*   Parkinson's disease
*   Hearing loss
* B_{12} and folate deficiencies
*   Trauma, especially with history of falls
*   Hypothyroidism
*   Infection
*   Cerebrovascular accident
*   Polypharmacy
*   Alcohol intoxication.

Psychiatric
*   Mood disorders (see Chapter 7)
*   Delirium (see above)
*   Anxiety disorders (see Chapter 8).

Clinical Management
General Considerations
*   Rule out or treat any conditions that may contribute to cognitive impairment.
*   Discontinue unnecessary medications, especially sedatives and hypnotics.

Pharmacological Management
*   Cognitive symptoms
    *   N-Methyl D-Aspartate Glutamate Receptor Antagonists
        *   Prevent overexcitation of glutamate receptors and stabilize the neurodegenerative process

- Memantine (Namenda; 10–20 mg bid)
  - May slow the degenerative process
  - Promotes synaptic plasticity
  - May be used in combination with cholinesterase inhibitors.

- Cholinesterase Inhibitors
  - May be initiated for mild to moderate Alzheimer's disease
  - Modest clinical improvement in some clients, with studies showing 2- to 3-point improvement in MSE testing
  - Treat only symptoms, slow loss of function, and may improve agitated behaviors
  - Do not prevent pathological progression of disease
  - Not effective in severe, end-stage disease
  - Should stop if side effects develop, usually nausea and vomiting
  - Commonly used agents:
    - Donepezil (Aricept; 5–10 mg/d)
      - Now first line
      - Best with mild symptoms
      - May elevate LFTs, so monitor.

    - Rivastigmine tartrate (Exelon; 1.5–6 mg bid; increase gradually to avoid nausea)
    - Best with moderate symptoms.

    - Tacrine (Cognex; 40–160 mg/d)
      - May elevate LFTs and cause liver toxicity, so monitor
      - Many drug interactions (Cummings, 2000).

- Psychosis and Agitation
  - Try nonpharmacological therapies first.
  - Use antipsychotic agents regularly for agitation or psychotic symptoms.
  - Use lowest effective dose and attempt to wean periodically.
  - Antipsychotics may cause many side effects of significance in the older adult:
    - EPS
    - Sedation
    - Postural hypotension
    - Anticholinergic side effects.

  - Benzodiazepines may be used for treating anxiety or infrequent agitation.
    - Are not as effective as antipsychotics for severe symptoms (Jervis, 2002).

- Depression
  - Treat clients with depressive symptoms:
    - Depressed mood
    - Insomnia
    - Fatigue
    - Irritability
    - Appetite loss.
  - Use lowest effective dose.
  - Treat for 6–12 months, then attempt to wean; depression may recur and require lifelong treatment.

- Patients may have less depression as the dementia progresses and they become less aware of their circumstances.
- SSRIs have fewer side effects than tricyclic antidepressants (Draper, 1999).

Nonpharmacological Management
- Educate client and family about the illness, treatment, and community resources.
- Assist with long-term planning, including financial, legal, and advanced directives.
- Assess home and driving safety.
- Use behavior therapy to identify causes of problem behaviors and change the environment to reduce the problem behaviors.
- Use recreational therapy, art, and pet therapy to reduce agitation and promote normalized behavior.
- Use reminiscence therapy to process through any unresolved issues and recollect the past.
- Maintain a simple daily routine for bathing, dressing, eating, toileting, and bedtime.
- Integrate cultural beliefs into the management of all clients with dementia (Cummings & Jeste, 1999).

Psychotherapeutic Approaches for HIV-Related Dementia
- Major psychodynamic themes for individuals with HIV-related dementia are issues of guilt, self-esteem, and fear of dying.
- Because the client may not be able to give a complete and accurate history, family or friends should be questioned about any unusual behavior or mental status changes.
- Changes in the level of activity, in interest in other people, or in personality are clues to an acute central nervous system disturbance.
- Some changes are directly due to brain dysfunction, while other changes are due to psychological distress over a systemic problem—for example, anxiety that the person is dying.
- The spectrum of neuropsychiatric and neurological manifestations depends on the severity of immunosuppression.
- Psychiatric disorders may preexist or result from HIV.

✓ Remember that even subtle neurocognitive impairment may affect psychological coping.

- Neuropsychiatric disorders are much more prevalent in late-stage illness.

Life Span Considerations
- Primarily a disease of older adults but can occur in children
  - Diagnosis based on impaired cognition; diagnosis not applicable until ages 4–6 years, when cognition can be fully assessed
  - Dementia in children usually presents as deterioration in functioning, such as school performance or delay in normal development.

Case Study

Rachael, a 59-year-old homemaker with a positive family history for Alzheimer's disease, has been very worried lately at her subjective belief that she is losing her memory. She has hesitated to go for an evaluation because of her concern and is very upset as she shares her beliefs with the PMHNP. She gives a social history of being happily married for the past 35 years and of having several children and two new grandchildren. She has had no recent stressors and has felt a slow decline in her memory for the past 2 years. She believes no one else has noticed, but recently it is harder to hide her deficit from her family.

She has been employed as a nurse for the past 25 years at the local hospital but has begun to notice a decline in her ability to keep track of all of the information needed to do her job well. She has a history of asthma and periodically uses a rescue inhaler and steroids to manage her asthma. She routinely takes one aspirin a day and uses over-the-counter kava kava when she feels stressed. She has been taking Pravachol 20 mg/day for her cholesterol level for the past 2 years. She has no significant physical findings but does show mild impairment in short-term memory testing during the mental status exam. There are many issues to consider in planning care with this client:

• What is the probable diagnosis at this time?

• What further assessment is needed?

• What role does the medication taken by the client play in decision making?

• Would you include the family at this time in the care planning?

• Are medications indicated at this time?

• What steps would you take to reduce the client's discomfort as she discusses her concerns?

Review Questions

1. Risk factors for the development of delirium include all of the following except

   a. Consistent use of aspirin-based products
   b. Age older than 50
   c. Substance abuse
   d. Multisystem illness

2. The most significant finding that should alert you to the possible diagnosis of delirium is

   a. Rapid onset of symptoms different from baseline functioning
   b. Slow, progressive onset of symptoms different from baseline functioning
   c. Presence of a strong family history suggesting vulnerability
   d. Rapid alteration in vital signs

3. Prevention and screening actions are essential in the identification of dementia because
   a. Early detection can prevent some of the deterioration of the illness
   b. Early recognition allows for ruling out reversible forms of dementia
   c. Medications are more effective in treating dementia if started later in the illness
   d. Comorbidities can be prevented by early recognition

4. The medication most commonly used to treat moderate cognitive deficits seen in dementia is
   a. Strattera (atomoxetine)
   b. Exelon (rivastigmine tartrate)
   c. Haldol (haloperidol)
   d. Celebrex (celecoxib)

References and Resources

American Geriatric Society. (1999). *Geriatric review syllabus*. New York: Kendall/Hunt.

American Psychiatric Association. (2000). *Diagnostic and statistical manual of mental disorders* (4th ed., text rev.). Washington, DC: Author.

Bickley, L. S. (2007). *Bate's guide to physical examination and history taking* (9th ed.). Philadelphia: Lippincott Williams & Wilkins.

Blessed, G., Tominson, B. E., & Roth, M. (1968). The association between quantitative measures of dementia and senile changes in cerebral gray matter of elderly subjects. *British Journal of Psychiatry, 114*, 797–811.

Burke, M., & Laramie, J. A. (2003). *Primary care of older adults* (2nd ed.). St. Louis, MO: Mosby.

Crum, R. M., Anthony, J.C., Bassett, S. S., & Folstein, M. F. (1993). Population-based norms for the Mini-Mental State Examination by age and education level. *Journal of the American Medical Association, 269*, 238–238.

Cummings, J. (2000). Cholinesterase inhibitors: A new class of psychotropic compounds. *American Journal of Psychiatry, 157*, 4–11.

Cummings, J., & Jeste, D. (1999). Alzheimer's disease and its management in the year 2010. *Psychiatric Services, 50*, 1173–1177.

Desai, A., & Grossberg, G. (1999). Risk factors and protective factors for Alzheimer's disease. *Clinical Geriatrics, 7*(11), 43–47.

Doornbos, M. M. (2002). Family caregivers and the mental health care system: Reality and dreams. *Archives of Psychiatric Nursing, 15*(4), 39–46.

Draper, B. (1999). The diagnosis and treatment of depression in dementia. *Psychiatric Services, 50*, 1151–1156.

Freidman, J. H. (1998). *Neurology in primary care*. Boston: Butterworth/Heinemann.

Jervis, L. L. (2002). Contending with problem behaviors in the nursing home. *Archives of Psychiatric Nursing, 15*(4), 32–38.

Pfeiffer, E. (1975). A short portable mental status questionnaire for the assessment of organic brain deficit in elderly patients. *Journal of American Geriatric Society, 23,* 433–441.

Uphold, C. R. (2003). *Clinical guidelines in family practice* (4th ed.). Gainesville, FL: Barmarrae Books.

Notes:

Substance-Related Disorders

Substance use, abuse, and dependence is one of the most common but least well-addressed class of disorders. Psychiatric–mental health nurse practitioners (PMHNPs) who work in primary psychiatric settings or primary care settings commonly deal with clients with substance-related disorders. These disorders can stand alone or be part of complex comorbid disorders with either general medical conditions or psychiatric disorders.

Many substances can be used and abused. No matter what the substance, two general categories of substance-related disorders exist: substance abuse and substance dependence. Although the specific drug of abuse will determine many of the physical, behavioral, and cognitive symptoms exhibited by the client, some commonalities exist for all drugs.

This chapter focuses on the PMHNP role in determining the presence of either substance abuse or substance dependence and the available clinical management and treatments. It also emphasizes alcohol abuse and dependency as the primary example of these two disorders. Alcohol is discussed because it is the most commonly abused agent, the most well-researched substance, and the substance PMHNPs will encounter most often in clinical settings. Much of what is known about abuse and dependence to alcohol is believed to be transferable to other substances.

Substance-Related Disorders

Description
- *Substance-related disorders* are a cluster of disorders in which cognitive, behavioral, and physical symptoms occur, indicating that an individual is experiencing the effects of a drug of abuse.
- Psychiatric symptom clusters may be related to substance use, discontinuation of substance use, or withdrawal from habitual substance use.
- The word *substance* can describe a drug of abuse, a medication, or a toxin that produces psychoactivation and alters cognitive, behavioral, and affective perceptions.
- *Addiction* historically has been conceptualized as a disease, yet little is known about its underlying pathophysiology.

Etiology

- Multiple theories ranging from psychological to neurobiological
- Probable multifactorial etiological profile
  - Two common types of theories—psychodynamic and biological
    - Psychodynamic Theory
      - Behaviors of abuse are seated in oral-stage fixation.
      - An individual seeks gratification through oral behaviors.
      - Maladaptive regressive behaviors can become overlearned, fixed, and reinforced through dysfunctional family patterns.
      - Sociocultural factors attempt to explain population-based differences in substance abuse rates
        - Gender differences
        - Ethnic differences.
    - Biological Theory
      - Genetic loading
        - Individuals with a strong genetic vulnerability to addiction are thought to have defects in the working of the reward center of the brain, which predisposes them to stronger-than-normal positive rewards that draw them to substance use.
        - This also predisposes them to stronger-than-normal negative rewards, making it more difficult to stop abuse once it has begun.

  - Involves two neurobiological processes:
    1. Reinforcement
       - Brain-based changes in structure and function can lead to addictive behavior.
       - The process of positive and negative rewards is physiologically linked to memory function.
       - Changes appear to occur with any drug of abuse.
       - Reinforcement results in "feel good" sensations when a drug of abuse is used and in "feel bad" sensations when the drug exits the body.
       - Positive rewards of reinforcement result in the social rewards commonly associated with drug use, such as disinhibition, euphoric mood, and anxiety reduction.
         - Mediated by dopamine (DA) pathways.
       - Negative rewards are aversive, such as increased anxiety and dysphoria.
         - Mediated by the gamma-amino-butyric acid (GABA) pathways.
       - Reinforcement occurs in the ventral tegmental area and the nucleus accumbens of the brain, collectively called the *reward center*.
       - DA release within the reward center is enhanced further by the release of natural morphine-like neurotransmitters called *neuropeptides* (enkephalins, beta-endorphins).
       - Neuropeptides further enhance the reinforcing pleasure experienced by the individual.
       - With repeated drug use, the DA system becomes increasingly sensitized.
       - Eventually, associated drug use stimuli (e.g., pictures of drug paraphernalia) can cause DA release, leading to reinforcement of use and often to increased drug use.

2. Neuroadaption
   - Brain-based changes in structure and function can lead to *tolerance* and *withdrawal.*
     - Drug-specific alterations in the normal level and function of neurotransmitters occur as the body adapts to the chronic presence of the substance of abuse.
     - Neuroadaptive processes become very significant when the individual stops substance use.
     - These processes become the basis for withdrawal symptoms, as adaptive responses are unopposed when the substance is no longer present.
     - Neuroadaptive changes may be more permanent in some individuals, possibly lasting for years, thus increasing their potential for relapse.
     - This concept helps to explain why, after a long period of sobriety, an individual who returns to substance abuse often picks up at the same level of tolerance and physical impact as experienced before sobriety.

Incidence and Demographics

- The United States has higher rates of substance abuse than any other developed country.
- More than 50% of U.S. clients with a psychiatric disorder also are experiencing substance abuse or dependence.
  - Individuals with schizophrenia are 4 times more likely to have a substance dependence comorbidity than the general population.
  - Individuals with bipolar affective disorder are 5 times more likely to have a substance dependence comorbidity than the general population.
- More than 2 million admissions annually are made to inpatient substance abuse treatment facilities.
  - Marijuana is the most commonly abused illegal drug.
  - Alcohol is the most commonly abused drug.
- Rates are higher in men than in women.
  - 90% of men have used alcohol.
  - 70% of women have used alcohol.
- Rates are highest in African Americans, Hispanics, and Native Americans; rates are lowest in Asian Americans.
- 55% of fatal driving accidents in the United States occur with a driver under the influence of alcohol.
- 50% of crimes committed in the United States are done under the influence of alcohol.
- The lifetime risk for alcohol dependence is 15% in the general U.S. population.

Risk Factors

- Genetic loading
  - Family history of substance abuse or major depressive disorder (MDD).
- Association with peer structure with heavy substance use or abuse
- Co-occurring psychiatric disorder
- Age and gender

- Existence of chronic pain
- Untreated chronic pathological-level anxiety.

Prevention and Screening

- At-risk family education
- Community education
  - Stigma reduction
  - Signs and symptoms of illness
  - Treatment potential for control of symptoms.

- Early recognition, intervention, and initiation of treatment to prevent disease development of complications of disorder
  - Use of professional nursing standards such as *Practice Guideline for the Advanced Practice Nurse: Alcohol Withdrawal in the Acute Care Setting* (ISPN, 2001).

- Implications of alcohol and other drugs of abuse during pregnancy:
  - Fetal alcohol syndrome (FAS)
  - Birth defects.

- Acute alcohol intoxication in nontolerant individuals such as teenagers:
  - Coma
  - Respiratory depression
  - Death.

- CAGE screening test most commonly used screening tool for alcohol abuse (see Table 11–1).

Table 11–1. CAGE Screening Test

C	Have you ever felt you ought to **cut down** on your drinking?
A	Have people **annoyed** you by mentioning your drinking?
G	Have you ever felt bad or **guilty** about your drinking?
E	Have you ever had a drink first thing in the morning to steady your nerves or get rid of a hangover **eye-opener**?

Adapted from D. Mayfield, G. McLeod, & P. Hall, (1974), The cage questionnaire: Validation of a new alcoholism instrument. *American Journal of Psychiatry, 131,* 1121–1123.

- Administered by asking the client four questions.
- Each positive answer scored as 1 point; negative answers receive no score.
- The more positive answers, the greater the probability of an alcohol abuse disorder.
- Clients scoring 0–2 are at mild to moderate risk for alcohol dependency.
- Clients scoring 3–4 are considered to be at high risk for alcohol dependency.

Assessment

History–Assess for the Following:
- Detailed history of present illness, including time frame, progression, and associated symptoms

- Social history, including present living situation; marital status; occupation; education; and alcohol, tobacco, or illicit drug use
- Medication use, including prescription, over-the-counter, alternative, supplements, and home remedies
- Initial and periodic functional history and assessment
- Validate history with a family member
- Identify category of drug abused by the client
  - Knowing category allows for anticipation of physical impact of drug and prediction of potential symptoms of withdrawal
  - Clients often abuse drugs from categories with similar pharmacological properties.
  - Categories of abused agents:
    - Alcohol
    - Amphetamines or similar sympathomimetics
    - Caffeine
    - Cannabis
    - Cocaine
    - Hallucinogens
    - Inhalants
    - Nicotine
    - Opioids
    - Phencyclidine (PCP) or similar arylcyclohexylamines
    - Sedatives
    - Hypnotics
    - Anxiolytics.

Assess for Presence of Substance Abuse

- Maladaptive pattern of substance use manifested by recurrent and significant adverse consequences related to repeated use of a substance
- Is *not* synonymous with *use, misuse,* or *hazardous use*
- Specific criteria needed to identify substance use as abuse
  - Maladaptive pattern of use occurring for at least a 12-month period of sustained abuse
  - Must be accompanied by repeated failure to fulfill major role obligation
  - Must be accompanied by use in situation that presents as physically hazardous, such as drinking and driving
  - Abuse continues despite multiple problems related to substance use patterns, such as legal, interpersonal, or social.

- Caffeine and nicotine use patterns not considered when determining presence of substance abuse.

Assess for Presence of Substance Dependence

- Cluster of cognitive, behavioral, and physiological symptoms indicating that the individual continues use of a substance despite significant substance-related problems
- Synonymous with *addiction*
- Pattern of repeated use that leads to clinically significant impairment or distress with three or more of the following symptoms within a 12-month period:
  - Tolerance
  - Withdrawal
  - Using larger amounts than intended
  - Persistent craving or unsuccessful attempts to cut down
  - Large amount of time spent obtaining substance, using substance, or recovering from effects
  - Activities decreased or given up because of use
  - Using despite consequences.

- Specify "with physiological dependence" or "without physiological dependence"
- Physiological dependence implies tolerance and withdrawal
- Symptoms of tolerance or withdrawal need not be present to meet criteria for substance dependence
- Degree of tolerance and withdrawal symptoms substance specific.
- *Tolerance*—Need for markedly increasing amounts of a substance to achieve desired effect
- *Withdrawal*—Maladaptive behavioral change with physiological and cognitive symptoms, occurring after blood or tissue concentrations of substance declines in an individual who has had prolonged heavy substance use
  - Can be physical, psychological, or both, depending on the substance
  - Withdrawal symptoms almost always the opposite of the acute action of the substance
  - Categories of abused substances with pronounced, *obvious withdrawal symptoms:*
    - Alcohol
    - Opioids
    - Sedatives
    - Hypnotics
    - Anxiolytics.
  - Categories of abused substances with less pronounced, *less obvious withdrawal symptoms:*
    - Stimulants
    - Nicotine
    - Cannabis.
  - Categories of abused substances with *little to no pronounced, obvious withdrawal symptoms:*
    - Hallucinogens
    - PCP.

Course Modifiers for Substance Dependence
- *Early Partial Remission*—One or more criteria (but not full criteria) have been met for substance dependence for at least 1 month but less than 12 months
- *Sustained Partial Remission*—One or more criteria (but not full criteria) have been met for substance dependence for 12 months or longer
- *Early Full Remission*—No criteria met for abuse or dependence for at least 1 month but less than 12 months
- *Sustained Full Remission*—No criteria met for abuse or dependence for 12 months or longer.

Assess for the Presence of Substance Withdrawal or Intoxication
- Clients abusing substances present for assessment either under the influence of the drug (intoxication) or experiencing problems related to cessation of substance use (withdrawal)
  - *Intoxication*—Reversible substance-specific syndrome due to recent ingestion of a psychoactivating substance
  - *Withdrawal*—Potentially nonreversible substance-specific syndrome due to cessation or significant reduction in heavy prolonged use of a substance.

- Blood alcohol level (BAL) determines presence of substance.
    - Tolerant individuals often have higher blood level with less impairment than nontolerant individuals.
    - Must interpret BAL of a client based on his or her degree of tolerance.

Diagnostic Criteria for Substance Withdrawal

- Cessation of or reduction in alcohol use that has been heavy or prolonged
- Two or more of the following symptoms within several hours or days of reduction or cessation:
    - Hand tremor
    - Insomnia
    - Autonomic hyperactivity (sweating, increased heart rate and blood pressure)
    - Nausea or vomiting
    - Hallucinations or illusions
    - Psychomotor agitation
    - Anxiety
    - Seizures.

- Structured interview (see Table 11–2) allows for assessment of the use patterns and consequences of an individual's substance use.
    - Assess for all dimensions of the impact of substance abuse/dependence on the individual.

Table 11–2. Structured Interview

Data Set	Potential Assessment Question
Current drug use	Please tell me about your use of [substance]. What prescribed and self-prescribed drugs do you take regularly? Do you think you have a drug problem? Does anyone important to you think you have a drug problem?
Patterns of use	Type/amount of drug consumption What is the longest period recently that you have gone without drug use? What happens when you go this long without [drug]? When was your last drug use? Have you had blackouts or memory loss during drug use? Is your drug use different now than it was 1 year ago? 5 years ago?
Social consequences	Have you ever been arrested related to your drug use (such as DUI)? Have you ever gotten into trouble at work/school because of your drug use? Have you ever behaved in a way you have regretted when using drugs?
Relational aspects	Have you ever gotten into arguments with your partner/spouse because of your drug use? Have you ever behaved toward your partner/spouse in a way you have regretted when using drug (such as being abusive)?

Continued on the next page

Table 11–2. Continued

Data Set	Potential Assessment Question
Sequelae of dependency	Has your physical health suffered because of your drug use? Have you suffered any injury or trauma related to your drug use? Have you ever not complied with recommended medical care because it would mean you had to be drug free?

Adapted from International Society of Psychiatric Mental Health Nurses (ISPN). (2001). *Practice guideline for the advanced practice nurse: Alcohol withdrawal in the acute care setting.* Philadelphia: International Society of Psychiatric Mental Health Nurses. Used with permission.

Physical Exam Findings

- Substance abuse/dependence produces many physical symptoms
- Usually a result of sequelae of use/abuse rather than findings specific to abuse/dependence
- Generally nonspecific when viewed in isolation
- Must be considered as a cluster of symptoms that raise an index of suspicion of addiction potential
  - Abdominal pain and tenderness
  - Nausea
  - Weight loss
  - Gastrointestinal bleeding
  - Hypertension
  - Anxiety
  - First episode seizure in adult.

- Physical findings (see Table 11–3) are drug specific; alcohol-induced physical findings are most well known.

Table 11–3. Physical Findings Suggestive of Alcohol Dependency

Organ System	Finding
Gastrointestinal	Abdominal tenderness Splenomegaly Hepatomegaly (in some cases, size decreases)
Dermatological	Diaphoresis Alopecia (especially distal extremity) Unexplained bruises Spider nevi, telangiectases, or angioma Palmer erythema Rosacea Superficial infections
Cardiovascular	Tachycardia Cardiomyopathy Arrhythmia Hypertension

Table 11–3. Continued

Organ System	Finding
Respiratory	Alcohol odor on breath
	Aspiration pneumonia
	Chronic upper respiratory infection
Neuropsychiatric	Depression
	Anxiety
	Nystagmus
	Ataxia
	Emotional lability
	Irritability
	Peripheral neuropathy
	Hallucinations (especially tactile)
Endocrine	Testicular atrophy
	Gynecomastia
	Sexual dysfunction

National Institute on Alcohol Abuse and Alcoholism (NIAAA) (1997). Alcohol's effect on organ function, *DHHS Publication, 21*(1), 5–93.

Mental Status Exam (MSE) Findings

• Nature of findings (see Table 11–4) depends heavily on whether the client is experiencing substance intoxication or withdrawal or is substance free at the time of assessment.

  • Index of suspicion for substance-related disorder should be raised if client presents differently during different periods of assessment.

Table 11–4. MSE Findings Consistent With Substance Abuse

Category of Abused Substance	Clinical Findings	
Stimulant agents	Anxiety	Irritability
	Agitation	Mood swings
	Restlessness	Hallucinations
	Aggression	Impotence
	Panic episodes	Dilated pupils
	Grandiosity	Chest pain
	Elated mood	
Depressant agents	Dysphoria	Impaired judgment
	Mood swings	Hallucinations
	Ataxia	Paranoia
	Aggression	Psychomotor retardation
	Lack of impulse control	Slurred speech
	Disinhibition	Drowsiness
	Impaired attention	Myalgia
	Impaired memory	

Continued on the next page

Table 11–4. Continued

Category of Abused Substance	Clinical Findings	
Hallucinogens	Mood swings	Tremors
	Ataxia	Impaired concentration
	Severe anxiety	Impaired memory
	Panic episodes	Impaired judgment
	Aggression	Inability to make decisions
	Hallucinations	Dilated pupils
	Paranoia	Nystagmus
	Flashbacks	
Cannabis	Paranoia	Confusion
	Time distortion	Hallucinations
Inhalants	Ataxia	Confusion
	Agitation	Stupor
	Irritability	Hallucinations
	Delirium	Illusions

Adapted from National Institute on Drug Abuse. (2005). *Medical consequences of drug abuse/mental health effects.* Available at www.drugabuse.gov/consequences/mortality.

Diagnostic and Laboratory Findings
- CBC, chemistry profile, thyroid function tests, and B_{12} level to rule out metabolic causes or unidentified conditions
- Drug toxicity screening, if indicated by history
- Alcohol dependence and abuse produce characteristic laboratory findings (see Table 11–5).

Table 11–5. Laboratory Findings Suggestive of Alcohol Dependence

Test	Abnormality Suggestive of Alcohol Dependence
BAL	>100 mg/dl at the time of routine examination >150 mg/dl without gross evidence of intoxication >300 mg/dl at any time
MCV	Elevated (present in 60% of clients with alcohol dependency)
GGT	Elevated 20% or more (present in 80% of clients with alcohol dependency)
AST	Elevated 40% or more
ALT	Elevated 20% or more
PT	Increased
Amylase	Elevated
WBC	Low
NA⁺	Hyponatremia
K⁺	Hypokalemia

Table 11–5. Continued

Test	Abnormality Suggestive of Alcohol Dependence
Serum lipids	Hyperlipidemia
Uric acid	Elevated
Triglycerides	Elevated

Adapted from Graham, A. W., & Schultz, T. K. (2007). *Principles of addiction medicine* (3rd ed.). Baltimore: American Society of Addiction Medicine.

Differential Diagnosis

- Endocrine disorders
  - Cushing's disease.

- Neurological disorders
  - Seizure disorders.

- Cardiovascular disorders
  - Myocardial infarction.

- Mood disorders
  - MDD
  - Bipolar (BP) disorder.

- Anxiety disorders
- Personality disorders
- Differential diagnostic consideration for acute alcohol withdrawal:
  - Many acute general health conditions can mimic symptoms of alcohol withdrawal.
  - In clients with a history of alcohol dependency, the PMHNP needs to consider not only withdrawal as a possible explanation for findings but also the possibility of a general medical condition that can mimic alcohol withdrawal, such as hepatic encephalopathy or hypoglycemia.

Clinical Management

- Rule out or treat any conditions that may contribute to clinical findings.
- *Note:* 80%–90% of individuals who require alcohol treatment do not get it.
  - Common reasons for failure to receive needed treatment:
    - Lack of diagnosis
    - Lack of referral
    - Lack of access to services
    - Resistance to treatment.

- The genetics of addiction vulnerability is becoming better known, which allows for preventive and early intervention treatments.
- The knowledge base of pathophysiology of dependence has promoted new somatically based interventions.
  - Psychopharmacology offers the promise of a new era in the treatment of addictions.

- Clinical management is different depending on the substance-related syndrome exhibited by the individual:
  - Acute withdrawal
  - Acute intoxication
  - Long-term sobriety maintenance
  - Relapse prevention.

- Alcohol withdrawal carries a high risk of mortality.
- Clinical management of alcohol withdrawal is a specialized treatment that requires specific experience in this type of care.
- Some clinical findings may assist in identification of clients at risk for severe alcohol withdrawal:
  - Agitation
  - Decreased short-term memory
  - Disorientation
  - Hallucinations
  - Irregular pulse
  - Opthalmoplegia

Clinical Institute Withdrawal Assessment for Alcohol (CIWA–Ar; Sullivan, Sykora, Schneiderman, Naranjo, & Sellers, 1989)

- Used to determine likelihood of withdrawal and delirium tremens (DTs), which usually occur within the first 24 to 72 hours after cessation of alcohol
- Assesses 10 common withdrawal symptoms:
  - Nausea/vomiting
  - Tremors
  - Paroxysmal sweats
  - Anxiety
  - Agitation
  - Tactile disturbances
  - Auditory disturbances
  - Visual disturbances
  - Headaches
  - Altered sensorium.

- Each symptom is graded on a 0–7 point scale with the exception of orientation and sensorium, which is graded on a 0–4 point scale. The higher the total score (maximum = 67), the more likely the individual will experience severe withdrawal and DTs: 0–8 = *mild withdrawal,* 9–15 = *moderate withdrawal,* >15 = *severe withdrawal and possible DTs.*

Pharmacological Management

- Pharmacological treatments are symptom specific.
- Clinical Management of *Acute Withdrawal*
  - Detoxification (detox) agents substitute uncontrolled use of substance with slow tapering of controlled substance to minimize neuroadaptive rebound.
    - Multiple daily doses of benzodiazepines are used according to a fixed schedule and gradually tapered down over a series of several days.
    - Examples include
      - Ativan (lorazepan)
      - Librium (chlordiazepoxide)

- Valium (diazepam)
- Serax (oxazepam).

- Polytherapy is a newer approach that matches drugs required for safe and effective withdrawal with neurotransmitter deficits created by substance use.
  - Selected serotonin reuptake inhibitors
  - Opioid antagonists Revex, Vivitrol, or Revia
  - N-methyl-D-aspartate (NMDA) agonists.

- Antiseizure medications such as Tegretol and Depakene are sometimes used to decrease the potential of seizures.
- Adrenergic medications are sometimes used to decrease blood pressure and pulse associated with withdrawal.

- Clinical Management of *Craving* (see Table 11–6)
  - Use anticraving medication such as Revia, Campral, Zofran, or Buprenex.
  - Use behavior treatment to help client learn substitute behaviors.

- Clinical Management and *Maintenance of Sobriety* (see Table 11–6)
  - Individual may require ongoing treatment for comorbid psychiatric disorder.
  - May use *aversion treatment* to avoid alcohol in individuals with alcohol dependence.
    - Disulfiram (Antabuse)
      - Do not administer until individual is alcohol free for at least 12 hours.
      - Advise client to refrain from using anything that contains alcohol (e.g., vinegar, aftershave lotion, perfumes, mouthwash, cough medication) while taking Antabuse and up to 2 weeks after discontinuing Antabuse.
      - Antabuse can elevate LFTs, so monitor.
      - Antabuse may potentially induce mania in individuals with BP disorder.
- General health maintenance medications to treat vitamin deficiencies in individuals with alcohol dependence include thiamine, folic acid, and B-complex vitamins.

Table 11–6. Pharmacological Useful in Treating Craving and Maintaining Drugs Sobriety from Abusive Substances

Pharmacological Drug	Chemical Category	Action	Effect
Celexa (citalopram)	Selective serotonin reuptake inhibitor	Augment central serotonergic function	Decreased desire and "liking"
Antabuse (disulfiram)	Aldehyde dehydrogenase inhibitor	Aversive therapy; inhibits enzyme aldehyde dehydrogenase	Causes symptoms of headache, nausea, vomiting, flushing if alcohol ingested

Continued on the next page

Table 11–6. Continued

Pharmacological Drug	Chemical Category	Action	Effect
Narcan (naloxone)	Opioid antagonist, antidote	Blocks effects of opioids	Used as an antidote for opioid overdose
Buprenex (buprenorphine)	Opioid partial agonist, opioid antagonist	Binds to opiate receptors in central nervous system (CNS), causing an analgesic effect; has agonist and antagonist activity	Decreases heroin craving and use of opiates
Suboxone (buprenorphine and naloxone)	Narcotic analgesic, opioid agonist, opioid antagonist	Binds to opiate receptor, causing an analgesic effect; acts as an opioid antagonist	Used in treatment of opioid dependence; must meet qualification criteria to prescribe
Dolophine (methadone)	Narcotic analgesic	Binds to opiate receptors in the CNS, producing an analgesic effect, thus decreasing withdrawal symptoms	Suppresses withdrawal symptoms from opiates; used as detox and maintenance treatment of narcotic addiction; must be part of FDA-approved program
Revex (nalmefene)	Opioid antagonist	Blocks ethanol-induced release of dopamine	Increases abstinence; decreases history of drinking days
Revia; Vivitrol (naltrexone) (extended release injectable)	Opioid antagonist	Blocks opioid receptors involved in rewarding effects of alcohol	Increases abstinence; decreases history of drinking days; assists with cravings
Campral (acamprosate)	Homotaurine	Agonist activity at GABA receptors and inhibitory activity at glutamate receptors	Increases abstinence through decreased alcohol craving; thought to alter development of tolerance
Zofran (onadesteron)	Selective inhibitor of serotonin ($5\text{-}HT_3$)	Selective inhibition of Type 3 serotonin ($5\text{-}HT_3$) receptors that exhibit anti-emetic activity	Increases abstinence; decreases craving

Adapted from Graham, A. W., & Schultz, T. K. (2007). *Principles of addiction medicine* (3rd ed.). Baltimore: American Society of Addiction Medicine.

Nonpharmacological Management
- Multimodality treatment needed.
- Lifetime treatment often required.
- Inpatient treatment usually needed for safe and effective withdrawal from alcohol.
- Indications for inpatient alcohol detoxification include history of severe withdrawal symptoms, seizures, or delirium tremens; multiple past detoxifications; additional medical or psychiatric illness; recent significant alcohol consumption; lack of reliable support system; and pregnancy (Myrick & Anton, 1998).
- Reduce central nervous system stimulation by maintaining a quiet environment; put client in room close to the nurses' station to facilitate frequent observation and monitoring; minimize abrupt changes in environment; decrease bright light and sharp, sudden noises; decrease room clutter; and do not restrain.
- Maintain hydration by monitoring intake and anticholinergic effects of benzo-diazepines. Frequently offer fluids.
- Before discharge from acute care setting, have a definite plan for follow-up treatment.
- Connect client and family with support groups.
  - 12-step groups in community
  - Concrete plan for first week of support group attendance (may need daily).

- Connect client with counseling or psychotherapy.
- Identify a primary health care provider.
- Note medical problems that will require further evaluation and potential treatment:
  - Neurological sequelae of chronic alcohol consumption
  - Nutritional deficiencies
  - Cardiomyopathy, hypertension, arrhythmias, ischemic heart disease
  - Blood dyscrasias
  - Gastrointestinal inflammations
  - Esophageal, liver, nasopharyngeal, and laryngeal cancers.

- Individual care needs
  - Substance-abuse education classes
  - Substance-abuse counseling program
  - Continued 12-step program involvement (e.g., Alcoholics Anonymous, Narcotics Anonymous)
  - Halfway housing
  - Cognitive–behavioral therapy.

- Family care needs
  - Current and understandable information about condition, progress, and treatment plan.
  - Connect family to community support groups such as Al-Anon and Alateen.
  - Management of feelings such as guilt and anger.
  - Referrals to community resources.
  - Specific considerations—Relationship with treatment team; role strain; financial stresses; social isolation and "code of silence"; family support systems; family violence/marital and family strife; family members' work and school functioning; and history of mental disorders, including substance-related disorders.
  - Assist family in coping with difficulties incorporating drinking member back into routines; encourage further counseling to resolve these difficulties.

- Refer for further treatment if family members report symptom clusters from anxiety and mood disorders, eating disorders, and addiction.

Life Span Considerations

Children and Adolescents
- Most common period to start drug use
- Significant impact of peer pressure on substance-use patterns
- 30%–40% of adolescents report drinking frequently
- 15% report binge-drinking patterns
- Approximately 50% of high school–age students report at least a one-time use of illicit drugs.

Older Adults
- Referral to specialized treatment program that emphasizes interventions to deal with losses
- Large-print psychoeducation materials
- Transportation to service locations
- Treatment with same-age peer group
- Adaptations to home environment to cope with physical disabilities
- Close collaboration with primary care physician for follow-up.

Case Study

Mrs. Day is a 61-year-old widow who has multiple health problems. She had been diagnosed with essential hypertension and chronic bronchitis and has non-insulin-dependent diabetes. She has been coming to your primary care clinic for 6 months, and before that she had been receiving her care from multiple other providers in the community, spending an average of 8 months with a practice group, then changing her care to another provider. She has CHAMPUS as her insurance and receives Social Security Disability Insurance.

Mrs. Day's chief complaint for the past few months has been stasis ulcers on her lower left leg, which have not healed well despite multiple approaches to care. She also complains of problems with her "nerves." She currently is taking

- Multivitamin daily

- Zantac 150 mg Q 12 hrs

- Xanax 1 mg bid

- Glucotrol 20 mg bid.

Mrs. Day is in today, and this is the first time you see her. On initial approach, she is hostile and difficult to get information from, stating "You should know all this; you have my chart right there in your hand." She states that today she wants a refill of all of her prescriptions, and she wants you to write a letter to her landlord to "stop harassing me." She reports that her landlord is insisting that she place her garbage in the containers in the parking lot of the complex. She feels that is too far for her to walk, and she wants a letter supporting her current practice of leaving her garbage bags in the hallway outside her apartment door.

She also is reporting that her nerves are worse, and the pain in her legs is worse as well. She also believes that she has had a return of "chronic bronchitis," and she is requesting an antibiotic. She is requesting that you increase her Xanax and add codeine or morphine or "any other thing like that" for her "constant pain." She states, "Just do this and get me out of here. I know what I need."

MSE

- *Appearance:* Moderately obese, well dressed with appropriate hygiene, poor eye contact
- *Motor:* Mild psychomotor restlessness, slightly ataxic gait, tremulous
- *Speech:* Underproductive
- *Affect:* Hostile
- *Mood:* Self-described as "cranky"
- *Thought Process:* Goal directed and organized without evidence of psychotic processing, but does show some mild thought blocking and tangentiality
- *Thought Content:* Thematic for mistrust of health providers and for fear of pain continuing
- *Memory:* One-third of objects after 15 minutes
- *Concentration:* Refuses to do numbers testing, stating "I was never good with book work or numbers."
- *Abstraction:* Is abstract on proverbs; asks, "You got any more dumb questions?"
- *Judgment:* Intact for self-welfare
- *Education:* Completed 12th grade and went to 2-year secretarial/business school
- *Employment History:* Was a medical claims clerk for 32 years at the VA Medical Center
- *Social History:* No children; lives by herself. History of two-pack-a-day smoker and "I drink a six-pack or so at night to relax myself—wouldn't you?"

Her physical exam is overall unremarkable. Her vital signs are within her documented baseline, with BP 132/88, P 96, RR 26, Temp 99°F, Weight 209 lbs. Her lungs are overall clear. On her left leg she has a stasis ulcer, which is circular and approximately 6 cm in circumference. It is open and oozing white–yellow liquid drainage, with redness around the borders. She reports it is painful to touch and increasingly painful when weight bearing. She is ordered silvadine treatments with cling wrap and hot soaks q 6 hours. She refuses to cover it because "It hurts when I remove the bandage" and is not very clear about whether or not she is doing the hot soaks. Recent labs are all within normal limits, including TSH, electrolytes, and CBC. There are many issues to consider in planning care with this client:

- What is the primary health care concern of this client?
- Is her use of potentially addictive prescription drugs warranted?
- What further assessment should be considered?
- If the client is unwilling to participate in further assessment, how will you deal with her health needs?

Review Questions

1. The concept of *substance abuse* implies that the individual is

    a. Having withdrawal and tolerance symptoms when not using substances

    b. Having psychoactive effects when using substances

    c. In denial about the impact of substance use on their life

    d. Having functional problems related to frequent or excessive substance use

2. To diagnose a person with substance dependence, you must determine the current or past presence of which of the following clinical findings during your assessment of the client?

    a. Addictive manipulative behaviors

    b. Denial and projection

    c. Tolerance and withdrawal signs and symptoms

    d. Mental illness

3. Many abused substances have questionable withdrawal symptoms. Whether or not a person dependent on a particular substance will have withdrawal symptoms depends on

    a. The biochemistry of the person

    b. The nature of the substance

    c. The biochemistry of the agent and the person

    d. Neither the person nor the agent but a combination of the two factors

4. John is dependent on Falvoxaz (Fabs), a new synthetic substance currently popular among high school–age children in your community. John comes into the ER after a car accident and admits to frequent, regular use of Falvoxaz. Because this drug is new, you are not familiar with the potential types of withdrawal symptoms. The best assessment question to ask to determine the nature of possible withdrawal symptoms from this drug is

    a. How do you feel when you take Fabs?

    b. What is the chemical name for Fabs?

    c. How many Fabs do you take a week?

    d. How long have you been using Fabs?

5. Medical detoxification from a substance is required *only* when the substance is known to produce

    a. Physical withdrawal symptoms

    b. Psychological withdrawal symptoms

    c. Both physical and psychological withdrawal symptoms

    d. Uncomfortable and unwanted withdrawal symptoms

References and Resources

Barker, L. R., Burton, J. R., & Zieve, P. D. (2006). *Principles of ambulatory medicine* (7th ed.). Philadelphia: Lippincott Williams & Wilkins.

Bayard, M., McIntyre, J., Hill, K., & Woodside, J. (2004). Alcohol withdrawal syndrome. *American Family Physician, 69,* 1443–1450.

Brown, V. B., Ridgely, M. S., Pepper, B., Levine, I. S., & Ryglewicz, M. N. (1989). The dual crisis: Mental illness and substance abuse. *American Psychologist, 44,* 565–560.

DePetrillo, P., & McDonough, M. (1999). *Alcohol withdrawal treatment manual.* Glen Echo, MD: Focused Treatment Systems.

DiClemente, C., Bellino, L., & Neavins, T. (1999). Motivation for change and alcoholism treatment. *Alcohol Research and Health, 23*(2), 86–92.

Evans, K., & Sullivan, J. M. (2001). *Dual diagnosis: Counseling the mentally ill substance abuser* (2nd ed.). New York: Guilford Press.

Fuller, R., & Hiller-Sturmhofel, S. (1999). Alcoholism treatment in the United States: An overview. *Alcohol Research and Health, 23*(2), 69–77.

Graham, A. W., & Schultz, T. K. (2007). *Principles of addiction medicine* (3rd ed.). Baltimore: American Society of Addiction Medicine.

Hasin, D. S. (2001). The epidemiology of alcohol use and abuse in the United States: A review. *Economics of Neuroscience, 3*(12), 38–46.

Humphreys, K. (1999). Professional interventions that facilitate 12-step self-help group involvement. *Alcohol Research and Health, 23*(2), 93–98.

International Society of Psychiatric Mental Health Nurses. (2001). *Practice guideline for the advanced practice nurse: Alcohol withdrawal in the acute care setting.* Philadelphia: Author.

Johnson, B., & Ait-Daoud, N. (1999). Medications to treat alcoholism. *Alcohol Research and Health, 23*(2), 99–106.

Kasper, D. (2005). *Harrison's principles of internal medicine* (16th ed.). New York: McGraw-Hill.

Lawson, A., & Lawson, G. (2004). *Alcoholism and the family: A guide to treatment and prevention* (2nd ed.). Gaithersburg, MD: Aspen.

Mayfield, D., McLeod, G., & Hall, P. (1974). The CAGE questionnaire: Validation of a new alcoholism instrument. *American Journal of Psychiatry, 131,* 1121–1123.

Miller, N., Gold, M., & Smith, D. (1997). *Manual of therapeutics for addictions.* New York: Wiley-Liss.

McCabe, S. (2000). Rapid detox: Understanding new treatment approaches for the addicted patient. *Perspectives in Psychiatric Care, 36,* 113–120.

McCabe, S., & Laraia, M. (2002). The neurobiology of medications to treat addictions. *APNA News, 14*(1), 12–14.

Minkoff, K., & Drake, R. (Eds.). (1991). *Dual diagnosis of major mental illness and substance disorder: New directions for mental health services.* San Francisco: Jossey-Bass.

Murray, C.J.L., & Lopez, A. D. (1996). *The global burden of disease: A comprehensive assessment of mortality and disability from diseases, injuries, and risk factors in 1990 and projected to 2020.* Cambridge, MA: World Health Organization & Harvard University School of Public Health.

Myrick, H., & Anton, R. (1998). Treatment of alcohol withdrawal. *Alcohol, Health, and Research World, 22(1),* 38–43.

Naegle, M. A., & D'Avanzo, C. E. (2001). *Addictions and substance abuse: Strategies for advanced practice nursing.* Upper Saddle River, NJ: Prentice Hall Health.

National Institute on Alcohol Abuse and Alcoholism. (1997). *Alcohol and health* (DHHS Publication No. 97-4017). Rockville, MD: Author.

National Institute on Alcohol Abuse and Alcoholism. (1997). Alcohol's effect on organ function. *DHHS Publication 21*(1), 5–93.

National Institute on Drug Abuse. (2005). *Medical consequences of drug abuse/mental health effects.* Available at www.drugabuse.gov/consequences/mortality.

Sciacca, K. (1987). New initiative in the treatment of the chronic patient with alcohol/substance abuse–use problems. *Tie-Lines, 3,* 5–6.

Sullivan, J. T., Sykora, K., Schneiderman, J., Naranjo, C. A., & Sellers, E. M. (1989). The clinical institute withdrawal assessment for alcoholism. *British Journal of Addictions, 84*(11), 1353–1357.

Swift, R. M. (2001). The pharmacotherapy of alcohol dependence: Clinical and economic aspects. *Economics of Neuroscience, 3*(12), 62–66.

Vogel-Sprott, M. (1992). *Alcohol tolerance and social drinking: Learning the consequences.* New York: Guilford Press.

West, S., Garbutt, J. C., & Carey, T. S. (1999). *Pharmacotherapy for alcohol dependence: Evidence report/technology assessment* (AHCPR Publication No. 99-E0004). Rockville, MD: Agency for Health Care Policy and Research.

Notes:

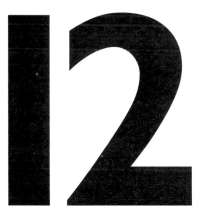

Personality Disorders

This chapter reviews a category of illnesses called personality disorders, common disorders that can affect the quality of the general health care that an individual receives. Although these disorders can create great difficulty for the individual, he or she remains able to perform routine daily functions. Often the individual does not recognize a problem or seek treatment.

This chapter briefly reviews the concept of *personality* and then its disorders. Assessment and clinical management features of personality disorders are discussed.

Personality

Description
- *Personality* is the sum total of all emotional, cognitive, and behavioral attributes of an individual.
- Personality involves an enduring pattern of perceiving, relating to, and thinking about the environment and oneself that are exhibited in a wide array of social and personal contexts.
- When healthy, personality structures allow for realistic, happy, and satisfying self-perceptions and interpersonal interactions.

Characteristics
- Personality is organized early in life and is dynamic and deeply ingrained; however, it can be altered.
- Patterns of behavior based on personality can be perceived by the individual as comfortable (*ego-syntonic*) or uncomfortable (*ego-dystonic*):
    - Ego-syntonic
        - Behavior consistent with personality
        - Causes little concern to the individual
        - Person generally fails to recognize problem
        - Person does not seek treatment.
    - Ego-dystonic
        - Behavior inconsistent with personality
        - Causes discomfort and concern to the individual

- Person generally recognizes problem
- Person often seeks treatment.

- Personality is reflected in behavioral traits habitually displayed by the individual:
  - Coping
  - Interpersonal or interactive style
  - Perceptions
  - Cognitive beliefs about events, individuals, and situations.

Personality Disorders

General Description

- Personality disorders are chronically maladaptive patterns of behaviors that cause functional impairment in work, school, or relationships.
- These disorders manifest as maladaptive patterns in four areas of functionality:
  1. Maladaptive *affective* traits, such as overly affectual patterns of response
  2. Maladaptive *behavioral* traits, such as poor impulse control patterns of response
  3. Maladaptive *cognitive* traits, such as unrealistic perceptual patterns of response
  4. Maladaptive *social* traits, such as maladaptive unsatisfying interpersonal patterns of response.
- These disorders can cause *subjective distress.*
- An individual is unlikely to recognize the problem and seek help if maladaptive patterns of behavior are ego-syntonic.
- An individual is more likely to recognize the problem and seek help if maladaptive patterns of behavior are ego-dystonic.
- Maladaptive patterns are *inflexible* and *pervasive* across most personal and social situations.
- These disorders are coded in the *DSM-IV-TR* (American Psychiatric Association, 2000) as Axis II disorders (see Table 12–1).
- Clients seldom fit neatly into one personality disorder diagnosis; rather, they often exhibit features of several similar disorders.
- For this reason, personality disorders often are referred to by the category of commonly manifesting symptom clusters (e.g., A, B, or C).

Table 12–1. Categories of Personality Disorders

Category	Characteristic Behavior	Disorders
Cluster A	Odd, unusual, eccentric, asocial	Paranoid personality disorder Schizoid personality disorder Schizotypal personality disorder
Cluster B	Dramatic, affective instability	Antisocial personality disorder Borderline personality disorder Histrionic personality disorder Narcissistic personality disorder

Table 12–1. Continued

Category	Characteristic Behavior	Disorders
Cluster C	Anxious	Avoidant personality disorder Dependent personality disorder Obsessive–compulsive personality disorder

Etiology

- Multiple theories ranging from psychological to neurobiological
- Probable multifactorial etiological profile
- Less empirical data available on neurobiological etiological factors
- Borderline personality disorder most well researched.

- Two common types of theories of personality disorders
  1. **Psychodynamic Theory**—primarily borderline personality disorder—Based on two etiological factors:
     - Early separation problems
       - Object Relations Theory
         - Internalized intrapsychic experiences of interpersonal relationships
         - Mental representation of the self in relation to others
         - Stability and depth of an individual's relationships
         - During development, child must accomplish two tasks: *separation* and *individuation.*
           - *Separation*—Develop intrapsychic self-representation distinct and separate from mother
           - *Individuation*—Form distinct identity with characteristics unique to the individual.
         - Four stages to process of separation–individuation (Mahler, Pine, & Bergman, 1975):
           1. Differentiation
           2. Practicing
           3. Rapprochement
           4. Object constancy.
              - Failure in separation–individuation is etiologically linked to development of personality disorders.
              - Different personality disorders linked to problems with different stages of the separation–individuation process.
     - Disturbed parental interaction
       - Family background assumed to be dysfunctional
         - Enmeshed family patterns
         - Role reversal patterns of child–parent interaction
         - Restricted involvement of family with the rest of the environment
         - Social isolation

- Confusion of parental authority and nurturing roles
- Blurred family boundaries.
  - Dysfunctional family patterns block separation–individuation processes; family rejection occurs if person attempts individuation.

2. **Biological Theory**
   - Genetic factors
     - Familial tendency
     - Genetic overlap between loading for some Axis I disorders and personality disorders.
   - Structural abnormalities
     - Reduced gray matter volume in prefrontal cortex
     - Limbic system deregulation.
   - Neurotransmitter dysfunction
     - Decreased levels of serotonin
     - Elevated levels of norepinephrine
     - Dysregulation of dopamine receptors.
   - Neurobiological impact of trauma
     - Most studied in borderline personality disorder
     - Assumes early childhood trauma alters basic brain patterns of response
     - In genetically susceptible individuals, may function as the environmental vulnerability that causes expression of genetic load.

Incidence and Demographics
- Difficult to estimate, as individuals with personality disorders are rarely hospitalized and often receive no treatment
- Incidence varies with disorder
- Generally assumed to be 0.5%–5.4% in the general U.S. population.

Risk Factors
- Genetic loading
- Dysfunctional family of origin.

Prevention and Screening
- At-risk family education
- Community education
  - Stigma reduction
  - Signs and symptoms of illness
  - Treatment potential for control of symptoms.
- Early recognition, intervention, and initiation of treatment
- Preventive work with young children in identified dysfunctional family settings.

Assessment
- Symptoms of personality disorder are enduring maladaptive patterns of behavior, generally seen as problems with living.
- Often several interviews are needed to clarify the diagnostic picture.

History–Assess for the Following:

- Detailed history of present illness, including time frame, progression, and associated symptoms
- Social history, including present living situation; marital status; occupation; education; and alcohol, tobacco, or illicit drug use
- Medication use, including prescription, over-the-counter, alternative, supplements, and home remedies
- Initial and periodic functional history and assessment
- Validate history with family member.

Long-Term Patterns of Functioning

- Stability of traits over time and across situations.

Cultural Issues vs. Maladaptive Personality Traits

- Issues of acculturation in new immigrants
- Cultural expression of habitual behavior
- Custom or religious practices.

Assessment for Cluster A Disorders

- Patterns of pervasive distrust and suspiciousness, with odd and unusual behavior
  - Present in a variety of contexts, even without supportive evidence.

- Distrust usually not at psychotic level but can display brief psychotic episodes under stress
- Significant history includes the following:
  - Limited social network
  - Poor interpersonal relationships
  - Limited disclosure or revealing of self to others, often refusing to answer personal questions
  - Compliments often misinterpreted
  - Pathological jealousy common
  - Difficult to get along with
  - Appearing cold and lacking in feelings
  - High control needs
  - Rigid and critical of others
  - Often highly litigious
  - Negatively perceive others; often biased and prone to stereotypes.

- Differences in Cluster A disorders are in degree of suspiciousness and mistrust and in behavioral manifestations of these traits (see Table 12–2).

Table 12–2. Characteristics of Cluster A Personality Disorders

Disorder	Characteristic
Paranoid personality disorder	Neither desires nor enjoys close relationships
	Chooses solitary activities
	Shows little to no interest in sexual activity with another person
	Derives no pleasure in social activities

Continued on the next page

Table 12–2. Continued

Disorder	Characteristic
Schizoid personality disorder	Lacks close friends or social supports
	Is indifferent of opinion of others
	Appears cold and detached
	Exhibits affective flattening
Schizotypal personality disorder	Ideas of reference
	Odd beliefs
	Magical thinking
	Unusual perceptual experiences
	Paranoid ideation
	Inappropriate or constricted affect
	Behavior overtly odd, eccentric, or peculiar
	Few or no close friends
	Excessive social anxiety

Assessment for Cluster B Disorders

- Patterns of pervasive affective and interpersonal disruption
  - Present in a variety of contexts, even without supportive evidence.

- Disturbance usually not at psychotic level but can display brief psychotic episodes under stress
- Of all clusters, disorders of Cluster B type may require hospitalization during period of active symptom expression and when client under significant levels of stress
- Significant history includes the following:
  - Fluctuating emotional states
  - Dramatic qualities to how the individual lives his or her life.

- Antisocial Personality Disorder
  - Usually diagnosed by age 18
  - More common in men
  - High substance abuse comorbidity
  - High impulsivity
  - Often diagnosed with conduct disorder as children.

- Borderline Personality Disorder
  - Predominantly in women
  - Often with positive history of significant childhood physical abuse, sexual abuse, neglect, or early parental separation or loss.

- Differences in Cluster B disorders are in degree of affective instability, type of interpersonal disruption, and behavioral manifestations of those traits (see Table 12–3).

Table 12–3. Characteristics of Cluster B Personality Disorders

Disorder	Characteristic
Antisocial personality disorder	Failure to conform to social norms Repeated acts that are grounds for arrest Deceitfulness, lying, and use of aliases for profit or pleasure Impulsivity and failure of future planning Reckless disregard for the welfare of others Consistent irresponsibility Lack of remorse; indifference to the feelings of others
Borderline personality disorder	Frantic efforts to avoid real or imagined abandonment Pattern of unstable, intense interpersonal relationships Identity disturbances Impulsivity, often with self-damaging behavior Recurrent suicidal behavior Chronic feelings of emptiness Inappropriate, intensified affective anger responses Transient psychotic symptoms of paranoia and dissociation
Histrionic personality disorder	Uncomfortable in situations in which he or she is not center of attention Interactions with others characterized by inappropriate seductive or sexualized or provocative behavior, rapid shifting, and shallow emotional responses Consistent use of physical appearance to draw attention to self Speech excessively impressionistic and lacking in detail Suggestible and easily influenced Relationships considered more intimate than they are
Narcissistic personality disorder	Grandiose sense of self-importance Preoccupation with fantasies of power, success, brilliance, and beauty Belief of self-importance and being special and unique Excessive admiration required Unreasonable expectations or sense of entitlement Interpersonally exploitative Empathy lacking Envy of others and belief that others envy him or her Arrogant and haughty behaviors

Assessment for Cluster C Disorders
- Patterns of pervasive anxiety and fear
  - Present in a variety of contexts, even without supportive evidence.
- Disturbance usually not at psychotic level but can display brief psychotic episodes under stress
- Significant history includes the following:
  - Avoidant behavior

- Procrastination
- Difficulty in following through
- Fearful of rejection and criticism
- Difficulty relaxing.

- Avoidant Personality Disorder
  - Must consider cultural variable when looking at avoidant behavior
  - Disorder equal for both genders.

- Dependent Personality Disorder
  - Most frequently diagnosed personality disorder
  - Rates higher in women than in men
  - Commonly diagnosed in individuals with history of chronic physical illnesses.

- Obsessive–Compulsive Personality Disorder
  - Predominantly in men
  - Symptoms similar to but less severe than obsessive–compulsive disorder

- Differences in Cluster C disorders are in the degree of anxiety and fear and in behavioral manifestations of those traits (see Table 12–4).

Physical Exam Findings
- Nonspecific.

Diagnostic and Laboratory Findings
- CBC, chemistry profile, and thyroid function tests to rule out metabolic causes or unidentified conditions
- Drug toxicity screening if indicated by history.

Table 12–4. Characteristics of Cluster C Personality Disorders

Disorder	Characteristic
Avoidant personality disorder	Avoidance of activities involving significant interpersonal contact Fear of criticism, disapproval, or rejection Unwillingness to be involved with people unless sure of being liked Restraint in intimate relationships for fear of being shamed Preoccupation with being criticized or rejected in social settings View of self as socially inept, personally unappealing, or inferior Unusual reluctance to take personal risks or engage in new activities
Dependent personality disorder	Difficulty making everyday decisions without excessive advice Needing others to assume responsibility for most areas of life Difficulty expressing disagreement Difficulty initiating projects Goes to excessive lengths to obtain nurturing and support from others Urgent seeking of another relationship if a close relationship ends Unrealistic preoccupation with fears of being left alone

Table 12–4. Continued

Disorder	Characteristic
Obsessive–compulsive personality disorder	Preoccupation with details, rules, order, and organization
	Perfectionism that interferes with task completion
	Excessive devotion to work and productivity
	Overly conscientious, scrupulous, and inflexible on issues of morality
	Inability to discard worn-out or worthless objects
	Reluctance to delegate tasks or work with others
	Adoption of a miserly spending style toward self and others
	Rigidity and stubbornness

Differential Diagnosis
- Mood disorders (see Chapter 7)
  - Affective instability of borderline personality disorder often mistaken for bipolar affective disorder
- Substance-induced disorders (see Chapter 11).

Clinical Management
- Rule out or treat any conditions that may contribute to cognitive impairment.
- Personality disorders are generally managed in a community setting.
- In some cases, hospitalization may be required (Clarkin, Foelsch, Levy, Hull, Delaney, & Kernberg, 2001).

Pharmacological Management
- No specific class of pharmacological agents used to treat personality disorders
- Individualized symptom control
  - Impulsivity
    - Selected serotonin reuptake inhibitors (SSRIs)
    - Anticonvulsant mood stabilizers.
  - Affective instability
    - SSRIs
    - Anticonvulsant mood stabilizers.
  - Anxiety
    - Non-benzodiazepine (BNZ) anxiolytics
    - SSRIs
    - BNZs (use with caution).

Nonpharmacological Management
- Most common form of treatment for personality disorders
- Focus on issues of limit setting, protection from self-harm, improved coping, and enhanced interpersonal functioning

- Multiple therapeutic interventions may be used, such as
  - Case management
  - Psychotherapy
    - Focus on individual gaining control
    - Improvement of interpersonal skill level
    - Enhanced coping
    - Alteration of problematic patterns of behavior
    - Forms of therapy:
      - Dialectical–behavioral therapy
      - Interpersonal therapy
      - Behavioral therapy
      - Cognitive–behavioral therapy.
  - Milieu therapy.

- Assist with realistic expectation formation.
- Structure environment.
- Improve realistic self-appraisal ability.

Life Span Considerations
Children
- Before diagnosis is determined, sufficient life experiences must occur so that chronicity of maladaptive patterns can be observed.
- Features of personality disorder usually become apparent during adolescence to early adulthood.
- It is unusual for person to be given personality disorder diagnosis before ages 16–18 (an exception is antisocial personality disorder, which often is observable by onset of puberty; however, diagnosis of antisocial personality disorder is not made until age 18).
- Separation anxiety and chronic physical illness often precede and predict onset of dependent personality disorder.

Follow-up
- These are chronic disorders, and clients may be resistant to change.
- Relapse is common and frequent.
- How long to treat and success rates vary with individual characteristics and motivation.
- Prognosis is poor without treatment.
- Prognosis improves if treatment started as early in life as possible.

Case Study

Mr. Jevers is a 42-year-old new client who seeks health care for a general physical exam. The family nurse practitioner who examines Mr. Jevers asks the psychiatric–mental health nurse practitioner (PMHNP) to speak with him because of his odd presentation. The client discusses with the PMHNP an unusual, recurrent experience he has been having.

Mr. Jevers lives in an apartment building downtown and works as a bartender in the late evening. He tells the PMHNP that every night as he walks home from work he watches to see if the wind "blows north to south or south to north." He relates that on the occasions that the wind goes north to south, he takes that as a sign that a woman will visit him. He tells of a woman who rides a bicycle down the road and, as she passes him, he receives a blessing from her that protects him from those who wish him harm. He believes the woman is a "spirit from the other side" and that no one but he can see the woman.

As Mr. Jevers tells his story, his affect is inappropriate, his mood pleasant and happy, and he exhibits some paranoid ideation as he worries that others will try to take away the spirit. His MSE shows ideas of reference and some magical thinking as he shares his "blessing" with customers in the bar, and he describes odd, eccentric, and peculiar behaviors. Mr. Jevers is not at all bothered by his unusual experience and seems to enjoy telling it to others. He considers himself lucky to have "special powers" and to see and understand things that others do not. He denies the presence of any typical manifestations of hallucinations or delusions, any mood disturbance or anxiety, and alcohol or other drug use. He reports having several close friends and a strong support network and is in general good health, but he does experience significant social anxiety. He does not believe his unusual experience is a symptom of an illness and wishes no intervention or assistance at this time. There are many issues to consider in planning care with this client:

- What is the most probable diagnosis for this client?

- What further assessment should occur?

- If the client desires no treatment, should the PMHNP attempt to follow up with him?

- What treatment should be suggested at this time?

Review Questions

1. Impulsivity is a common behavioral manifestation of personality disorders. The PMHNP working with a client with high impulsivity should consider which of the following pharmacological interventions?

    a. Use of a TCA agent

    b. Use of a benzodiazepine agent

    c. Use of an antipsychotic agent for its sedative effect

    d. Use of an SSRI agent

2. The affective instability common in some personality disorders can be clinically managed with all of the following except:

    a. Anticonvulsant agents

    b. SSRI agents

    c. MAOI agents

    d. Antipsychotic agents

3. The cluster of personality disorders that manifest with dramatic, overly affective behavior is

    a. Cluster A
    b. Cluster B
    c. Cluster C

4. Etiological models that attempt to explain the development of personality disorders include which of the following?

    a. Object loss theory
    b. Object relations theory
    c. Situation crisis development
    d. Object adjustment theory

References and Resources

Alper, G., & Peterson, S. J. (2001). Dialectical behavior therapy for patients with borderline personality disorder. *Journal of Psychosocial Nursing and Mental Health Services, 39*(10), 38–45.

American Psychiatric Association. (2000). *Diagnostic and statistical manual of mental disorders* (4th ed., text rev.). Washington, DC: Author.

Burke, M., & Laramie, J. A. (2003). *Primary care of older adults* (2nd ed.). St. Louis, MO: Mosby.

Clarkin, J. F., Foelsch, P. A., Levy, K. N., Hull, J. W., Delaney, J. C., & Kernberg, O. F. (2001). The development of a psychodynamic treatment for patients with borderline personality disorder: A preliminary study of behavioral change. *Journal of Personality Disorders, 15,* 487–495.

Daghestani, A. N., Dinwiddie, M. D., & Hardy, D. W. (2001). Antisocial personality disorder in and out of correctional and forensic settings. *Psychiatric Annals, 31,* 441–446.

Feinstein, R. E. (2000). Personality disorders in the primary care setting: Diagnosis, management, and intervention. *Resident and Staff Physician, 11,* 47–56.

Freidman, J. H. (1998). *Neurology in primary care.* Boston: Butterworth/Heinemann.

Keltner, N., Schwecke, L. H., & Bostrom, C. E. (2006). *Psychiatric nursing* (5th ed.). St. Louis, MO: Mosby.

Mahler, M., Pine, F., & Bergman, A. (1975). *The psychological birth of the human infant: Symbiosis and individuation.* New York: Basic Books.

Parker, L. (2001). Dialectical behavioral therapy: A working perspective. *Nursing Times, 9* (4), 38–39.

Schmahl, C. G., McGlashan, T., & Bremner, J. D. (2002). Neurobiological correlates of borderline personality disorder. *Psychopharmacology Bulletin, 36*(2), 69–78.

Stone, M. H. (2000). Clinical guidelines for psychotherapy for patients with borderline personality disorder. *Psychiatric Clinics of North America, 23,* 193–210.

Stuart, G. W., & Laraia, M. (2004). *Principles and practice of psychiatric nursing* (8th ed.). St. Louis, MO: Mosby.

Uphold, C. R. (2003). *Clinical guidelines in family practice* (4th ed.). Gainesville, FL: Barmarrae Books.

Notes:

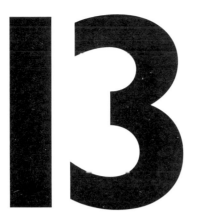

Disorders of Childhood and Adolescence

Disorders first diagnosed in infancy, childhood, or adolescence, such as conduct disorder, oppositional defiant disorder, attention-deficit/hyperactivity disorder, Asperger's disorder, Rett's disorder, autistic spectrum disorder, eating disorders, and mental retardation, are considered brain-based illnesses and have many similarities to disorders diagnosed more commonly in adulthood. In addition, these disorders often are missed during childhood and adolescent years and are therefore not identified until early adulthood.

The disorders in this category differ in presentation, in developmental age of common onset, and in gender factors. Assessment, treatment planning, and therapeutic interventions for these disorders must always occur within the context of the family and assume a multimodal, systems-oriented approach to care. In addition, assessment of children is different from assessment of adults. Therefore, psychiatric–mental health nurse practitioners (PMHNPs) must apply principles of child assessment to effectively care for the client and family experiencing or at risk for these disorders.

Assessment and Care Planning for Children and Adolescents

Requires alteration in assessment process
- Generally takes more time
- Must develop trusting relationship with the child to put him or her at ease
- Need to separate the young child from the parents for assessment and thus deal effectively with separation and stranger anxiety
- Must attend to developmental needs and interests of the child
- Must attend to the cognitive and language abilities of the child.

Mental Status Examination
- Modified to reflect developmental and other age-related issues in children
- Often requires establishment of play environment to open communication with the child.

Appearance

- Conclusions must consider age and developmental processes (e.g., dressing in all-black clothing may be developmentally appropriate for an adolescent but not for a preschooler)
- Gait and motor skills assessed on expected normative behaviors for age.

Speech

- Assessed on expected normative behaviors for age in comprehension, word selection, and range of vocabulary.

Thought Process

- Assessed on expected normative behaviors for age in degree of organization, goal orientation, and ability to focus.

Abstraction

- Assessed on expected normative behaviors for age
- Children ages 12 or younger not expected to have abstractive thought abilities
- Proverb testing and similarity testing require prior exposure to concept, word choices, and ability to think abstractly.

Therapeutic Care Planning

- Variety of effective treatments commonly used with children and adolescents:
  - Play therapy
  - Game therapy
  - Art therapy
  - Bibliotherapy
  - Orative therapy (e.g., storytelling, family narrative therapy)
  - Behavioral therapy
  - Milieu therapy
  - Pharmacotherapy.

Conduct Disorder

Description

- *Conduct disorder* is a persistent pattern of behavior in which the rights of others or societal norms or rules are violated.

Etiology

- No single factor accounts for presentation.
- Etiology is largely unknown.
- Many biopsychosocial factors contribute to the development.

Incidence and Demographics

- Conduct disorder is more common in children of parents with antisocial personality disorder, alcohol dependence, mood disorders, or schizophrenia than in the general population.

- It affects 1%–10% of general U.S. population, 6%–16% of boys and 2%–9% of girls.
- Onset is earlier for boys (10–12 years) than girls (16 years).

Risk Factors
- Genetic loading
- Dysfunctional family patterns
- Substance abuse.

Prevention and Screening
- At-risk family education
- Community education
  - Stigma reduction
  - Signs and symptoms of illness
  - Treatment potential for control of symptoms.

- Early recognition, intervention, and initiation of treatment
  - Secondary prevention is important in younger clients.

Assessment
- Detailed history of present illness, including time frame, progression, and associated symptoms
- Social history, including present living situation; education; and alcohol, tobacco, or illicit drug use
- Medication use, including prescription, over-the-counter, alternative, supplements, and home remedies
- Initial and periodic functional history and assessment
- Developmental history
- Validate history with a family member.

History–Assess for the Following:
- Four categories of behaviors:
  - Aggression toward people and animals
  - Destruction of property
  - Deceitfulness or theft
  - Serious violation of rules.

- Must have three or more symptoms of the disorder in the past year and at least one symptom in the past 6 months
- Significant impairment in social, academic, and occupational functioning
  - Childhood Onset
    - At least one criterion characteristic present before age 10 years

  - Adolescent Onset
    - No criteria characteristic present before age 10 years

Physical Exam Findings
- Nonspecific.

Mental Status Exam Findings

Affect
- Irritable
- Angry
- Uncooperative.

Mood
- Anger.

Thought Content
- Lack of empathy or concern for others.

Concentration
- Distractible.

Insight
- Poor.

Diagnostic and Laboratory Findings
- No specific laboratory tests
- Drug screening to rule out possible substance abuse
- CBC, chemistry profile, thyroid function tests, and B_{12} level to rule out metabolic causes or unidentified conditions.

Differential Diagnosis
- Attention-deficit/hyperactivity disorder (ADHD; see below)
- Oppositional defiant disorder (ODD; see below)
- Mood disorders (see Chapter 7)
- Substance abuse disorders (see Chapter 11).

Clinical Management
- Rule out or treat any conditions that may contribute to current symptom manifestation.

Pharmacological Management
- No specific pharmacological interventions
- Aggression and agitation treated with antipsychotics, mood stabilizers, selective serotonin reuptake inhibitors (SSRIs), and alpha agonists.

Nonpharmacological Management
- Multimodality treatment programs that use all available family and community resources
- Behavioral therapy is mainstay.
  - Individual therapy
  - Family therapy
  - Classroom assistance.

Life Span Considerations

- May be diagnosed in clients age 18 years or older if criteria for antisocial personality disorder not met.

Oppositional Defiant Disorder (ODD)

Description

- *Oppositional defiant disorder* (ODD) is an enduring pattern of negativistic, defiant, disobedient, hostile, and defiant behaviors, usually directed at an authority figure.

Etiology

- No single factor accounts for presentation.
- Etiology is largely unknown.
- Many biopsychosocial factors contribute to the development.

Incidence and Demographics

- ODD is more common in children of parents with a history of ODD, conduct disorder, ADHD, antisocial personality disorder, mood disorders, or substance abuse disorder.
- It affects 2%–16% of the general U.S. population.
- Boys with the disorder are more prevalent than girls before puberty; after puberty, the boy-to-girl ratio is equal.

Risk Factors

- Genetic loading.

Prevention and Screening

- At-risk family education
- Community education
  - Stigma reduction
  - Signs and symptoms of illness
  - Treatment potential for control of symptoms.

- Early recognition, intervention, and initiation of treatment
  - Secondary prevention important in younger clients

Assessment

- Detailed history of present illness, including time frame, progression, and associated symptoms
- Social history, including present living situation; education; and alcohol, tobacco, or illicit drug use
- Medication use, including prescription, over-the-counter, alternative, supplements, and home remedies
- Initial and periodic functional history and assessment
- Validate history with a family member.

History–Assess for the Following:
- Criteria behaviors persisting for *at least 6 months* and including *at least four* of the following:
  - Often loses temper
  - Often argues with adults
  - Often actively defies or refuses to comply with adults' requests or rules
  - Often deliberately annoys people
  - Often blames others for his or her mistakes or misbehavior
  - Often is touchy or easily annoyed by others
  - Often is angry and resentful
  - Often is spiteful or vindictive.

Physical Exam Findings
- Nonspecific.

Mental Status Exam Findings
Mood
- Lability.

Concentration
- Impaired.

Thought Content
- Low frustration tolerance.

Diagnostic and Laboratory Findings
- No specific laboratory tests
- CBC, chemistry profile, thyroid function tests, and B_{12} level to rule out metabolic causes or unidentified conditions
- Drug toxicity screening, if indicated by history
  - Toxicology screen to rule out a substance abuse disorder.

Differential Diagnosis
- ADHD (see below)
- Mood disorders (see Chapter 7)
- Substance-abuse disorders (see Chapter 11)
- Mental retardation (see below)
- Conduct disorder (see above)
- Psychotic disorders (see Chapter 9).

Clinical Management
- Rule out or treat any conditions that may contribute to current symptom manifestation.

Pharmacological Management
- Nonspecific.

Nonpharmacological Management
- Behavioral therapy is mainstay.
  - Individual therapy
  - Family therapy, with emphasis on child management skills.

Attention-Deficit/Hyperactivity Disorder (ADHD)

Description
- *Attention-deficit/hyperactivity disorder* (ADHD) is a persistent pattern of inattention or hyperactivity/impulsivity, or both, that is more frequent and more severe than that typically observed in individuals of the same developmental level.

Etiology
- Many biopsychosocial factors contribute to the development.
- Polygenic neurobiological deficits are associated with ADHD.
  - Problems with executive functioning
  - Abnormalities of fronto–subcortical pathways
    - Frontal cortex
    - Basal ganglia.

  - Abnormalities of reticular activating system
  - Structural abnormalities producing neurotransmitter abnormalities
    - Dopamine dysfunction
    - Norepinephrine dysfunction.

Incidence and Demographics
- 3%–5% of U.S. children have ADHD.
- It is much more common in boys than girls.
- Average age of onset is 3 years; mean age of diagnosis is 9 years.
- Approximately 60% of clients have symptoms persisting into adulthood.
  - Inattention symptoms are more persistent than hyperactivity/impulsivity symptoms.

Risk Factors
- Genetic loading
  - ADHD
  - Mood disorders
  - Anxiety disorders.

- Pregnancy and perinatal complications
- Family conflict.

Prevention and Screening
- At-risk family education
- Community education
  - Stigma reduction
  - Signs and symptoms of illness
  - Treatment potential for control of symptoms.

- Early recognition, intervention, and initiation of treatment
  - Secondary prevention is important in young patients.

Assessment

History–Assess for the Following:

- Because of high genetic link, history of attention and impulse problems in client's parents and grandparents
- History of criteria symptoms in client
  - Inattention
    - Inattention to details
    - Careless mistakes
    - Difficulty sustaining attention
    - Seeming not to listen
    - Failure to finish tasks
    - Difficulty with organizing
    - Avoidance of tasks requiring sustained attention
    - Loss of things
    - Distractibility
    - Forgetfulness.

  - Hyperactivity/impulsivity
    - Blurting out answers before question is finished
    - Difficulty awaiting his or her turn
    - Interrupting or intruding on others
    - Fidgeting
    - Inability to stay seated
    - Inappropriate running or climbing
    - General restlessness
    - Difficulty engaging in leisure activities
    - Always "on the go"
    - Excessive talking.

- Variations in pervasiveness, frequency, and degree of impairment
- Subtypes
  - ADHD—Inattentive
    - Inattentive symptoms dominate.
    - Lack of criterion symptoms for hyperactivity/impulsivity.

  - ADHD—Hyperactive
    - Hyperactivity/impulsivity symptoms dominate.
    - Lack of criterion symptoms for inattention.

  - ADHD—Combined
    - Criterion symptoms met for inattention and hyperactivity/impulsivity.

Physical Exam Findings

- Nonspecific
- Minor physical anomalies at higher rates in people with ADHD than in general population
  - Hypertelorism

- • Highly arched palate
- • Low-set ears.
- • Higher-than-average accidental injury rates.

Mental Status Exam Findings
- • Restlessness
- • Inattention
- • Distractible speech patterns
- • Overproductive speech patterns
- • Affective lability
- • Poor memory
- • Poor concentration.

Diagnostic and Laboratory Findings
- • Nonspecific.

Common Comorbidities
- • Major depressive disorder (MDD; see Chapter 7)
- • Bipolar (BP) disorder (see Chapter 7)
- • Anxiety disorders (see Chapter 8)
- • Obsessive–compulsive disorder (OCD; see Chapter 8)
- • Substance abuse disorders (see Chapter 11)
- • Learning disorders.

Differential Diagnosis
- • Under stimulated home environment
- • Substance abuse
- • MDD
- • BP disorder
- • Stereotypic movement disorder.

Clinical Management
Pharmacological Management
- • Most commonly used agents (see Table 13–1) are stimulants (Schedule II)—Controlled substances, carry risk for abuse.

Table 13–1. Most Commonly Used Agents for ADHD

Drug	Dosage
Ritalin (methylphenidate hydrochloride), Schedule II	5–40 mg/d
Ritalin LA/Ritalin SR (methylphenidate hydrochloride), Schedule II	10–60 mg/d
Metadate CD (methylphenidate hydrochloride), Schedule II	10–60 mg/d
Metadate ER (methylphenidate hydrochloride), Schedule II	10–60 mg/d
Concerta (methylphenidate hydrochloride), Schedule II	18–72 mg/d
Methylin (methylphenidate hydrochloride), Schedule II	5–60 mg/d

Continued on the next page

Table 13–1. Continued

Drug	Dosage
Methylin ER (methylphenidate hydrochloride), Schedule II	10–60 mg/d
Dexadrine (dextroamphetamine), Schedule II	2.5–20 mg/d
Adderall (amphetamine, dextroamphetamine), Schedule II	5–40 mg/d
Adderall XR (amphetamine, dextroamphetamine), Schedule II	5–60 mg/d
Focalin/Focalin XR (dexmethylphenidate), Schedule II	2.5–20 mg/d
Vyvanse (lisdexamfetamine dimesylate), Schedule II	30–70 mg/d
Strattera (atomoxetine hydrochloride), not a controlled substance	10–100 mg/day

- Monitor for side effects and adverse effects of stimulants:
  - GI upsets
  - Cramps
  - Anorexia nervosa
  - Weight loss
  - Growth suppression
  - Cramps
  - Headache
  - Dizziness
  - Irritability
  - Psychosis (rare).

Nonpharmacological Management
- Behavioral therapy
- Psychoeducation
- Treatment of learning disorders
- Family therapy and education
  - Parents of children with ADHD have many difficult emotions
    - Stress
    - Self-blame
    - Social isolation
    - Embarrassment
    - Depressive reaction
    - Marital discord.

  - Typical family concerns
    - Stigma
    - Anger
    - Concerns over treatment options
    - Presence of controversial information in media
    - Claims of dietary causes of disorder
    - Belief in family etiological factors.

  - Family educational needs
    - Environmental structuring
    - Psychiatric comorbidities
    - School issues and concerns
    - Peer relationship building
    - Smoking and substance-abuse rates
    - Stress management.

Follow-up
- Monitor clinical progress over time.
- Use standardized rating scales such as
  - Conner's Parent and Teacher Rating Scales (Conners, 1969).
- Monitor growth and development milestone attainment.
  - Use of stimulants can adversely affect development.
- Symptoms may persist into adulthood.
  - Plan for long-term needs.

Asperger's Disorder

Description
- *Asperger's disorder* is severe, sustained impairment in social interaction and restricted, repetitive patterns of behavior, interests, and activities.

Etiology
- No single factor can account for presentation.
- Etiology is largely unknown.
- Many biopsychosocial factors contribute to the development.

Incidence and Demographics
- The disorder appears to be more common among family members who have the disorder or who have autistic spectrum disorder (ASD).
- Prevalence is not known, but the disorder is more common in boys.

Risk Factors
- Genetic loading.

Prevention and Screening
- At-risk family education
- Community education
  - Stigma reduction
  - Signs and symptoms of illness
  - Treatment potential for control of symptoms.
- Early recognition, intervention, and initiation of treatment
  - Secondary prevention is important in young clients.

Assessment
- Detailed history of present illness, including time frame, progression, and associated symptoms
- Social history, including present living situation; marital status; occupation; education; and alcohol, tobacco, or illicit drug use
- Medication use, including prescription, over-the-counter, alternative, supplements, and home remedies

- Initial and periodic functional history and assessment
- Validate history with a family member.

History–Assess for the Following:
- Qualitative impairment in social interaction
- Restricted, repetitive, and stereotyped patterns of behavior, interests, and activities
- Significant impairment in social, occupational, or other areas of functioning
- Diagnostic criteria very similar to autism, except no clinically significant delay in language, cognitive development, or adaptive behavior.

Physical Exam Findings
- Nonspecific.

Mental Status Exam Findings
Appearance
- Stereotypic or repetitive motor mannerisms
- Poor eye contact.

Affect
- Flat.

Reaction to Interview
- Lack of emotional reciprocity.

Diagnostic and Laboratory Findings
- No laboratory tests
- CBC, chemistry profile, thyroid function tests, and B_{12} level to rule out metabolic causes or unidentified conditions
- Drug toxicity screening, if indicated by history.

Differential Diagnosis
- ASD (see below)
- Rett's disorder (see below)
- Childhood disintegrative disorder (marked deterioration of functioning after a period of at least 2 years of normal functioning and development)
- Schizophrenia (see Chapter 9)
- Schizoid personality disorder (see Chapter 12).

Clinical Management
- Rule out or treat any conditions that may contribute to current symptom manifestation.

Pharmacological Management
- Nonspecific
- Treat symptoms as indicated.

Nonpharmacological Management
- Multimodality treatment
  - Behavioral therapy
  - Appropriate school placement
  - Occupational therapy
  - Physical therapy
  - Speech therapy.

Rett's Disorder

Description
- *Rett's disorder* is the development of specific deficits following a period of normal functioning after birth.

Etiology
- Etiology is unknown.
- There is a known, progressive, and deteriorating course after an initial normal period.
- It is compatible with probable metabolic disorder.
- Suspected genetic mutation exists.

Incidence and Demographics
- The disorder occurs primarily in girls.
- It is usually associated with severe or profound mental retardation (see below).

Risk Factors
- Mental retardation
- Seizure disorder.

Prevention and Screening
- At-risk family education
- Community education
  - Stigma reduction
  - Signs and symptoms of illness
  - Treatment potential for control of symptoms.

- Early recognition, intervention, and initiation of treatment
  - Secondary prevention is important in young clients.

Assessment
- Detailed history of present illness, including time frame, progression, and associated symptoms
- Social history, including present living situation; marital status; occupation; education; and alcohol, tobacco, or illicit drug use
- Medication use, including prescription, over-the-counter, alternative, supplements, and home remedies

- Initial and periodic functional history and assessment
- Validate history with a family member.

History–Assess for the Following:
- Normal prenatal and perinatal development
- Normal psychomotor development through the first 5 months after birth
- Normal head circumference at birth
- Onset of all of the following after the period of normal development:
  - Deceleration of head growth between age 5 and 48 months
  - Loss of previously acquired purposeful hand skills between ages 5 and 30 months, with the subsequent development of stereotypic hand movements
  - Early loss of social engagement
  - Appearance of poorly coordinated gait or trunk movements
  - Severely impaired expressive- and receptive-language development with severe psychomotor retardation.

Physical Exam Findings
- Associated features:
  - Seizures
  - Irregular respirations
  - Scoliosis
  - Loss of purposeful hand skills
  - Stereotypic hand movements.

Mental Status Exam Findings
Appearance
- Stereotypic hand movements.

Speech
- Expressive- and receptive-language impairment.

Affect
- Flat or blunted.

Diagnostic and Laboratory Findings
- No specific laboratory or diagnostic findings
- CBC, chemistry profile, thyroid function tests, and B_{12} level to rule out metabolic causes or unidentified conditions
- Drug toxicity screening, if indicated by history
- EEG and nonspecific abnormalities on brain imaging.

Differential Diagnosis
- ASD (see below)
- Childhood disintegrative disorder (see above)
- Mental retardation (see below)
- Asperger's disorder (see above).

Clinical Management
- Rule out or treat any conditions that may contribute to current symptom manifestation.

Pharmacological Management
- Nonspecific.

Nonpharmacological Management
- Multimodality treatment
- Treatment aimed at symptomatic intervention.

Autistic Spectrum Disorder (ASD)

Description
- *Autistic spectrum disorder* (ASD) involves the marked impairment of social and cognitive abilities.

Etiology
- Imbalances of glutamate, serotonin, and gamma-aminobutyric acid (GABA) are thought to be implicated in causation.
- Brain-imaging studies (Gillberg, 1999) of children with autism reveal microscopic and macroscopic abnormalities of the amygdala, hippocampus, and cerebellum.
- Decreased numbers of Purkinje cells in the cerebellum are thought to play a role in the development.

Incidence and Demographics
- ASD is more common in children with a family history of pervasive developmental disorders.
- The concordant rate for an identical twin with autism is 60%.
- The incidence is 2–5 cases per 10,000 in the United States.
- The male-to-female ratio is 4:1.
- 75% of children with autism have mental retardation.
- Onset of symptoms is before age 3 years.

Risk Factors
- Male
- Severe mental retardation
- Genetic loading.

Prevention and Screening
- At-risk family education
- Community education
  - Stigma reduction
  - Signs and symptoms of illness
  - Treatment potential for control of symptoms.

- Early recognition, intervention, and initiation of treatment
- Secondary prevention is important in young clients.

Assessment

History–Assess for the Following:

- Impairment with social interaction, communications, and behavior
  - Impaired social interactions such as abnormal gaze, posture, and expression in social interactions.
- Lack of peer relationships, emotional reciprocity, and spontaneous seeking of enjoyment
- Impaired communication, such as a delay in or lack of the development of spoken language, impaired ability to initiate and sustain conversations, repetitive and stereotypic use of language, and inability to play with others
- Restricted repetitive and stereotypic patterns of behavior, interests, and activities, such as inflexible adherence to specific nonfunctional routines and repetitive, stereotypic motor mannerisms (e.g., hand or finger flapping, rocking, swaying)
- Parents may report any of the following symptoms:
  - No cooing by age 1 year, no single words by age 16 months, no two-word phrases by age 24 months
  - Loss of language skills at any time
  - No imaginary play
  - Little interest in playing with other children
  - Extremely short attention span
  - No response when called by name
  - Little or no eye contact
  - Intense tantrums
  - Fixations on single objects
  - Unusually strong resistance to changes in routines
  - Oversensitivity to certain sounds, textures, or smells
  - Appetite or sleep–wake disturbance, or both
  - Self-injurious behavior.

Physical Exam Findings

- Nonspecific.

Mental Status Exam Findings

- Little or no eye contact
- Flat or blunted affect
- Lack of emotional reciprocity
- Stereotypic or repetitive motor mannerisms
  - Expressive- and receptive-language impairment.

Diagnostic and Laboratory Findings

- No specific laboratory tests.

Differential Diagnosis

- Rett's disorder (see above)
- Asperger's disorder (see above)

- Childhood disintegrative disorder (see above)
- Mental retardation (see below)
- Hearing impairment
- Developmental language and speech disorders
- Tic disorders
- Stereotypic movement disorder
- Schizophrenia (see Chapter 9)
- Cluster A personality disorders (see Chapter 12).

Clinical Management

Pharmacological Management
- No specific pharmacological interventions.
- Antipsychotics effective for symptoms such as tantrums; aggressive behavior; self-injurious behavior; hyperactivity; and repetitive, stereotypic behaviors
- Antidepressants, naltrexone, clonidine, and stimulants used to diminish self-injurious and hyperactive and obsessive behaviors.

Nonpharmacological Management
- Behavioral therapy to improve cognitive functioning and reduce inappropriate behavior
- Occupational therapy to improve sensory integration and motor skills
- Speech therapy to address communication and language barriers
- Appropriate school placement with a highly structured approach.

Eating Disorders

Description
- *Eating disorders* are characterized by disordered patterns of eating, accompanied by distress, disparagement, preoccupation, and a distorted perception of one's body shape.
- Common forms of eating disorder
  - *Anorexia Nervosa*
    - Clients refuse to maintain a normal body weight
    - Restrict caloric intake
    - Have an intense fear of gaining weight because of a distorted body image.

  - *Bulimia Nervosa*
    - Clients engage in binge eating
    - Combined with inappropriate ways of stopping weight gain
      - Associated with efforts made to lose weight.

  - *Binge Eating Disorder*
    - Recurrent episodes of binge eating with lack of control
    - Occurs at least 2 days weekly for 6 months
    - Not regularly associated with compensatory behaviors
    - Suggested for possible inclusion in *DSM-IV-TR* (American Psychiatric Association, 2000), but still undergoing research.

Etiology

- Etiology is multifactorial, with biological, social, and psychological factors implicated in causation.
- Biological factors include decreased hypothalamic norepinephrine activation, dysfunction of lateral hypothalamus, and decreased serotonin.

Incidence and Demographics

- Incidence is more common in girls, with 85%–95% of occurrences.
- Anorexia nervosa affects approximately 0.28% of the general U.S. population.
- Bulimia nervosa affects approximately 1.0% of the general U.S. population.
- Onset is typically between ages 14 and18 years.

Risk Factors

- Genetic loading
- Increased risk of eating disorders among first-degree biological relatives of individuals with certain other psychiatric disorders:
  - Eating disorders
  - Mood disorders
  - Substance abuse disorders.

Prevention and Screening

- At-risk family education
- Community education
  - Stigma reduction
  - Signs and symptoms of illness
  - Treatment potential for control of symptoms.

- Early recognition, intervention, and initiation of treatment
  - Secondary prevention is important in young clients.

Assessment

- Detailed history of present illness, including time frame, progression, and associated symptoms
- Social history, including present living situation; marital status; occupation; education; and alcohol, tobacco, or illicit drug use
- Medication use, including prescription, over-the-counter, alternative, supplements, and home remedies
- Initial and periodic functional history and assessment
- Validate history with a family member.

History–Assess for the Following:

- Anorexia Nervosa
  - Refusal to maintain a minimally normal body weight
  - Weight less than 85% of expected weight
  - Fear of gaining weight or becoming fat
  - Distorted body image
    - *Restricting Type*—During the current episode, the person has not regularly engaged in binge eating or purging behavior.

- *Binge Eating/Purging Type*—During the current episode, the person has regularly engaged in binge eating or purging behavior.
- Bulimia Nervosa
    - Recurrent, episodic binge eating
    - Both binge eating and inappropriate compensatory behaviors occur at least twice weekly for 3 months
    - Recurrent, inappropriate compensatory behaviors to prevent weight gain
        - Self induced vomiting
        - Laxatives
        - Enemas
        - Diuretics
        - Stimulants
        - Abuse of diet pills
        - Fasting
        - Excessive exercise.

    - Self-evaluation unduly influenced by body shape and weight
        - *Purging Type*—During the current episode, the person regularly has engaged in purging or the misuse of laxatives, enemas, or diuretics.
        - *Nonpurging Type*—During the current episode, the person has used other inappropriate compensatory behaviors, such as fasting or excessive exercise, but has not regularly engaged in purging or misuse of laxatives, enemas, or diuretics.

Physical Exam Findings

Anorexia Nervosa

- Low body mass index (BMI)
- Amenorrhea
- Emaciation
- Bradycardia
- Hypotension
- ECG changes
    - Inversion of T-waves
    - ST segment depression
    - Prolonged QT interval.
- Hypothermia

- Yellow skin secondary to carotenemia
- Dry skin
- Brittle hair and nails
- Lanugo growth on face, extremities, and trunk
- Peripheral edema
- Hypertrophy of the salivary glands
- Erosion of dental enamel
- Russell's sign—Scarring or calluses on the dorsum of the hand secondary to self-induced vomiting.

Bulimia Nervosa

- Weight usually within normal range
- Erosion of dental enamel
- Russell's sign
- Hypertrophy of salivary glands
- Rectal prolapse.

Mental Status Exam Findings

Appearance

- Emaciated appearance with anorexia nervosa.

Affect
- Lability
- Anxiety
- Constricted and sad.

Mood
- Dysphoric mood.

Thought Content
- Preoccupation with food and body weight
- Suicidal ideation
- Low self-esteem.

Concentration
- Decreased concentration.

Judgment
- Impaired for self-welfare.

Insight
- Impaired.

Diagnostic and Laboratory Findings
- CBC, chemistry profile, thyroid function tests, and B_{12} level to rule out metabolic causes or unidentified conditions
- Drug toxicity screening, if indicated by history
- *Anorexia Nervosa*
  - No definitive laboratory tests
  - Laboratory changes
    - Normochromic, normocytic anemia
    - Leukopenia
    - Neutropenia
    - Anemia
    - Thrombocytopenia
    - Hypokalemia
    - Hypomagnesemia
    - Hypoglycemia
    - Decreased luteinizing hormone (LH) and follicle-stimulation hormone (FSH).

- *Bulimia Nervosa*
  - No definitive laboratory tests
  - Laboratory changes
    - Hypotension
    - Bradycardia
    - Hypokalemia
    - Hyponatremia
    - Hypochloremia
    - Hypomagnesemia

- Metabolic acidosis or alkalosis
- Elevated serum amylase.

Differential Diagnosis
- General medical condition
- Mood disorders (see Chapter 7)
- Cluster B personality disorders (see Chapter 12)
- OCD (see Chapter 8)
- Schizophrenia (see Chapter 9).

Clinical Management
- Rule out or treat any conditions that may contribute to current symptom manifestation.

Pharmacological Management
- Medication management as adjunctive therapy to psychotherapy
- No specific medication therapy for anorexia nervosa
- Fluoxetine FDA-approved for bulimia nervosa
- SSRIs and tricylic antidepressants (TCAs) effective in reducing the frequency of bingeing and purging
- Treat associated symptoms, such as depression and anxiety, with appropriate pharmacological therapy.

Nonpharmacological Management
- Multimodal treatment
  - Medical and nutritional stabilization
    - Weight restoration
    - Correction of electrolyte disturbance
    - Vitamin supplementation
    - Nutrition counseling.

  - Dental care
    - Psychotherapeutic interventions
    - Individual psychotherapy
    - Behavioral therapy
    - Cognitive–behavioral therapy
    - Family therapy
    - Group therapy.

  - Community resources
    - Eating disorder support groups
    - 12-step programs.

Mental Retardation

Description

- *Mental retardation* is subaverage general intellectual functioning based on a standardized intelligence test.
- Onset must occur before age 18 years.
- IQ is below 70.
- Concurrent impairment exists in adaptive functioning in at least two of the following areas:
  - Communication
  - Self-care
  - Home living
  - Social or interpersonal skills.

Etiology

- Heredity accounts for 5% of cases
  - Inborn metabolism errors (e.g., Tay–Sachs disease)
  - Single-gene abnormalities (e.g., tuberous sclerosis)
  - Chromosomal aberrations (e.g., translocation of chromosome 21 [Down syndrome] and X-linked gene of FMR-1 [fragile X syndrome]).

- Early alterations in embryonic development account for 30% of cases.
  - Prenatal exposure to toxins (e.g., maternal alcohol consumption, infections).

- Pregnancy and perinatal problems account for 10% of cases
  - Fetal malnutrition
  - Premature birth
  - Fetal hypoxia
  - Birth trauma.

- General medical conditions acquired during infancy or childhood contribute to approximately 5% of cases
  - Infections
  - Brain trauma
  - Exposure to toxins (e.g., lead poisoning).

- No clear etiology can be found in 30%–50% of cases.
- The most preventable cause of mental retardation is fetal alcohol syndrome.
- Characteristics of fetal alcohol syndrome include
  - Epicanthal skin folds
  - Low nasal bridge
  - Short nose
  - Indistinct philtrum
  - Small head circumference
  - Small eye openings
  - Wide-set eyes
  - Thin upper lip.

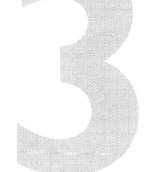

Risk Factors

- Genetic loading
- Adverse birth events.

Incidence and Demographics

- Between 1% and 3% of the general population.

Assessment

History—Assess for the Following:

- Mild Mental Retardation (IQ range, 50–55 to 70)
  - Accounts for 10% of cases
  - Can develop social and communication skills
  - Minimal sensorimotor abnormalities
  - Can acquire academic skills up to approximately 6th-grade level
  - Can achieve social and vocational skills adequate for minimum self-support
  - Can live successfully in the community independently or in supervised settings.

- Moderate Mental Retardation (IQ range, 35–40 to 50–55)
  - Accounts for 10% of cases
  - Limited social awareness
  - Can acquire some communication skills
  - May benefit from vocational training
  - Seldom advances academically beyond the 2nd-grade level
  - Can be trained to care for most personal needs
  - Can perform unskilled or semiskilled work in sheltered job placements
  - Can live in the community but usually in a supervised setting such as a group home.

- Severe Mental Retardation (IQ range, 20–25 to 35–40)
  - Accounts for 3%–4% of cases
  - Slow and poor motor development
  - Little or no communicative speech
  - May be able to learn to sight-read some survival words such as *stop* and *exit*
  - May be able to perform simple tasks in closely supervised settings
  - Can live in the community in group homes unless some other disability requires specialized nursing care.

- Profound Mental Retardation (IQ below 20–25)
  - Accounts for 1%–2% of cases
  - Minimal capacity for sensorimotor functioning
  - Poor cognitive and social capacities
  - Speech often absent
  - May develop minimal motor skills, self-care skills, and communication skills if appropriate training provided
  - May live in group homes or intermediate care facilities
  - May be able to perform simple tasks in a closely supervised and sheltered setting.

Physical Exam Findings

- Oblique eye folds
- Small, flattened skull
- Large tongue
- Broad hands with stumpy fingers
- Single transverse palm crease
- High cheekbones
- Small height
- Brushfield spots on iris
- Abnormal finger and toe prints
- Cryptorchidism
- Congenital cardiac defects
- Early dementia
- Hypothyroidism.

Mental Status Exam Findings

- Communication deficits
- Dependency
- Passivity
- Poor self-esteem
- Low frustration tolerance
- Aggressiveness
- Stereotypic, repetitive motor movement
- Self-injurious behavior.

Diagnostic and Laboratory Findings

- No specific laboratory findings
- Some laboratory findings associated with a variety of causes of mental retardation (e.g., metabolic disturbances).

Differential Diagnosis

- Borderline intellectual functioning
- Learning and communication disorders
- Pervasive developmental disorder (PDD)
  - 75% of individuals with a PDD have comorbid mental retardation.
- ADHD (see above)
- Stereotypic movement disorder
- General medical condition.

Clinical Management

Pharmacological Management

- Pharmacological treatment is symptom specific.
  - Treat concomitant psychopathology (e.g., ADHD, depressive disorder, anxiety disorder, schizophrenia).
  - Aggressive or self-injurious behavior may be controlled with antipsychotics and mood stabilizers.

Nonpharmacological Management

- Therapy
- Behavioral therapy
- Group therapy
- Family therapy.

- Community Resources
  - Day-care settings
  - Sheltered workshops
  - Group homes.

Case Study

The parents of a child with attention-deficit/hyperactive disorder (ADHD) ask to speak to you privately after your assessment of their child is complete. They tell you they have several questions that they want answered, and they want to ask you to keep the answers to yourself and not tell their son what they ask. Their first question is about diet. They have read that ADHD can be managed by dietary therapy instead of medications, and they want your opinion about trying this strategy with their child. They also want to know how likely it is that their son will eventually "outgrow" the disorder. You have many issues to consider before answering the parents' questions.

- What is the most accepted theory of etiology regarding ADHD?

- What is the empirical database for dietary treatment in ADHD clients?

- What is the natural course of this illness? Is it likely that the son's symptoms will improve as he ages?

- What are the other issues to consider regarding the parents' request to keep confidential the concerns that they are expressing?

Review Questions

1. A diagnosis of mental retardation is made when a person has significantly below-average intelligence accompanied by impaired adaptive functioning. The IQ range for consideration of mental retardation is an

   a. IQ below 70
   b. IQ below 60
   c. IQ below 50
   d. IQ below 40

2. Most of the stimulants commonly used to treat ADHD are classified as Schedule II controlled substances. The exception is

   a. Ritalin
   b. Dexedrine
   c. Adderall
   d. Strattera

3. A child presents with a behavioral pattern of negative, defiant, disobedient, and hostile behavior, especially toward adults in authority roles. The most likely diagnosis for this child is

   a. ADHD

   b. Rett's disorder

   c. Antisocial personality disorder

   d. Oppositional defiant disorder

4. Which of the following is not required to make a diagnosis of conduct disorder?

   a. Destruction of property

   b. Aggression toward people and animals

   c. Poor interpersonal relationships with limited peers

   d. Deceitfulness or theft

References and Resources

American Psychiatric Association. (2000). *Diagnostic and statistical manual of mental disorders* (4th ed., text rev.). Washington, DC: American Psychiatric Association.

American Psychiatric Association. (2001). Practice parameters for the assessment and treatment of children and adolescents with suicidal behavior. *Journal of the American Academy of Child and Adolescent Psychiatry, 4*(Suppl. 7), 245–478.

Barkley, R. (2005). *Attention deficit hyperactivity disorder: A handbook for diagnosis and treatment* (3rd ed.). New York: Guilford Press.

Barlow, D. A., & Durand, V. M. (2004). *Abnormal psychology* (4th ed.). Pacific Grove, CA: Brooks/Cole.

Bernstein, G. A., & Shaw, K. (1997). Practice parameters for the assessment and treatment of children and adolescents with anxiety disorders. *Journal of the American Academy of Child and Adolescent Psychiatry, 36*(Suppl. 69), 80S–84S.

Blazer, D. G., & Kaplar, B. H. (2000). Controversies in community-based psychiatric epidemiology: Let the data speak for themselves. *Archives of General Psychiatry, 57,* 227.

Bremner, J. D. (1999). Devastating effects and clinical implications of childhood abuse. *Directions in Psychiatry, 19,* 147–160.

Conners, C. K. (1969). A teacher rating scale for use in drug studies with children. *American Journal of Psychiatry, 126,* 884–888.

Cyranowski, J. M., Frank, E., Young, E., & Shear, M. K. (2000). Adolescent onset of the gender difference in lifetime rates of major depression. *Archives of General Psychiatry, 57,* 21–27.

DelCarmen-Wiggins, R., & Carter, A. S. (2001). Assessment of infant and toddler mental health: Advances and challenges. *Journal of the American Academy of Child and Adolescent Psychiatry, 40*(1), 8–10.

Dohenwend, B. P. (1998). A psychosocial perspective on the past and future of psychiatric epidemiology. *American Journal of Epidemiology, 147,* 222–231.

Frances, A. (1998). Problems in defining clinical significance in epidemiologic studies. *Archives of General Psychiatry, 55,* 119.

Frankel, F. D. (2001). Common peer relationship problems in childhood. *Primary Psychiatry, 8*(12), 25–31.

Gadow, K., Sprafkin, J., & Nolan, E. (2001). DSM-IV symptoms in community and clinic preschool children. *Journal of the American Academy of Child and Adolescent Psychiatry, 40,* 1383–1392.

Gillberg, C. (1999). Neurodevelopmental processes and psychological functioning in autism. *Developmental and Psychopathology, 11,* 567–587.

Halmi, K. A., & Romano, S. J. (2001). Anorexia nervosa: An overview. *Primary Psychiatry, 6*(2), 35–56.

Harrison, P. L. (1999). Assessment and treatment of children with autism in the schools. *School Psychology Review, 28,* 533–693.

House, A. E. (2002). *DSM-IV diagnosis in the schools* (rev. ed.). New York: Guilford Press.

Kashani, J. H., & Orvaschel, H. (1990). A community study of anxiety in children and adolescents. *American Journal of Psychiatry, 147,* 313–318.

Kazdin, A. E. (2000). Developing a research agenda for child and adolescent psychotherapy. *Archives of General Psychiatry, 57,* 829–835.

McClellan, J., & Werry, J. S. (1997). Practice parameters for the assessment and treatment of children and adolescents with bipolar disorder. *Journal of the American Academy of Child and Adolescent Psychiatry, 36*(Suppl.), 157S–176S.

Nolan, E., Gadow, K., & Sprafkin, J. (2001). Teacher reports of DSM-IV ADHD, ODD, and CD symptoms in school children. *Journal of the American Academy of Child and Adolescent Psychiatry, 40,* 241–249.

Reiger, D. A. (2000). Community diagnosis counts. *Archives of General Psychiatry, 57,* 223.

Reiger, D. A., Kaelber, C. T., Rae, D. S., Farmer, M. E., Knauper, B., Kessler, R. C., et al. (1998). Limitations of diagnostic criteria and assessment instruments for mental disorders: Implications for research and policy. *Archives of General Psychiatry, 55,* 109–115.

Romano, S. J., & Quinn, L. (2001). Evaluation and treatment of bulimia nervosa. *Primary Psychiatry, 6*(2), 57–62.

Rush, A. J., & Frances, A. (2000). Expert consensus guidelines series: Treatment of psychiatric and behavioral problems in mental retardation. *American Journal of Mental Retardation, 105,* 161–228.

Shaffer, D., Fisher, P., Dulcan, M., Davies, M., Piacentini, J., Schwab-Stone, M. E., et al. (1996). The NIMH diagnostic interview schedule for children: Description, acceptability, prevalence rates, and performance in the MECA study. *Journal of the American Academy of Child and Adolescent Psychiatry, 35,* 865–877.

Spitzer, R. (1998). Diagnosis and need for treatment are not the same. *Archives of General Psychiatry, 55,* 120.

Spencer, T., Biederman, J., & Wilens, T. (1999). Attention-deficit/hyperactivity disorder and comorbidity. *Pediatric Clinics of North America, 46,* 573–579.

U.S. Department of Health and Human Services. (2000). *Mental health: A report of the Surgeon General.* Washington, DC: U.S. Department of Health and Human Services.

Notes:

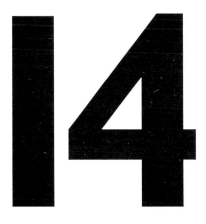

Other Conditions, Disorders, and Frequently Encountered Clinical Problems

This chapter deals with common conditions, disorders, and clinical problems frequently encountered by psychiatric–mental health nurse practitioners (PMHNPs), including sleep and insomnia, domestic violence, sexual assault and abuse, and grief and bereavement. These conditions and clinical problems may co-occur with the disorders already discussed or may present in clients with no other identifiable psychiatric or mental health problems. They also may be frequent findings in primary care settings while working with clients with general medical conditions.

Sleep

General Considerations
- Must be systematically assessed
- Comparison of present level of sleep to historical baseline
- Can be measured by polysomnography
- Rapid eye movement (REM) alternating with four distinct non-rapid eye movement stages (NREM).
  - Stage I
    - NREM
    - Transitional stage from wakefulness to sleep
    - 5% of total normal sleep cycle.

  - Stage II
    - NREM
    - Specific EEG waveforms
    - 50% of total sleep cycle.

  - Stages III and IV
    - NREM
    - Slow-wave sleep period
    - Deepest level of sleep
    - 20%–25% of total sleep cycle.

- Sleep stages organized and sequential during sleep period
  - Stages III and IV tend to occur in first one-third to one-half of sleep period.

- REM occurs cyclically throughout the night, alternating with NREM on average every 80–100 minutes.
    - REM increases in duration toward morning.
- Sleep patterns varying with age
    - Children and adolescents have large amounts of slow-wave sleep.
    - Sleep continuity and depth decrease with age.
    - Consider age when assessing for sleep–rest problems.

- Sleep patterns varying with medication use
    - Many medications and agents of abuse affect sleep cycle.
    - Assess recent changes in medication or drug use in individual presenting with sleep pattern disturbances.

Insomnia

Description
- *Insomnia* is the inability to get the amount of sleep needed to function efficiently during the day.
- It is not a specific disease, is commonly associated with several disorders, and commonly occurs with mood disorders.
- It is associated with increased mortality, poor career performance, overeating, and increased hospitalization.

Etiology
- Dysfunction in sleep–wake circuits of the brain stem
- Neurochemical imbalances impinging on these circuits
- May be stress related in brief episodic insomnia.

Incidence and Demographics
- 35% of Americans have difficulty sleeping.
- 18% of Americans have serious sleep problems.
- 4% of Americans take prescription medications to help them sleep.

Risk Factors
- Age
- History of insomnia
- Significant stress
- Forced pattern changes
    - Working alternating shifts
    - Swing-shift work patterns
    - Travel across time zones.

- High-use patterns of medications, drugs, or substances known to affect sleep cycles
    - Caffeine
    - Alcohol
    - Benzodiazepines (BNZs).

Prevention and Screening
- At-risk family education
- Limits on shift work
- Avoidance of medications known to affect sleep patterns
- Good sleep hygiene patterns
- Avoidance of stimulants late in the day
- Early recognition, intervention, and initiation of treatment
  - Routine screening at all health care settings.

Assessment
- Detailed history of present illness, including time frame, progression, and associated symptoms
- Social history, including present living situation; marital status; occupation; education; and alcohol, tobacco, or illicit drug use
- Medication use, including prescription, over-the-counter, alternative, supplements, and home remedies
- Initial and periodic functional history and assessment
- Validate history with family member.

History–Assess for the Following:
- Sleep–wake patterns
  - Number of hours in usual sleep pattern
  - Sleep aids
    - Position
    - Pillow.

  - Environmental regulation
    - Temperature
    - Sound control
    - Light control.

- Duration of sleep disturbance
  - Transient insomnia
    - Can be caused by stress, jet lag, or physical environment
    - May last several days
    - Generally can be relieved by exercise, a hot bath, warm milk, and changing bedroom environment.

  - Short-term insomnia
    - Result of stress, illness, or bereavement
    - May linger for up to 3 weeks.

  - Long-term insomnia
    - Lasts for more than 3 weeks
    - Calls for an extensive diagnostic examination.

  - Insomnia related to another psychiatric disorder
    - More than 50% of insomnia cases related to primary psychiatric disorder
      - Mood disorders (see Chapter 7)
      - Anxiety disorders (see Chapter 8)
      - Substance-related disorders (see Chapter 11).

- Early-morning wakefulness a possible sign of depression
- Sudden, dramatic decrease in sleep a sign of possible mania or schizophrenia
- Poor sleep a sign of possible obsessive–compulsive disorder
- Panic and anxiety episodes during sleep a sign of possible panic disorder
- Alcohol causes numerous awakenings during the night for long periods of time.

Physical Exam Findings

- Nonspecific
- Sleep often a manifestation of an underlying disorder
- Patients with insomnia should have full exam.

Mental Status Exam (MSE) Findings

- Nonspecific
- Depending on duration of sleep deprivation, many areas of MSE may be affected.

Diagnostic and Laboratory Findings

- CBC, chemistry profile, thyroid function tests, and B_{12} level to rule out metabolic causes or unidentified conditions
- Drug toxicity screening, if indicated by history.

Differential Diagnosis

- Cardiac illnesses
- GI disorders
- Chronic obstructive pulmonary disease
- Medication side effects
- Sleep apnea
- Anxiety
- Depression
- Stress reaction
- Active substance abuse
- Drug use
  - Caffeine
  - Stimulants.

Clinical Management

- Rule out or treat any conditions that may contribute to current symptom manifestation.

Pharmacological Management

- Benzodiazepines (BNZs)
  - Benzodiazepine agents that may be used to promote sedation and rest:
    - Dalmane (flurazepam)
      - Long-lasting agent
      - May cause excess drowsiness.

    - Restoril (temazepam)
      - Intermediate-acting agent.

- Halcion (triazolam)
  - Short-acting agent
  - Little to no excess sedation.
- Common side effects:
  - Impaired memory
  - Poor learning for new information
  - Efficacy decreases over time
  - Should not be used on a long-term basis or for longer than 2 weeks.

- Antidepressants
  - Used for sedating properties
    - Elavil
    - Remeron
    - Trazadone.

- Sleep Agents
  - Work on sleep architecture and not just by causing sedation
    - Sonata (zaleplon)
    - Ambien/Ambien CR (zolpidem)
    - Lunesta
    - Rozerem.

Nonpharmacological Management
- Sleep Hygiene Practices
  - Establish a bedtime routine.
  - Have a regular time to sleep and wake.
  - Never lie in bed for more than 15 minutes if not able to sleep.
  - Reduce stress.
  - Do stress-reduction activities before bedtime.
  - Avoid late-in-the-day exercise.
  - Avoid late-in-the-day stimulant use, such as caffeine in coffee.
  - Do not lie in bed other than to sleep (e.g., avoid watching TV in bed).

- Psychotherapy
  - Cognitive therapy.

- Relaxation Therapies
  - Abdominal breathing
  - Progressive muscle relaxation
  - Meditation
  - Imaging
  - Hypnosis
  - Biofeedback
  - Stimulus control
  - Sleep curtailment
  - Light therapy.

- Somatic and Other Therapies
  - Exercise
  - Hot bath

- Warm milk
- Changing bedroom environment.

Life Span Considerations

Insomnia in Children
- This is most commonly related to stress.
- Children with insomnia often have been poor sleepers since birth.
- Pharmacological treatment is not recommended for most children.

Insomnia in Older Adults
- If first presentation is in older years, insomnia often is the result of changes in chronobiological rhythms.
- It may indicate the following underlying psychiatric disorders:
  - Mood disorders
  - Anxiety disorders.

- It is a common finding in Alzheimer's disease.
- Elderly people often manifest confusion and restlessness as aspects of insomnia.
- A careful, complete assessment is necessary when pharmacological interventions are planned.

Domestic Violence

Description
- *Domestic violence* is physical, emotional, economic, or sexual pain and injury that is intentionally inflicted.
- The goals of domestic violence are to
  - Establish power
  - Manipulate the other individual
  - Intimidate the other individual
  - Control the other individual.

Etiology

Characteristics of Abusers
- Personality disorders
  - Antisocial personality disorder
  - Narcissistic personality disorder
  - Borderline personality disorder.

- Environmental stressors
  - Financial difficulties
  - Ending of a relationship
  - Unemployment.

Incidence and Demographics
- Domestic violence is the leading cause of injury to women ages 15–44.
- 1 in 4 pregnant women have a history of domestic violence.

- 15%–25% of pregnant women are physically abused.
- 22%–35% of all women seen in emergency rooms experience injuries as a result of domestic violence; 50% of homeless women experience domestic violence.
- 63% of men incarcerated between the ages of 11 and 20 have murdered their mother's abuser.
- 33% of male abusers are well educated and include men in professional jobs.

Risk Factors

For Abusers
- Exposure to violence at an early developmental age
- Low self-esteem
- Social isolation
- Lack of support
- Cognitive impairment
- Physical, financial dependency.

Prevention and Screening
- Public education and awareness
- Social programs
- At-risk family education
- Community education
  - Stigma reduction
  - Signs and symptoms of illness
  - Prevention programs
  - Treatment potential for control of symptoms.
- Early recognition, intervention, and initiation of treatment
  - Routine screening at all health care settings.

Assessment
- Interview the individual who has experienced the violence alone.
- Determine primary caregivers, living arrangements, legal custodian, and power of attorney.

History—Assess for the Following:
- Determine recurrent history of medical treatment consistent with abuse.
  - Accidents
  - Fractures
  - Physical injuries
  - Traumas
  - Refusal of ongoing treatment or follow-up
  - Missed medical appointments.
- Determine environmental, psychosocial, and financial stressors.

Physical Exam Findings
- Monitor nutritional status for dehydration and malnutrition.
- Look for lacerations, bruises, wounds, burns, or fractures.
- Look for poor skin and personal hygiene.

Mental Status Exam Findings

- Findings of traits and behaviors suggestive of experiencing abuse:
  - Fearful
  - Evasive
  - Guarded
  - Depressed
  - Passive
  - Dependent.

Diagnostic and Laboratory Findings

- Nonspecific to abuse
- Determine general health and nutritional status.

Differential Diagnosis

- Accidental injuries
- Mood disorders (see Chapter 7)
- Anxiety disorders (see Chapter 8)
- Substance abuse (see Chapter 11).

Clinical Management

- Most state laws mandate reporting of suspected abuse and neglect of vulnerable populations:
  - Elderly people
  - People with disabilities
  - Children.

Pharmacological Management

- Nonspecific to condition.

Nonpharmacological Management

- The safety and medical well-being of the individual experiencing the abuse is most important.
- Refer the individual to a domestic abuse shelter when feasible.
- Help the individual develop a safety plan.
  - Assist client in developing a "code word" for family or other support system as an attempt to inform them that the individual is in need of help.
  - Advise client to tell one person in his/her support system about the situation.
  - Advise client to pack an "emergency bag" and hide it in case of need to leave quickly.
  - Advise client to keep the domestic violence hotline and other telephone numbers (e.g., police department, counselor, shelter) in a secure place.
- Monitor medical status as symptomatology presents.
- Monitor nutritional status and vital signs.
- Suggest psychotherapy to assist in gaining insight and developing new coping skills.
- Suggest hospitalization when in the best interest of the individual.

Sexual Assault and Abuse

Description
- *Sexual assault or abuse* is any sexual act or penetration committed through coercion or physical force.
- This includes rape, incest, sodomy, oral and anal acts, or use of a foreign object.
- It is an act of violence and humiliation expressed through sexual means.
- It is used to express power or anger.

Etiology
For Abusers
- Character disorders
- Behavioral act of violence is reinforcing.
  - Once done, likely to repeat.

- Social exposure to violence in culture, media, and home.

Incidence and Demographics
- Women have a greater incidence of being assaulted than men.
- Sexual assault is the most common form of abuse.
  - Men are more frequently perpetrators than women.
  - The assaults are committed by fathers and stepfathers, uncles, older siblings, and men that women are dating.

- Incestuous behavior is reported more frequently among families with low socioeconomic status.
- Alcohol is involved in 34% of all forcible rapes.
- Only 1 in 4 rapes are reported.

Risk Factors
For Abusers
- Substance abuse disorders
- Psychiatric disorders
- Divorce
- Pregnancy
- Family or personal history of physical or sexual abuse
- Long-term exposure to violence
- Social isolation and lack of support systems
- Environmental stressors such as unemployment or financial difficulty.

Prevention and Screening
- Public education and awareness campaigns
- Community resources and support
- Community emergency shelters, help lines, and safe houses
- Assertiveness training and self-defense
- At-risk family education

- Community education
  - Prevention programs
  - Treatment potential for control of symptoms.

- Early recognition, intervention, and initiation of treatment
  - Routine screening at all health care settings.

Assessment

- Interview individuals who have experienced the assault alone when possible.
- Establish a safe, trusting relationship to promote sharing.

History–Assess for the Following:

- Include questions concerning domestic violence in medical history.
- Interview alone and not in presence of family, friend, or partner.
- Interview for social history, including history of living arrangements and relationships.

Physical Exam Findings

- Nonspecific.
- Presentation of traits and behaviors consistent with potential for abuse
  - Withdrawn
  - Frightened appearance
  - Hyperreactive to touch.

- *Associated Findings*
  - Unexplained bruises, abrasions, cuts, laceration, burns, soft-tissue swellings, and hematomas
  - Sexually transmitted diseases
    - Genital rash or discharge
    - Rectal tissue swelling or discharge.

- Physical signs that are *strongly suggestive of sexual abuse in children:*
  - Lacerations, ecchymosis, and newly healed scars of the hymen or posterior fourchette
  - No hymenal tissue from 3–9 o'clock area
  - Healed hymenal transactions, especially in the above area
  - Perianal lacerations.

✓ Remember that any child presenting with concerning physical signs should be evaluated by a sexual abuse expert. A complete history and a sexual abuse examination need to take place.

Mental Status Exam Findings

- Withdrawn
- Frightened
- Anxious
- Scattered appearance
- Hyperreactive to touch.

Diagnostic and Laboratory Findings

- Nonspecific
- Assessment and documentation labs
  - Forensic specimens
  - Pregnancy tests
  - Rectal, throat, and vaginal cultures
  - Veneral Disease Research Laboratory (VDRL), HIV
  - Herpes B, herpes simplex
  - Human papillomavirus
  - Trichomonas vaginalis.

Differential Diagnosis

- Accidental injuries
- Consensual sexual activity
- Lichen sclerosis
- Posttraumatic stress disorder
- Anxiety disorder (see Chapter 8).

Clinical Management

- Use sensitivity and respectful care.
- Be aware of legal reporting requirements.
- Utilize available community resources.

Pharmacological Management

- Emergency contraception
  - Diethylstilbestrol (DES), 25 mg bid for 5 days within 48 hours of incident
  - Norgestrel, .5 mg, and ethinyl estradiol, .05 mg (Ovral), 2 tablets within 72 hours of incident
  - Norgestrel, .3 mg, and ethinyl estradiol, .03 mg (Lo/Ovral), 4 tablets within 72 hours of incident with 4 tablets 12 hours later.

- If required, clinical management of anxiety.

Nonpharmacological Management

- Ensure safety and well-being.
- Ensure confidentiality.
- Complete accurate documentation.
- Assess for potential suicidal ideation if the individual is showing any depressive symptoms.
- Suggest cognitive–behavioral therapy (CBT).
- Offer support groups and community resources.
- Assist with access to criminal and legal supports.

Grief and Bereavement

Description

- *Grief and bereavement* involve a wide range of normal responses that can become abnormal and excessive.

- They involve normative emotional, cognitive, and behavioral reactions to death or loss of a significant individual or object.
- They involve nonnormative psychological responses to an identifiable stressor that can result in the development of clinically significant emotional or behavioral symptoms.
  - Stressor encompassing elements of perceived loss
  - Develops *within 3 months* of stressor
    - *Single Event*
      - End of relationship
      - Death of relative or partner.
    - *Recurring Event*
      - Living with individual with terminal illness.
    - *Developmental Event*
      - Leaving home to go away to school
      - Getting married
      - Becoming a parent
      - Retiring from work.
- PMHNP assessment is needed to separate normal healthy grieving from pathological grieving.
  - Severity of response
  - Duration of response
  - Effects of response on normal daily functioning
  - Individual's perceptions of impact of stressor.
- When severity or duration is excessive, the grieving may be abnormal.
- In the absence of other significant clinical symptoms, grief usually is classified as *adjustment disorder.*
  - Adjustment disorder with depressed mood
  - Adjustment disorder with anxiety
  - Adjustment disorder with mixed anxiety and depression
  - Adjustment disorder with disturbed conduct.

Etiology
- Significant loss
- Limited coping skills
- Limited social supports.

Incidence and Demographics
- Normal grief is universally experienced.
- Grief is common in elderly people as their social sphere begins to decrease.
- 20% of elderly individuals who lose a spouse experience depression within the first year of that loss.
- 2%–8% of people in the U.S. will develop an adjustment disorder in their lifetime.
- Grief occurs in 12% of general hospital clients.
- Grief occurs in 50% of cardiac clients after cardiac surgery.

Risk Factors
- Limited social network
- Poor physical health
- Limited coping skills.

Prevention and Screening
- Ask about losses.
- Identify at risk individuals
- Do preventive counseling.
- Begin early recognition, intervention, and initiation of treatment.
  - Routine screening at all health care settings.

Assessment
- Often clients will not disclose grieving or bereavement issues unless directly asked.

History–Assess for the Following:
- Recent losses
- Anniversary dates of past losses
- Reaction to loss
- Functional impairment
- Social and family support systems
- Presence of dysfunctional coping
  - Suicidal thoughts
  - Substance abuse
  - Denial.

Physical Exam Findings
- Nonspecific
- Insomnia
- Anorexia.

Mental Status Exam Findings
- Depressed mood
- Anxious affect
- Crying uncontrollably.

Diagnostic and Laboratory Findings
- CBC, chemistry profile, thyroid function tests, and B_{12} level to rule out metabolic causes or unidentified conditions
- Drug toxicity screening, if indicated by history.

Differential Diagnosis
- Normal grieving
- Major depressive disorder (MDD; see Chapter 7)
- Anxiety disorders (see Chapter 8)
- Substance-related disorders (see Chapter 11).

Clinical Management

Pharmacological Management

- If needed
  - Short-term use of anti-anxiety agents
    - BNZs

  - Short-term use of sleep-induction agents
    - BNZs
    - Tricyclic antidepressants
    - Antihistamines.

Nonpharmacological Management

- Encourage expression of grief and loss.
- Use support groups.
- Offer community resources.
- Offer psychoeducation on grief reactions and responses.
- With significant functional impairment, consider psychotherapy (e.g., crisis therapy, brief solution-focused therapy, CBT).

Life Span Considerations

- Can occur at any age
- Older adults at greater risk because of higher numbers of losses that may become cumulative in their impact.

Follow-up

- Follow up weekly during acute period.
- Monitor for development of MDD.
- Monitor for impact on general health state.
- Maintain supportive follow-up over time.
- Be sensitive to nontraditional losses that may be significant to the individual:
  - Loss of a pet
  - Loss of status in work or school setting.

Case Study

Mrs. Jones, a 43-year-old receptionist, presents at your clinic with a primary complaint of insomnia. She reports lifelong problems with sleeping that "come and go" depending on her stress level and general health. She has been experiencing a 4- to 5-day period of poor sleeping, reporting only 3–4 hours of sleep and early-morning awakening. She has tried over-the-counter medication and has received no relief. She reports that her health is generally good but states that she is a two-pack-a-day smoker and has increased her recreational use of alcohol to one–two drinks a night in the past few weeks in order to get to sleep.

Her insomnia is now beginning to impair her daily functioning and her interest in social activities. She reports an irritable mood since her sleep has been difficult and problems with memory and concentration in the morning after she has slept poorly. She denies depression or any other mood problem and currently is taking no routine medication. Her physical exam is unremarkable, and routine lab studies, including TSH, CBC, and electrolytes, are all normal. There are many issues to consider in planning care with this client:

- What is the most likely diagnosis for this client at this time?

- What further assessment would you make?

- What treatment would you consider?

- Is medication warranted at this time to induce sleep?

Review Questions

1. In evaluating a client for insomnia, which of the following is most consistent with a presentation of transient insomnia?

   a. Usually caused by stress, jet lag, or physical environmental concerns

   b. Lasts for 3 or more weeks

   c. May linger for up to 3 weeks

   d. Calls for a complete evaluation and diagnostic work up

2. Insomnia is a common finding in clients with psychiatric disorder and is most commonly found in clients diagnosed with

   a. Mood disorders

   b. Schizophrenic disorders

   c. Substance abuse disorders

   d. Anxiety disorders

3. Insomnia in children is most often caused by

   a. Illness

   a. Family stress

   a. School performance problems

   a. Substance abuse

4. A PMHNP is working with a woman whom she suspects is in a violent domestic relationship. The client denies this and refuses to discuss her home life. She continues to present at the clinic for treatment of minor injuries and always is brought by her boyfriend. The client refuses to discuss abuse as a cause of her injuries, simply stating "I'm just clumsy." The best initial intervention for the PMHNP to take is

   a. Report the suspected abuse to the police

   b. Confront the client's boyfriend during the next clinic visit

   c. Spend a long time with the client building a trusting relationship

   d. Refer the client to social services for follow-up

References and Resources

American Nurses Association. (2000). *Scope and standards of psychiatric–mental health clinical nursing practice.* Washington, DC: Author.

American Psychiatric Association. (2000). *Diagnostic and statistical manual of mental disorders* (4th ed., text rev.). Washington, DC: Author.

Brown, D. B. (1999). Managing sleep disorders: Solutions in primary care. *Clinical Reviews, 9* (10), 51–69.

Davidson, J. R. (2000). Trauma: The impact of post-traumatic stress disorder. *Journal of Psychopharmacology, 14* (Suppl. 1), 5–12.

Eddy, M. (1999). Insomnia. *American Family Practice, 1,* 11–16.

Edmunds, M. W., Horan, N. M., & Mayhew, M. S. (2000). *Adult nurse practitioner review manual.* Washington, DC: American Nurses Association.

National Center on Sleep Disorders, Research Working Group. (1999). Recognizing problem sleepiness in your patients. *American Family Physician, 15,* 11–13.

Nettina, S. M., & Knudtson, M. (2001). *The family nurse practitioner review manual.* Washington, DC: American Nurses Association.

Rajput, V., & Johnson, R. (1999). Chronic insomnia: A practical review. *American Family Practice, 11,* 1–6.

Shea, C. A., Pelletier, L., Poster, E. C., Stuart, G. W., & Verhey, M. P. (1999). *Advanced practice nursing in psychiatric mental health care.* St. Louis, MO: Mosby.

U.S. Department of Health and Human Services. (2000). *Mental health: A report of the Surgeon General.* Washington, DC: Author.

Notes:

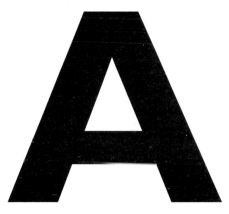

Discussion of Case Studies and Answers to Review Questions

Note. Discussion of the questions posed by the case studies is in *italics*; the correct answers to review questions are in **bold**.

Chapter 1

Case Study

Karen Harris is a newly graduated psychiatric–mental health nurse practitioner (PMHNP). She worked as a psychiatric nurse for 5 years before going to graduate school. She is considering a job at the local community mental health center. The director of the center has told her that her role would consist of seeing mainly adult clients with serious, chronic, and persistent mental illness.

On occasions when the psychiatrist is "busy," Ms. Harris is told she may be expected to see a few children in addition to adults. The director expects Ms. Harris to provide medication management to well-known clients and occasionally to assist in diagnostic evaluations of new clients or clients in crisis. He also expects that she will "from time to time" meet the emergent medical needs of clients who have limited access to primary care providers, including the routine, ongoing care of nonpsychiatric disorders such as diabetes, hypertension, and chronic pain. Ms. Harris has many issues to consider before deciding to take or not take the position:

- Would Ms. Harris be legally authorized to treat both children and adults?

    To be able to correctly answer this question depends on attending to the key word legally. *Professional standards and scope of practice documents suggest what is reasonable and prudent practice. Professional nursing organizations will provide information on what is seen as acceptable educational preparation for practice. But the individual legislative regulations of each state will determine what constitutes legal practice for each individual PMHNP.*

- What regulation, rule, or standard should Ms. Harris consult to determine if she is legally allowed to treat both children and adults?

    The Nurse Practice Act and related legislation of the state in which the PMHNP practices will delineate the legal boundaries of the PMHNP's practice.

- What regulation, rule, or standard should Ms. Harris consult to determine if she is legally allowed to treat both physical and psychiatric disorders?

  Professional standards and scope-of-practice documents would suggest what is reasonable and prudent practice. Professional nursing organizations will provide information and policy statements about what is seen as acceptable practice roles for PMHNPs. But the individual legislative regulations of each state will determine what constitutes legal practice for each individual PMHNP.

- What is the role of professional psychiatric nursing organizations in assisting Ms. Harris to determine the scope of practice that is appropriate for her as a new graduate?

  Professional nursing organizations will provide information and policy statements about what is seen as acceptable practice roles for PMHNPs.

Ms. Harris decides not to take that job and instead has been working for about a year as a PMHNP in a nurse-managed primary mental health clinic. One day she is asked to assess a client who is clearly psychotic, experiencing hallucinations and delusions, and expressing verbal threats against many individuals at another clinical practice in town who had "malpracticed me." The client is adamant that he does not wish any treatment and that he is not ill. To care for this client, Ms. Harris has many issues to consider:

- Is Ms. Harris able to treat the client if he is not consenting to care?

  Any client, including a psychiatric client, has the right to refuse treatment, and Ms. Harris is legally and ethically bound to honor that right.

- What legal standards must be met if she is to involuntarily treat this client?

  Ms. Harris must meet the legal standard in the state where she practices in order to treat the client against his or her wishes. This usually entails performing the legal task of committing a client and, in most states, ensuring that the following criteria are met:
  - *Individual has a diagnosed psychiatric disorder*
  - *Individual is unaware or unwilling to accept the nature and severity of disorder*
  - *Treatment is likely to improve functioning*
  - *Individual is harmful to self or others as a consequence of the disorder.*

About 5 weeks later, the above-mentioned client returns to the clinic for follow-up care. He is clinically stable, on medication, and showing no active symptoms. He is interested in developing a relapse prevention plan and asks Ms. Harris to assist him in this process. Ms. Harris has many issues to consider:

- Is the inclusion of a durable power of attorney an appropriate strategy in relapse planning for this client?

  A durable power of attorney allows individuals to choose, when they are healthy, an individual to act on their behalf should they become unable to make their own health care decisions. Because this client has a chronic illness that has the potential to render him unable to make his own health care decisions, a durable power of attorney document should be part of relapse planning.

- What quality indicators should be considered in planning his care with the client?

  Standardized client assessment and rating scales, evidence-based standards of care, measures of quality including client and family satisfaction measures.

- What risk management and liability issues should Ms. Harris consider?

  Adhere to standards and scope of practice, identify factors specific to this client that increase liability exposure.

Review Questions

1. The purpose of the American Nurses Association's *Scope and Standards of Psychiatric–Mental Health Clinical Nursing Practice* is to

   a. **Define the role and actions for the NP** *(Correct. The scope and standards reflect the activities and accountabilities of the psychiatric nurse, the "who, what, when, where, and how of practice.")*

   b. Establish the legal authority for the prescription of psychotropic medications

   c. Define the legal statutes of the role of the PMHNP

   d. Define the differences between the physician role and the NP role

2. The trend in legal rulings on cases involving mental illness over the past 25 years has been to:

   a. Encourage juries to find defendants not guilty by reason of insanity

   b. **Protect the individual's freedoms or rights when he or she is committed to a mental hospital** *(Correct. Identifies the trend of ensuring the protection of individual civil liberties for psychiatric clients.)*

   c. Place increasing trust in mental health professionals to make good and ethical decisions

   d. Decrease all the "red tape" associated with commitments so that commitments are faster and easier

3. A community has an unusually high incidence of depression and drug use among the teenage population. The public health nurses decide to address this problem, in part, by modifying the environment and strengthening the capacities of families to prevent the development of new cases of depression and drug use. This is an example of:

   a. **Primary prevention** *(Correct. This action focuses on interventions designed to reduce the incidence of new cases of disease.)*

   b. Secondary prevention

   c. Tertiary prevention

   d. Protective factorial prevention

4. Mrs. Kemp is voluntarily admitted to the hospital. After 24 hours she states she wishes to leave because "this place can't help me." The best nursing action that reflects the legal right of this client is:

    a. To discharge the client

    b. **Explain that the client cannot leave until you can complete further assessment** (*Correct. Almost every state allows for a brief period of detainment to assess a client for dangerousness to self or others before allowing the client to leave a hospital setting, even if the admission was voluntary.*)

    c. Allow the client to leave but have her sign forms stating she is leaving against medical advice

    d. Immediately start the paperwork to commit the client and to allow you to treat her against her wishes

Chapter 2

Case Study

Thomas Jones is a 19-year-old college freshman. During the second week of classes, he presented to the student health services clinic of the college he attends seeking help for "shyness." As the PMHNP working the day Mr. Jones presented for care, you are responsible for assessment and care planning with this client.

As you are working with him, he gives a chief complaint of feeling uncomfortable around all of the strangers he is meeting and of a desire to return home and drop out of school. There are several issues for you to consider as you begin to work with Mr. Jones.

- Chronologically, what stage of development should Mr. Thomas be experiencing?

    Adolescence.

- What are the tasks of this stage?

    Identity vs. role confusion.

- How would you assess the actual developmental issues that he is experiencing?

    Assess the degree of development of his personal sense of identity.

- What factors do you need to consider to determine whether he is experiencing normative or non-normative behaviors?

    The PMHNP must have an awareness of the normal milestones of development and the behaviors that indicate failure of developmental stages. Client's history and behaviors are then matched to the known norm for comparison.

- What characteristic do you as the PMHNP need to display to establish a therapeutic relationship with him?

    Genuineness, acceptance, nonjudgmental attitude, authenticity, empathy, and respect professional boundaries.

Mr. Jones reported that he has not been sleeping well, has experienced a decrease in appetite, and just wants to talk to someone about his problems in adjusting to school. In planning the follow-up care for Mr. Jones, you have many issues to consider.

- What would be the goal of continued work with Mr. Jones?

    Assisting the individual to establish insight into behaviors and to increase range and maturity of coping behaviors.

- If you were to start therapy with him, what kind of therapy would you consider?

    Several appropriate options that depend on factors such as the client's goals, motivation, past experiences with counseling, expectations for therapy, and resources.

- Would you consider him to have a mentally illness?

    Mental illness *can be defined as any disruption in the usual constitutions of mental health. Mental illness assumes an underlying psychopathology and can be defined as a clinically significant behavioral/psychological syndrome or pattern that occurs in an individual and that is associated with persistent distress or disability or with a significant increased risk of death, pain, disability, or an important loss of freedom. Mr. Jones appears to be experiencing mental health concerns but does not, based on available data, fit the definition of mental illness.*

Review Questions

1. The *DSM-IV-TR* provides for holistic client assessment by using a multiaxial assessment format. The general medical conditions experienced by a client that may influence treatment of his or her psychiatric disorders are coded on which of the five axes of the *DSM?*

    a. Axis I
    b. Axis II
    c. **Axis III *(Correct. Medical conditions are coded on this axis.)***
    d. Axis IV

2. Mrs. French has been in individual therapy for 3 months. She has shown much growth and improvement in her functioning and insight and is to discontinue services within the next few weeks. In the next session, after you discuss service termination, she suddenly begins to demonstrate the original symptoms that had brought her to treatment initially. She is now hesitant to discharge, wants to continue services, and is displaying an increase in regressive defense mechanisms. The best explanation of Mrs. French's behavior is

    a. An exacerbation of her symptoms related to stress
    b. The normal cyclic nature of chronic mental health symptoms

    c.   **A sign of normal resistance to termination seen in the termination phase of the nurse–client relationship** *(Correct. Clients frequently display resistance and regression at the termination of a meaningful therapeutic process. The PMHNP is responsible for planning an effective termination and monitoring clients during the termination period.)*

    d.   A sign of pathological attachment to the therapist that must be addressed

3. An example of a mature, healthy defense mechanism is

    a.   Denial

    b.   Rationalization

    c.   Repression

    d.   **Suppression** *(Correct. The only defense mechanism listed in which the client channels conflicting energies into growth-promoting activities.)*

4. A man thinks to himself that his wife is really ugly as he sees her at the breakfast table one morning. He doesn't tell her his thinking because he doesn't want to hurt her feelings. Later in the day he gets a sudden unexplainable urge to send his wife flowers. The best explanation for his unconscious action is

    a.   **Undoing** *(Correct. Undoing is the act of negating or undoing intolerable thoughts or feelings.)*

    b.   Suppression

    c.   Denial

    d.   Repression

Chapter 3

Case Study

Ms. Franklin is a 24-year-old sales clerk. She has a strong family history of mental illness and is worried that she may experience some problems in her life because of her family history. She presents to her local primary care provider complaining of the following symptoms:

- Hyperalertness
- Increased startle response
- Concern that people are staring at her and watching what she eats
- Decreased appetite
- Sedation
- Impaired memory.

Ms. Franklin is trying to determine if these experiences are normal or are the beginning of a mental illness. She wants to have a brain scan done to determine the answer. She also is getting married soon and wants to know what the risk is that her future children will experience mental illness, as she believes it runs in her family. In working with Ms. Franklin, the PMHNP must consider many issues.

- Are the symptoms described by Ms. Franklin consistent with a psychiatric disorder?

  More assessment would be needed to determine this, but they may be consistent with an anxiety or mood disorder.

- Do psychiatric disorders run in families, as Ms. Franklin believes?

  Most psychiatric illnesses have been shown to have, in part, a genetic link and, therefore, do tend to run in families.

- Do the symptoms as described by Ms. Franklin link with any known neuroanatomical or neurophysiologic deficit?

  Ms. Franklin's symptoms are consistent with excessive levels of norepinephrine.

- Is a brain scan warranted for Ms. Franklin?

  No. There is insufficient data presented to warrant the cost of such a procedure at this time.

- Can the risk of Ms. Franklin's children developing psychiatric disorders be determined?

  Yes, but only if Ms. Franklin is diagnosed as experiencing an actual psychiatric illness. Once this is determined, the genetic risk to her children can be identified through the use of such things as concordant rate tables.

Review Questions

1. The role of neurotransmitters in the central nervous system is to function as

   a. **A communication medium** *(Correct. Neurotransmitters are responsible for the communication of information between neurons.)*
   b. A gatekeeper for transmissions
   c. A building block for amino acids
   d. A agent to break down enzymes

2. Serotonin is produced in which of the following locations:

   a. Locus ceruleus
   b. Nucleus basalis
   c. **Raphi nuclei** *(Correct. Serotonin is produced in the raphi nuclei.)*
   d. Substantia nigra

3. A client presents with complaints of changes in appetite, feeling fatigued, problems with sleep–rest cycle, and changes in libido. The neuroanatomical area of the brain responsible for the normal regulation of these functions is the

    a. Thalamus
    b. **Hypothalamus** *(Correct. The hypothalamus is the brain's alarm system and plays a key role in regulatory functions such as thirst, hunger, water balance, circadian rhythms, etc.)*
    c. Limbic system
    d. Hippocampus

4. In considering whether of not to order an MRI for a client with suspected psychiatric disorders, which of the following would be a contraindication to this diagnostic test:

    a. Prosthetic limb
    b. History of head trauma
    c. **Pacemaker** *(Correct. MRIs are not to be used for individuals with pacemakers or implants of ferromagnetic metals.)*
    d. Pregnancy

Chapter 4

Case Study

A 22-year-old college student presents to the clinic for assistance with complaints of frequent headaches, generalized body aches, difficulty concentrating, and insomnia. She has been losing weight over the past few weeks and is unable to study or concentrate in class. She states that she feels "sick" but denies any other recent illnesses. She has an unremarkable history, has no chronic illnesses, and takes no routine medications. She is a moderate social drinker and does not smoke. Recent stressors include a heavy course load and a recent disappointment at failing to be accepted for membership in a sorority on campus. She denies family history for mental illness and talks at great length about why she believes she is "sick, not crazy." There are many issues to consider in assessing this patient.

- What additional assessments would you make at this time?

    Physical assessment, mental status exam, and diagnostic and lab testing.

- What specific diagnostic and laboratory tests would you order, and why?

    To evaluate the possibility of a psychiatric disorder, a thyroid panel should be obtained, as symptoms of thyroid disorder can mimic symptoms of depressive disorders. Electrolyte panel and CBC may be indicated as well for similar reasons. If there are any other clinical indications, a drug screening may be indicated.

- What, if any, specific physical findings would you look for?

  Should look for the presence of the physical findings suggestive of mood disorders and inconsistent with any other specific physical disorder.

- What communication strategies would you use to facilitate assessment of this patient?

  Broad opening statements, accepting, exploring, and clarifying.

- What milieu considerations would precede your interactions with her?

  Patient comfort level, low sensory stimulus area, private but safe area, with access to supplies or other staff if needed.

Review Questions

1. The concept of target symptom identification is best explained as

    a. Identification of the major clinical presentation of the client

    b. **Identification of specific, precise, and individualized symptoms reasonably expected to improve with medication** *(Correct. Must have the target symptoms identified to determine patient outcomes to care.)*

    c. Identification of the secondary messenger system syndrome

    d. Intentional modulation of synaptic pathways

2. Mr. Johnson is a newly admitted client to an inpatient psychiatric hospital. The PMHNP on call at the facility plans to perform the initial intake assessment and diagnostic process. Mr. Johnson asks to please talk in his room because, he says, "People make me nervous." His room at the end of the hallway and is the farthest away from the nursing station. The PMHNP's action should be based on awareness that the best location to do the assessment is

    a. In Mr. Johnson's room, because it is least noisy and most comfortable for him, thus facilitating data collection

    b. In the dayroom, which is full of people, to observe his interactions with other individuals

    c. **In a quiet place but public enough to get assistance with patient care should it be required during the assessment** *(Correct. One PMHNP role is to control the milieu as an aspect of assessment.)*

    d. In the treatment room with the door closed, a neutral location

3. In assessing a client, you ask him the meaning of the proverb "People who live in glass houses shouldn't throw stones." He replies, "Because it will break the windows." The correct interpretation of this findings is

   a. Client has a probable mood disorder
   b. Client has a probable anxiety disorder
   c. Client has limited intellectual ability
   d. **Unable to interpret the finding without knowing the client's age** *(Correct. The answer demonstrates concrete thought processes, which are normal in individuals younger than age 12 but are abnormal after age 12. To interpret the finding, the PMHNP must know the age of the client.)*

4. The PMHNP is planning to work with a client using an individual therapy model of care. During the first session, the client makes the following statement: "This is the third time my son has run away. I've grounded him, taken away his bike, even tried cutting of his allowance and locking him in his room. What should I do now?" The most therapeutic response for the PMHNP to make is

   a. "I wonder if locking him in his room was abusive."
   b. **"Maybe that depends on what you are trying to accomplish."** *(Correct. This statement allows the client to be in a partnership with the clinician and an active participant in his/her own treatment. This is the MOST therapeutic response.)*
   c. "Perhaps talking to his friends and teachers would help."
   d. Remain silent

5. Mrs. Shea has come to the mental health center seeking treatment for depression. She has a history of a suicide attempt by overdose 1 month ago. She was started on imipramine (TCA) after that event but stopped taking the medication 1 week later because it "did no good." The PMHNP meets with Mrs. Shea to plan care with her. Which of the following is the most appropriate initial action?

   a. **Asking Mrs. Shea how to help her** *(Correct. An aspect of assessment—all other answers are aspects of interventions, which are not initial actions of the PMHNP.)*
   b. Providing client teaching about the long time frame for TCAs to work
   c. Contracting with Mrs. Shea for 6 sessions of individual therapy
   d. Providing Mrs. Shea with feedback about how suicide might affect her family

Chapter 5

Case Study

Jane, a 74-year-old client who the PHMNP has been seeing for depression, presented at her appointment with complaints of tremors, diaphoresis, headache, and nausea over the past week. She is currently being prescribed Amitriptyline (50 mg q HS), which was increased at her last visit, and Zoloft (100 mg qd). She denies depression but admits to increased confusion and memory problems.

- What is your biggest pharmacological concern at this point with the combination of medication the client is being prescribed?

   Your biggest concern is that the SSRI is potentially increasing the concentration of the TCA to possibly toxic blood levels.

- What would be your plan of action?

   Check a blood level of amitriptyline, and decrease the dosage. Afterward, consider tapering the client off the TCA.

- What pharmacokinetics should you keep in mind when treating elderly people?

   Elderly people have greater body fat content, and because psychotropic drugs are lipophilic, they have an increased risk of toxicity. They also have decreased gastric acid secretion, which can slow the absorption of medications. Older people metabolize drugs slowly, which also can predispose them to toxicity. They are more prone to anticholinergic toxicity and orthostatic hypotension.

Review Questions

1. Sarah presents for her initial intake appointment with complaints of depression. She is being treated for hypertension and asthma by her primary care provider. Knowing that certain medications may cause or exacerbate depression, you obtain a complete medication history. Which of the following medications is known to exacerbate or cause depression?

   a. Prilosec

   b. **Propranolol** *(Correct. Beta blockers can cause or exacerbate depression.)*

   c. Synthroid

   d. Biaxin

2. When treating elderly people, you should keep in mind that they are more sensitive to issues of drug toxicity because of which of the following reasons?

   a. Decreased body fat

   b. Increased liver capacity

   c. **Decreased protein binding** *(Correct. Elderly people usually have decreased protein levels. Most psychotropic medications are highly protein bound. It is the unbound [free] concentration of the drug that is active; the bound concentration of the drug is inert. Thus, with decreased protein available for binding, there exists more free [active] drug, which then predisposes elderly people to toxicity.)*

   d. Increased muscle concentration

3. Which known teratogenic effects can be caused by the common psychotropic medications of Depakote and Lithium?

    a. Depakote—Epstein anomaly; Lithium—Cleft palate

    b. **Lithium—Epstein anomaly; Depakote—Spina bifida** *(Correct. Lithium during pregnancy is known to cause a cardiac defect called Epstein anomaly and Depakote during pregnancy is known to cause neural tube defects such as spina bifida.)*

    c. Depakote—Limb malformations; Lithium—Seizure disorder

    d. Lithium—Spina bifida; Depakote—Mental retardation

4. The study of what the body does to drugs is called

    a. Pharmacodynamics

    b. Pharmacology

    c. **Pharmacokinetics** *(Correct. This is the study of what the body does to drugs.)*

    d. Distribution

Chapter 6

Case Study

You are an existential therapist are in session with Bill, who has anxiety and states, "No one really understands me or cares about me. That is why I have low self-esteem and feel 'less than.' That is why I act the way I do." He has been self-medicating with alcohol and illicit drugs.

*   Using an existential style, how would you respond Bill's statement above?

    You would respond to Bill by gently confronting his attempt to escape his freedom through alcohol and drug use. You could convey to him that it is his passivity that is keeping him unfree.

*   What existential tenet does your response display?

    Humans are responsible for our actions and free to make a choice.

*   According to existential theory, how do you view Bill's anxiety?

    You would not see Bill's anxiety as something to be cured but rather as a vital part of living with uncertainty and freedom. To some degree, anxiety is healthy.

Review Questions

1. Group therapy is beneficial because it

    a. Increases social skills

    b. Is cost effective

    c. Enables participants to acquire the curative factors

    d. **All of the above** *(Correct. Groups are beneficial because they increase social skills, produce universality, are cost effective, and enable participants to acquire Yalom's curative factors.)*

2. You are using Beck's cognitive–behavioral therapy and know that this will help the client

    a. **Recognize and change his or her automatic thoughts** *(Correct. Cognitive behavioral therapy is based upon the theory that one's thoughts can determine one's feelings and behavior. If we recognize self-defeating thoughts, we can in turn change feelings and behavior.)*

    b. See reality as you see it

    c. Change his or her reality by changing his or her environment

    d. Recognize and accept that automatic thoughts suggest delusional thinking

3. Homeostasis in a family refers to

    a. Choices a family makes to keep the peace

    b. **Balance or stability that the family returns to despite its dysfunction** *(Correct. Homeostasis is the tendency of families to resist change in order to maintain a steady state of equilibrium.)*

    c. Need for change and balance in a family

    d. Calm in a family that returns after a crisis

4. In an attempt to bring the client toward the goal he or she is working on, you ask the client, "If a miracle were to happen tonight while you slept, and you awoke in the morning and the problem no longer existed, how would you know, and what would be different?" This technique is used in which type of therapy?

    a. Behavioral therapy

    b. **Solution-focused therapy** *(Correct. Miracle questions are used in solution-focused therapy.)*

    c. Adlerian therapy

    a. Existential therapy

Chapter 7

Case Study

Mary, a 35-year-old homemaker and mother of two children, presents to her primary care provider accompanied by her husband with complaints of lack of energy and inability to sleep that are getting progressively worse. The symptoms are affecting her ability to take care of her children and the household. Her husband reports that she often has crying spells, is not eating well, and cannot seem to concentrate. When questioned further, her husband said that she has mentioned not wanting to live, but he thought that she was just having a bad day.

Past Medical History

- Seasonal allergies and stress-induced asthma
- No significant surgical history, except for a tonsillectomy when she was a child
- Normal pregnancies and deliveries
- No chronic health problems identified.

Family History
- Significant for grandmother and father, who had "breakdowns."
- Father had alcoholism.

Social History
Mary is a homemaker and has two children, ages 8 and 10. She and her husband moved to the area 6 months ago. She does not smoke or use drugs but drinks socially. She has an MA degree in English and had planned to go back to school to get her teaching certificate when her children began high school.

Mental Status Exam
Client appears clean but somewhat disheveled. Hair is not combed or washed. She appears very tired. She avoids eye contact, talks very softly, and is slow to respond to questions. She hardly moves during the interview. Affect is constricted and sad. She says has no energy, and her mood is "very sad." She does not hear voices or have hallucinations. Her thoughts are appropriate and organized. She does admit to having episodic thoughts of suicide and has a vague plan to ingest an overdose of aspirin, acetaminophen, and alcohol when the children are with their father but has no clear timeline or planned intent. She is unable to do serial number testing and shows impaired short-term memory. She exhibits a few problems with immediate recall. She has difficulty concentrating but no difficulty with abstractions. She is oriented times 3, and shows good judgment and insight. She has above-average intelligence.

Current Medications
Mary takes Zyrtec for allergies and is now on Ortho-Tri-Cyclin contraceptive pills.

Labs
Platelets 230/mm
WBC 6,000/mm
Hematocrit 33%, hemoglobin 8.0 gm/dl
NA 140, K 4.0, Cl 101, CO_2 26, BUN 15, Creatinine 0.9, Glucose 102
TSH 1.1, T3 179, T4 1.3.

There are several issues to consider in planning care for Mary:

- What is the most probable diagnosis?

    This client's presentation is consistent with the symptoms of major depression.

- What further assessment is needed?

    Need to ensure that client meets the DSM-IV criteria for major depression. Should complete physical assessment and use common symptom rating scale such as Beck's Depression Inventory or Zung's Depression Self-Rating Scale. Should also complete assessment for any other physical health states.

- What target symptoms does patient display that are consistent with the probable diagnosis?

    Depressed mood most of the day, nearly every day, lack of energy, suicidal ideation, MSE findings consistent with MDD.

- What medications would be considered?

  SSRIs often are considered the first-line agents for the treatment of MDD.

- If client had psychotic features with her depression, how would this change the treatment plan?

  Clinical management often includes the short-term use of an antipsychotic agent to control psychotic symptoms. If used, an atypical antipsychotic is usually best tolerated.

- How would the plan differ if client had a heart condition and was taking no other medications?

  Would need to look at issues of compatibility of the various pharmacological agents that the client may be placed on, ensure that the medications used to treat the MDD did not have significant risk of adverse cardiac side-effects, ensure that appropriate and complete patient teaching occurred.

Review Questions

1. Mrs. Thomas has been diagnosed with MDD and is placed on Serzone 20 mg for her depression. For the PMHNP to effectively monitor this client's use of the medication, which of the following actions should be part of ongoing care?

   a. **Use of a standardized rating scale of depression *(Correct. The use of a standardized rating scale will allow the PMHNP to monitor the level of client symptoms and to evaluate the efficacy of the medication.)***
   b. Monitoring for potential abuse of the medication
   c. Monitoring of baseline labs of renal functioning
   d. Monitoring for potential cardiac side-effects

2. A 23-year-old female in brought into the ER after attempting suicide by cutting her wrists. Which nursing action by the PMHNP would be of highest priority initially?

   a. Assess her coping behaviors
   b. Assess her current level of suicidality
   c. **Take her vital signs *(Correct. Need to ensure that her suicide attempt has not led to medical instability.)***
   d. Assess her health history

3. The TCA class of medications can be characterized by all of the following properties *except*

   a. **Safety in overdose *(Correct. TCAs are generally unsafe in overdose.)***
   b. Inexpensive cost of medications
   c. Significant side-effect concerns
   d. Long half-life

4. For the PMHNP to provide a client with an adequate trial on an antidepressant medication, what time period of continuous medication use is required?

   a. **6 weeks of continuous medication use** *(Correct. Six to eight weeks is considered an adequate trial.)*

   b. 6 months of continuous medication use

   c. 3 weeks of continuous medication use

   d. 10 weeks of continuous medication use

Chapter 8

Case Study

John, a 47-year-old teacher, has a long-standing history of GAD. He had been doing well until about 4 weeks ago. At that time he was traveling overseas with his church group, participating in a caring mission in South America. He began to feel more and more depressed and anxious as he saw the "poverty and despair" in developing countries. He has started not sleeping and having "bad dreams" whenever he did try to sleep. He is beginning to think he is physically sick, as his anxiety is now beginning to interfere with work, and he is worried that he may need to be in the hospital to find out "what's wrong with me."

One week ago he began to feel overwhelmingly anxious, was convinced he was dying, and had his first of 6 discrete episodes he calls "panic attacks." He went to the local ER and was diagnosed with anxiety and given Valium 5 mg #30 to use prn. He at first felt like the Valium was helping, but now he is feeling "like nothing helps." He is increasingly despondent, sure he is dying and that no one will believe him, and has contemplated suicide. He says he would not do it but is bothered by thinking about suicide. He is having increased tremors with anxiety, headaches, and nausea, which the ER diagnosed as anxiety reaction. His wife agrees that it all of his symptoms are anxiety, but she reports that he is sure he is dying of cancer and no one will tell him the truth.

MSE

- *Appearance:* Well-nourished, well-dressed
- *Motor:* Some motor restlessness
- *Speech:* Some slowing and underproduction
- *Affect:* Anxious
- *Mood:* Depressed
- *Thought process/content:* Thematic for fear of becoming sicker and of dying early. Some vague suicidality without intent or plan; denies delusions or hallucinations.
- Abstractive on proverbs
- *Memory:* Impaired
- *Concentration:* Impaired.

Social History

- Married and has 3 children
- Works as high school gym teacher
- Overweight at 280 lbs., with sedentary lifestyle

- Smokes 2 packs a day
- Does not drink alcohol for religious reasons
- Wife very concerned and supportive.

Past Psychiatric History
- Hospitalized in 1998 for "nerves"
- At that time started on Paxil 20 mg/d
- After 3 months, dose raised to 40 mg/d; has been doing well until recently
- Has had no significant exacerbation of symptoms since initial treatment.

Past Medical History
- History of seizure disorder since childhood; well controlled with meds
- Recent exposure to tuberculosis during international travel.

Current Medications
- Isoniazid for prophylaxis treatment for 6 months
- Paxil 40 mg
- Valium 5 mg po prn q 4 hrs.

Labs
- All labs within normal limits.

Screening Tools
- BAI: Severe score range.

In planning care for this client, the PMHNP has many issues to consider:

- What is the most likely diagnosis?

    Panic disorder; also must be assessed for mood disorder.

- How will you separate comorbidity from complications of current diagnosis?

    Need to perform a complete assessment on the client, including physical examination, MSE, and lab studies. The client's current medications should be examined, and the chronology of symptoms should be compared to any changes in his health status.

- What medication adjustments would you make?

    Need to consider changing the client's antidepressant medication. Decision should be based on results of complete assessment, final diagnostic impressions, and input from the client and his family. Long-term use of a potentially addictive drug such as Valium needs to be examined carefully.

- How will you address the family issues?

    Several approaches might be appropriate. Using psychoeducation for the family, providing supportive counseling, or involving the family in family therapy are possible strategies.

- How often will you plan to see the client?

  Client should be seen frequently until symptoms are stable. Seeing the client weekly initially is ideal. If medication adjustments have been made, client should return for evaluation at intervals consistent with the pharmacodynamics of the medication in order for the PMHNP to assess the effects of medication treatment.

Review Questions

1. The psychodynamic theory of anxiety states that the etiology of anxiety is

   a. **Conflict between the id and superego** *(Correct. According to Freud, anxiety resulted from psychic conflict between the unconscious sexual or aggressive wishes and the corresponding threats from the superego.)*
   b. Conflict between the ego and the id
   c. Interpersonal conflict between significant others
   d. Perceived disapproval from significant others

2. The interpersonal theory of anxiety states that the etiology of anxiety is

   a. Conflict between the id and superego
   b. Conflict between the ego and the id
   c. Distortions in perceived interpersonal relationships with significant others
   d. **Perceived disapproval from significant others** *(Correct. According to Harry Stack Sullivan's interpersonal theory, the perceived disapproval from significant others in relationships with the individual is a main cause of anxiety.)*

3. Mr. Zimms is admitted to the hospital with a diagnosis of OCD. He exhibits high use of defense mechanisms; has automatic behavior, physical discomfort, and feelings of dread and horror and is trembling and ritualistically washing his hands. You would assess his level of anxiety as

   a. Mild
   b. Moderate
   c. **Severe** *(Correct. Severe symptoms of anxiety include autonomic nervous system triggered, flight-or-fight response, pupils dilated, vital signs increased, diaphoresis, muscles rigid, hearing decreased, pain threshold increased, urinary frequency, and diarrhea.)*
   d. Panic

4. Which of the following levels of anxiety is considered normal and useful in motivating a person to action:

   a. **Mild** *(Correct. Mild anxiety can be adaptive and have lifesaving qualities when it occurs as a warning of an external or internal threat.)*
   b. Moderate
   c. Severe
   d. Panic

Chapter 9

Case Study

Jim is a 28-year-old client newly diagnosed with schizophrenia. He initially experienced a psychotic episode while serving in the military and now is living at home with his parents. Jim is still reluctant to accept his diagnosis and continues to believe that he "got bad weed" in the service and that he will be fine once the weed is out of his body. He has been noncompliant with treatment, and his parents are threatening to evict him from the house if he does not start accepting treatment.

Jim has a history of juvenile-onset diabetes and has struggled to maintain a diabetic diet and to control his weight. When asked to identify his current goals, Jim will state only that he wishes to find a good wife and settle down to a normal life. There are many issues to consider in planning care with this client.

- What is the top priority for the PMHNP?

    To help the client develop a plan that addresses his multiple health needs and that he feels he can comply with and manage with some assistance from the PMHNP.

- What medications are reasonable to consider for the client at this time?

    Given his young age and probable lifelong need for medication, the atypical class of antipsychotics is most indicated, but his medications will need to be managed carefully given his history of diabetes.

- What is the relationship between his diabetes and schizophrenia?

    Both disorders are well known to produce concerns with compliance, have multiple complications, and affect many areas of a patient's life. Diabetes is a common comorbid disorder with schizophrenia, complicating the clinical management of patients with both disorders.

- How will his comorbid illness affect your care planning?

    The client's diet, weight management, exercise, and activity tolerance all must be considered in planning care for this client. Both disorders are chronic in nature, and long-term planning will be needed to consider relapse prevention and crisis care.

- What routine ongoing monitoring will he require?

    The PMHNP needs to be alert and monitor the client for common complication of both disorders. The PMHNP needs to be able to separate clinical findings of both disorders and to be aware of the complex interplay of the two disorders on the functioning of the client.

Review Questions

1. The neurotransmitter deregulations theory of the etiology of psychotic disorders such as schizophrenia support that psychosis is caused, in part, by

   a. **An excess of dopamine** *(Correct. Psychotic symptoms are partially caused by too much dopamine in the mesolimbic dopamine pathway.)*
   b. A deficiency of dopamine
   c. Poor acetylcholine regulation
   d. Poor synaptic uptake of serotonin receptors

2. The positive–negative model of classifying the symptoms of schizophrenia describes positive symptoms as

   a. **Symptoms that positively respond to antipsychotic medication** *(Correct. This definition was initially developed prior to the invention of the 2nd generational antipsychotics.)*
   b. Symptoms that are less serious to experience
   c. Symptoms that are less socially stigmatizing
   d. Symptoms that positively correlate to drug abuse

3. Mrs. Jay suffers from schizophrenia and is taking Navane 15 mg/d. During her appointment with the PMHNP, she complains of feelings of inner restlessness, tremors, drooling, and stiff muscles. The best explanation of these is

   a. **Extrapyramidal side effects of Navane** *(Correct. Extrapyramidal symptoms can include akathisia, postural tremors, dystonia, drooling.)*
   b. Anticholinergic side effects of Navane
   c. Atypical side effects of Navane
   d. Psychosomatic side effects

4. As part of treatment planning, the PMHNP places a note on Mrs. Jay's chart about seizure precautions. The client notices the note and states that she doesn't understand and that she has no history of seizures. The PMHNP explains that

   a. It is a clerical error, and she will correct it
   b. Seizures are common in mental illness, and the note is just a precaution
   c. Reactions to psychotropic medications are unpredictable
   d. **Typical antipsychotic medications can lower seizure threshold** *(Correct. All antipsychotics lower the seizure threshold, therefore precautions should be taken.)*

5. Mrs. Anders, a client with delusional disorder, has been started on Haldol 5 mg po bid, Tylenol 2 tabs po prn, Cogentin 1 mg po prn, and Ativan 2 mg prn for agitation. She is complaining of a sudden painful stiff neck and jaw muscles that started a few hours after she took her medication. These symptoms are most likely related to

   a. Akinesia
   b. Akathisia

c. **Dystonia** *(Correct. Dystonias are brief or sustained contractions of muscles, spasms, thickened or slurred speech due to enlarged tongue, oculogyric crises, unusual posturing of limbs.)*

d. Somatic delusions

6. The most appropriate PMHNP action to help relieve Mrs. Anders's pain and stiff muscles is

a. Switch to an NSAID to control her pain

b. **Increase her Cogentin dose** *(Correct. Anticholinergic drugs such as Cogentin are used for dystonias.)*

c. Teach her relaxation techniques

d. Work her up for a muscular–skeletal problem

7. After a few weeks, you see Mrs. Anders again. She is refusing to take Haldol because of continued problems with stiff muscles and blurred vision. She tells you that she has not taken her medication for 1 week, and the stiffness and blurred vision are better but still a problem. Mrs. Anders says, "Something else must be seriously wrong with me. I stopped the Haldol, and I'm still not okay." Your best explanation is that Mrs. Anders is

a. Fixated on her medications

b. Experiencing an unusual reaction to Haldol

c. **Experiencing a lipophilic reaction to Haldol** *(Correct. After the depot injection, the active ingredient is slowly absorbed in the bloodstream, and effects will last for 3-4 weeks following the injection.)*

d. Experiencing some problem other than a side effect of Haldol

Chapter 10

Case Study

Rachel, a 59-year-old homemaker with a positive family history for Alzheimer's disease, has been very worried lately at her subjective belief that she is losing her memory. She has hesitated to go for an evaluation because of her concern and is very upset as she shares her beliefs with the PMHNP. She gives a social history of being happily married for the past 35 years and of having several children and two new grandchildren. She has had no recent stressors and has felt a slow decline in her memory for the past 2 years. She believes no one else has noticed, but recently it is harder to hide her deficit from her family.

She has been employed as a nurse for the past 25 years at the local hospital but has begun to notice a decline in her ability to keep track of all of the information needed to do her job well. She has a history of asthma and periodically uses a rescue inhaler and steroids to manage her asthma. She routinely takes one ASA a day and uses over-the-counter kava kava when she feels stressed. She has been taking Pravachol 20 mg/day for her cholesterol level for the past 2 years. She has no significant physical findings but does show mild impairment in short-term memory testing during the MSE exam. There are many issues to consider in planning care with this client:

- What is the probable diagnosis at this time?

   Although complete assessment needs to be done, given client's family history and current clinical presentation, dementia must be considered.

- What further assessment is needed?

   Full physical exam, MSE, diagnostic and lab tests, determination of memory and cognitive functioning of the patient.

- What role does the medication taken by the patient play in decision making?

   Must consider effects of Pravachol and kava kava use on current clinical presentation. Can cause confusion and memory problems in some clients. Timeline of symptoms should be compared to medication use history.

- Would you include the family at this time in the care planning?

   Although the client's wishes should be honored, involvement of the family may decrease client's concerns and increase support and assistance during this difficult time for her.

- Are medications indicated at this time?

   Only once diagnostic clarity is reached. At that time, if dementia is the diagnosis, the use of cholinesterase inhibitor such as Aricept may be indicated. Discontinuation of kava kava is indicated as well.

- What steps would you take to reduce the client's discomfort as she discusses her concerns?

   Pay attention to milieu considerations, allow client to ventilate concerns, provide information to reduce anxiety, and use therapeutic communication strategies.

Review Questions

1. Risk factors for the development of delirium include all of the following except

   a. **Consistent use of aspirin-based products** *(Correct. All of the answers below are risk factors for delirium. Use of aspirin is not.)*
   b. Age older than 50
   c. Substance abuse
   d. Multisystem illness

2. The most significant finding that should alert the PMHNP to the possible diagnosis of delirium is

   a. **Rapid onset of symptoms different from baseline functioning** *(Correct. The onset of delirium is usually rapid, whereas the onset of dementia is gradual)*
   b. Slow, progressive onset of symptoms different from baseline
   c. Presence of a strong family history suggesting vulnerability
   d. Rapid alteration in vital signs

3. Prevention and screening actions by the PMHNP are essential in the identification of dementia because

   a. **Early detection can prevent some of the deterioration of the illness** *(Correct. Progression and deterioration of dementia can be delayed; however, dementia is not reversible. Medications are more effective if started early in the process.)*

   b. Early recognition allows for ruling out reversible forms of dementia

   c. Medications are more effective in treating dementia if started later in the illness

   d. Comorbidities can be prevented by early recognition

4. The medication most commonly used to treat moderate cognitive deficits seen in dementia is

   a. Strattera (atomoxetine)

   b. **Exelon (rivastigmine tartrate)** *(Correct. Exelon is a cholinesterase inhibitor which is used in the treatment of dementia.)*

   c. Haldol (haloperidol)

   d. Celebrex (celecoxib)

Chapter 11

Case Study

Mrs. Day is a 61-year-old widow who has multiple health problems. She had been diagnosed with essential hypertension and chronic bronchitis and has non-insulin-dependent diabetes. She has been coming to your primary care clinic for 6 months, and before that she had been receiving her care from multiple other providers in the community, spending an average of 8 months with a practice group, then changing her care to another provider. She has CHAMPUS as her insurance and receives Social Security Disability Insurance.

Mrs. Day's chief complaint for the past few months has been stasis ulcers on her lower left leg, which have not healed well despite multiple approaches to care. She also complains of problems with her "nerves." She currently is taking

- Multivitamin daily
- Zantac 150 mg Q 12 hrs
- Xanax 1 mg BID
- Glucotrol 20 mg BID.

Mrs. Day is in today, and this is the first time you see her. On initial approach, she is hostile and difficult to get information from, stating "You should know all this; you have my chart right there in your hand." She states that today she wants a refill of all of her prescriptions, and she wants you to write a letter to her landlord to "Stop harassing me." She reports that her landlord is insisting that she place her garbage in the containers in the parking lot of the complex. She feels that is too far for her to walk, and she wants a letter supporting her current practice of leaving her garbage bags in the hallway outside her apartment door.

She also is reporting that her nerves are worse, and the pain in her legs is worse as well. She also believes that she has had a return of "chronic bronchitis," and she is requesting an antibiotic. She is requesting that you increase her Xanax and add codeine or morphine or "any other thing like that" for her "constant pain." She states "Just do this and get me out of here. I know what I need."

MSE

- *Appearance:* Moderately obese, well-dressed with appropriate hygiene, poor eye contact
- *Motor:* Mild psychomotor restlessness, slightly ataxic gait, tremulous
- *Speech:* Underproductive
- *Affect:* Hostile
- *Mood:* Self-described as "cranky"
- *Thought Processes:* Goal directed and organized without evidence of psychotic processing but does show some mild thought blocking and tangentiality
- *Thought Content:* Thematic for mistrust of health providers and of fear of pain continuing
- *Memory:* One-third of objects after 15 minutes
- *Concentration:* Refuses to do numbers testing, stating "I was never good with book work or numbers."
- *Abstraction:* Is abstract on proverbs: asks; "You got any more dumb questions?"
- *Judgment:* Intact for self-welfare
- *Education:* Completed 12th grade and went to 2-year secretarial/business school
- *Employment History:* Was a medical claims clerk for 32 years at the VA Medical Center
- *Social History:* No children; lives by herself. History of 2-pack-a-day smoker and "I drink a six-pack or so at night to relax myself—wouldn't you?"

Her physical exam is overall unremarkable. Her vital signs are within her documented baseline, with BP 132/88, P 96, RR 26, Temp 99° F, Weight 209 lbs. Her lungs are overall clear. On her left leg she has a stasis ulcer, which is circular and approximately 6 cm in circumference. It is open and oozing white–yellow liquid drainage, with redness around the borders. She reports it is painful to touch and increasingly painful when weight bearing. She is ordered silvadine treatments with cling wrap and hot soaks q 6 hours. She refuses to cover it because "It hurts when I remove the bandage" and is not very clear about whether or not she is doing the hot soaks. Recent labs are all within normal limits, including TSH, electrolytes, and CBC.

- What is the primary health care concern of this client?

  Although the client has multiple health needs, her current noncompliance and self-medication with alcohol are of primary concern.

- Is her use of potentially addictive prescription drugs warranted?

  Although the client has a significant wound, and the probability is that she is in pain, her reliance on potentially addictive drugs is of concern, and alternative treatments should be considered.

- What further assessment should be considered?

    The client's psychiatric history and family history should be established. The reason she has frequently changed providers should be explored. The client's social supports and her substance use/abuse history should be assessed as well.

- If the client is unwilling to participate in further assessment, how will you deal with her health needs?

    Careful establishment of a rapport with this client will increase the likelihood of engaging her in treatment. The principles of therapeutic relationship building must be utilized, and careful use of therapeutic communication will increase the likelihood that she will remain in treatment.

Review Questions

1. The concept of *substance abuse* implies that the individual with it is

    a. Having withdrawal and tolerance symptoms when not using substances

    b. Having psychoactive effects when using substances

    c. In denial about the impact of substance abuse on their life

    d. **Having functional problems related to frequent or excessive substance use (Correct. The DSM-IV criteria for substance abuse states that there is recurrent use despite persistent social/interpersonal problems, legal problems, and failure to fulfill major role obligations.)**

2. To diagnose a person with substance dependence, you must determine the current or past presence of which of the following clinical findings during your assessment of the client:

    a. Addictive manipulative behaviors

    b. Denial and projection

    c. **Tolerance and withdrawal signs and symptoms (Correct. Tolerance and/or withdrawal are possible criteria for substance dependence. The other answers are not diagnostic criteria.)**

    d. Mental illness

3. Many abused substances have questionable withdrawal symptoms. Whether or not a person dependent on a particular substance will have withdrawal symptoms depends on

    a. The biochemistry of the person

    b. **The nature of the substance (Correct. Substance withdrawal is the development of a substance specific syndrome.)**

    c. The biochemistry of the agent and the person

    d. Neither the person nor the agent but a combination of the two factors

4. John is dependent on Falvoxaz (Fabs), a new synthetic substance currently popular among high school–age children in your community. John comes into the ER after a car accident and admits to frequent, regular use of Falvoxaz. Because this drug is new, you are not familiar with the potential types of withdrawal symptoms. The best assessment question to ask to determine the nature of possible withdrawal symptoms from this drug is

    a. **"How do you feel when you take Fabs?"** *(Correct. Knowing the action of the drug allows the PMHNP to infer that withdrawal symptoms will be the opposite of the effects of the agent.)*
    b. "What is the chemical name for Fabs?"
    c. "How many Fabs do you take a week?"
    d. "How long have you been using Fabs?"

5. Medical detoxification from a substance is required *only* when the substance is known to produce

    a. **Physical withdrawal symptoms** *(Correct. Physical withdrawal symptoms are the priority because they can lead to autonomic instability, seizures, and death in some instances.)*
    b. Psychological withdrawal symptoms
    c. Both physical and psychological withdrawal symptoms
    d. Uncomfortable and unwanted withdrawal symptoms

Chapter 12

Case Study

Mr. Jevers is 42-year-old new client who seeks health care for a general physical exam. The FNP who examines Mr. Jevers asks the PMHNP to speak with him because of his odd presentation. The client discusses with the PMHNP an unusual, recurrent experience he has been having.

Mr. Jevers lives in an apartment building downtown and works as a bartender in the late evening. He tells the PMHNP that every night as he walks home from work he watches to see if the wind "blows north to south or south to north." He relates that, on the occasions that wind goes north to south, he takes that as a sign that a woman will visit him. He tells of a woman who rides a bicycle down the road and, as she passes him, he receives a blessing from her that protects him from those who wish him harm. He believes the woman is a "spirit from the other side" and that no one but he can see the woman.

As Mr. Jevers tells his story, his affect is inappropriate, his mood pleasant and happy, and he exhibits some paranoid ideation as he worries that others will try to take away the spirit. His MSE shows ideas of reference and some magical thinking as he shares his "blessing" with customers in the bar, and he describes odd, eccentric, and peculiar behaviors. Mr. Jevers is not at all bothered by his unusual experience and seems to enjoy telling it to others. He considers himself lucky to have "special powers" and to see and understand things that other do not. Mr. Jevers denies the presence of any typical manifestations of hallucinations or delusions, any mood disturbance or anxiety, and alcohol or other drug use. He reports having several close friends, a strong support network, and is in general good health but does experience significant social anxiety. He does not believe his unusual experience is a symptom of an illness and wishes no intervention or assistance at this time.

• What is the most probable diagnosis for this client?

  Schizotypal personality disorder.

• What further assessment should occur?

  A complete assessment of the client should occur, including a physical exam, full MSE, and diagnostic and lab studies. In addition, a full history of this presentation and the health habits of the client are needed.

• If the client desires no treatment, should the PMHNP attempt to follow up with him?

  Personality disorders are chronic conditions with recurrent behaviors. The PMHNP should work on the development of a therapeutic relationship with the client to work toward assisting the client to identify his psychiatric health needs and to assist him to optimize his daily social and occupational functioning.

• What treatment should be suggested at this time?

  Personality disorders most often are treated with nonpharmacological interventions such as psychotherapy.

Review Questions

1. Impulsivity is a common behavioral manifestation of personality disorders. The PMHNP working with a client with high impulsivity should consider which of the following pharmacological interventions:

   a. Use of a TCA agent

   b. Use of a benzodiazepine agent

   c. Use of an antipsychotic agent for its sedative effect

   d. **Use of an SSRI agent** *(Correct. SSRIs improve the depressed mood and have successfully modulated impulsive behavior. It is important though to rule out bipolar-related impulsivity first.)*

2. The affective instability common in some personality disorders can be clinically managed with all of the following except:

   a. Anticonvulsant agents

   b. SSRI agents

   c. MAOI agents

   d. **Antipsychotic agents** *(Correct. Antipsychotics are useful to control anger and brief psychotic episodes.)*

3. The cluster of personality disorders that manifest with dramatic, overly affective behavior is

    a. Cluster A

    b. **Cluster B** *(Correct. These are antisocial, borderline, histrionic, and narcissistic personality disorders.)*

    c. Cluster C

4. Etiological models that attempt to explain the development of personality disorders include which of the following:

    a. Object loss theory

    b. **Object relations theory** *(Correct. During one's development, patterns of oneself are internalized in relation to others. Persons with personality disorders manifest particular patterns of interpersonal relatedness that stem from object relations.)*

    c. Situation crisis development

    d. Object adjustment theory

Chapter 13

Case Study

The parents of a child with attention-deficit/hyperactive disorder (ADHD) ask to speak to you privately after your assessment of their child is complete. They tell you they have several questions that they want answered, and they want to ask you to keep the answers to yourself and not tell their son what they ask. Their first question is about diet. They have read that ADHD can be managed by dietary therapy instead of medications, and they want your opinion about trying this strategy with their child. They also want to know how likely it is that, when their son grows up, he will "outgrow" the disorder. You have many issues to consider before answering the parents' questions.

- What is the most accepted theory of etiology regarding ADHD?

    Polygenic deficits leading to problems with executive functioning and abnormalities of fronto–subcortical pathways, especially with dopamine and norepinephrine functioning.

- What is the empirical database for dietary treatment in clients with ADHD?

    Empirical evidence suggests no association between dietary alteration and improvement in symptoms of ADHD.

- What is the natural course of this illness? Is it likely that the son's symptoms will improve as he ages?

    Hyperactivity symptoms tend to improve as child ages, but inattentive symptoms may persist into adulthood.

- What are the other issues to consider regarding the parent's request to keep confidential the concerns that they are expressing?

  Treatment of ADHD requires significant family involvement. Parental counseling to deal with issues often is very helpful. In addition, parents are an integral aspect of the behavioral therapy commonly used to treat ADHD symptoms. Working with the parents is an essential role for the PMHNP.

Review Questions

1. A diagnosis of mental retardation is made when a person has significantly below-average intelligence accompanied by impaired adaptive functioning. The IQ range for consideration of mental retardation is an

   a. **IQ below 70** *(Correct. An IQ of 50–70 signifies mild mental retardation; an IQ of 35–50 signifies moderate mental retardation; an IQ of 20–35 signifies severe mental retardation; and an IQ below 20 signifies profound mental retardation.)*
   b. IQ below 60
   c. IQ below 50
   d. IQ below 40

2. Most of the stimulants commonly used to treat ADHD are classified as Schedule II controlled substances. The exception is

   a. Ritalin
   b. Dexedrine
   c. Adderall
   d. **Strattera** *(Correct. Strattera was the first non-stimulant medication FDA approved for ADHD.)*

3. A child presents with a behavioral pattern of negative, defiant, disobedient, and hostile behavior, especially toward adults in authority roles. The most likely diagnosis for this child is

   a. ADHD
   b. Rhett's disorder
   c. Antisocial personality disorder
   d. **Oppositional defiant disorder** *(Correct. The diagnostic criteria for ODD is a pattern of negativistic, hostile, and defiant behavior. The child may often lose his/her temper, argue with adults, actively defy rules, deliberately annoy others, become angry and resentful, and act spitefully.)*

4. Which of the following is not required to make a diagnosis of conduct disorder:

    a. Destruction of property

    b. Aggression toward people and animals

    c. **Poor interpersonal relationships with limited peer supports** (*Correct. Although poor interpersonal relationships can be a consequence of the conduct disorder, it is not a required diagnostic criteria.*)

    d. Deceitfulness or theft

Chapter 14

Case Study

Mrs. Jones, a 43-year-old receptionist, presents at your clinic with a primary complaint of insomnia. She reports lifelong problems with sleeping that "comes and goes" depending on her stress level and general health. She has been experiencing a 4- to 5-day period of poor sleeping, reporting only 3–4 hours of sleep and early-morning awakening. She has tried over-the-counter medication and has received no relief. She reports that her health is generally good but states that she is a 2-pack-a-day smoker and has increased her recreational use of alcohol to 1–2 drinks a night in the past few weeks in order to get to sleep.

Her insomnia is now beginning to impair her daily functioning and her interest in social activities. She reports an irritable mood since her sleep has been difficult and problems with memory and concentration in the morning after she has slept poorly. She denies depression or any other mood problem and currently is taking no routine medication. Her physical exam is unremarkable, and routine lab studies, including TSH, CBC, and electrolytes, are all normal.

- What is the most likely diagnosis for this client at this time?

    Transient insomnia.

- What further assessment would you make?

    Identify life stressors, complete full psychiatric assessment, identify any other mental health needs.

- What treatment would you consider?

    Assist client to manage her sleep; use effective sleep hygiene strategies; encourage change in diet, reduction of smoking, and use for alcohol for sleep induction.

- Is medication warranted at this time to induce sleep?

    Short-term use of sleep induction medications such as Remeron or Elavil would provide relief with little risk to the client and may help her reduce current reliance on alcohol.

Review Questions

1. In evaluating a client for insomnia, which of the following is most consistent with a presentation of transient insomnia?

    a. **Usually caused by stress, jet lag, or physical environmental concerns** *(Correct. A brief period of insomnia is usually associated with anxiety, anticipation or consequences of a stressful experience, or jet lag.)*

    b. Lasts for 3 or more weeks

    c. May linger for up to 3 weeks

    d. Calls for a complete evaluation and diagnostic work-up

2. Insomnia is a common finding in clients with a psychiatric disorder and is most commonly found in clients diagnosed with

    a. **Mood disorders** *(Correct. Although insomnia can occur as a consequence of any of the listed disorders, research has found that mood disorders are most commonly found in individuals with insomnia.)*

    b. Schizophrenic disorders

    c. Substance abuse disorders

    d. Anxiety disorders

3. Insomnia in children is most often caused by

    a. Illness

    b. **Family stress** *(Correct. Although the other listed issues may cause insomnia, the most common cause of childhood insomnia is stress within the family.)*

    c. School performance problems

    d. Substance abuse

4. A PMHNP is working with a woman whom she suspects is in a violent domestic relationship. The client denies this and refuses to discuss her home life. She continues to present at the clinic for treatment of minor injuries and always is brought by her boyfriend. The client refuses to discuss abuse as a cause of her injuries, simply stating "I'm just clumsy." The best initial intervention for the PMHNP to take is

    a. Report the suspected abuse to the police

    b. Confront the client's boyfriend during the next clinic visit

    c. **Spend a long time with the client building a trusting relationship** *(Correct. Once rapport and trust is built, the client may feel safer and more comfortable to open up.)*

    d. Refer the client to social services for follow-up

Notes:

Index

Note: Page references in *italics* refer to tables.

About the Author

Karen Guess is a full-time nurse practitioner at a public mental health clinic in Dallas, Texas. She earned a Master of Science in Nursing at The University of Texas at Arlington and is board certified as both an Adult Nurse Practitioner and a Psychiatric Mental Health Nurse Practitioner with prescriptive authority. Past experience includes work in private outpatient psychiatry, operating room, emergency services, nursing education, and college health. Karen also served in the United States Air Force as a member of the medical team in the Middle East during the Desert Storm Gulf War. She has been published in a well-known professional journal and teaches psychiatric nurse practitioner review seminars for the American Nurses Credentialing Center. Karen is committed to keeping abreast of relevant scientific and technical developments and providing high-quality mental health care with the mission of attaining the highest standards of practice.